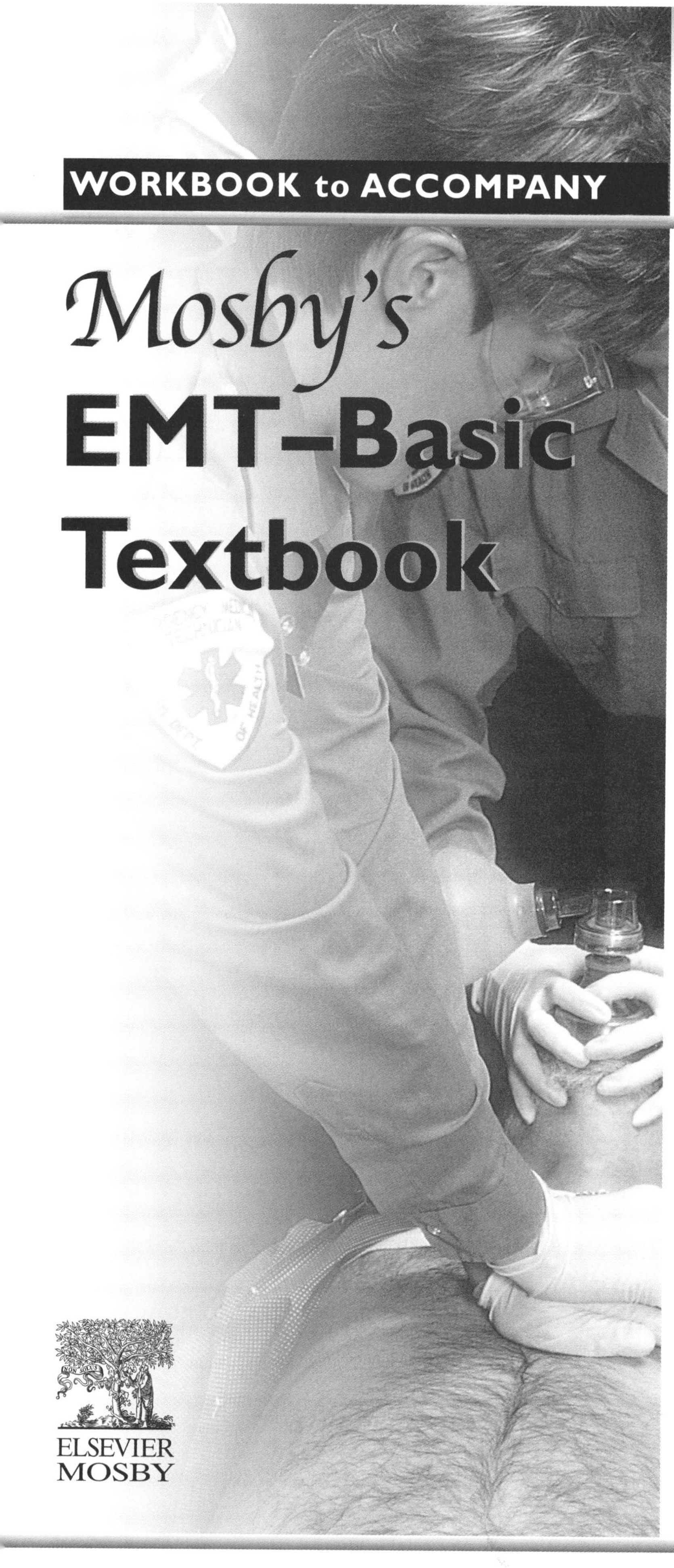

WORKBOOK to ACCOMPANY

# Mosby's EMT–Basic Textbook

**Walt Alan Stoy,** PhD, EMT-P, CCEMT-P
Professor and Director, Emergency Medicine Program
School of Health and Rehabilitation Sciences
Research Professor of Emergency Medicine
School of Medicine, Department of Emergency Medicine
University of Pittsburgh
Director, Office of Education and International Emergency Medicine
Center for Emergency Medicine
Pittsburgh, Pennsylvania

**Thomas E. Platt,** MEd, NREMT-P, CCEMT-P
Assistant Professor and Vice Program Director
Emergency Medicine Program
School of Health and Rehabilitation Sciences
University of Pittsburgh
Associate Director
Office of Education and International Emergency Medicine
Center for Emergency Medicine
Pittsburgh, Pennsylva

**Debra A. Lejeune,** MEd, NREMT-P
Instructor
Emergency Medicine Program
School of Health and Rehabilitation Sciences
University of Pittsburgh
Education Coordinator
Office of Education and International Emergency Medicine
Center for Emergency Medicine
Pittsburgh, Pennsylvania

ELSEVIER
MOSBY

ELSEVIER
MOSBY
11830 Westline Industrial Drive
St. Louis, Missouri 63146

WORKBOOK TO ACCOMPANY
MOSBY'S EMT–BASIC TEXTBOOK

ISBN-13: 978-0-323-04763-0
ISBN-10: 0-323-04763-7



NOTICE

Emergency Medicine is an ever-changing field. Standard safety precautions must be followed, but as new research and clinical experience broaden our knowledge, changes in treatment and drug therapy may become necessary or appropriate. Readers are advised to check the most current product information provided by the manufacturer of each drug to be administered to verify the recommended dose, the method and duration of administration, and contraindications. It is the responsibility of the licensed prescriber, relying on experience and knowledge of the patient, to determine dosages and the best treatment for each individual patient. Neither the publisher nor the author assumes any liability for any injury and/or damage to persons or property arising from this publication.

ISBN-13: 978-0-323-04763-0
ISBN-10: 0-323-04763-7

*Acquisitions Editor:* Linda Honeycutt
*Developmental Editor:* Katherine Tomber
*Publishing Services Manager:* Julie Eddy
*Project Manager:* Rich Barber

Printed in the United States of America

Last digit is the print number: 9 8 7 6 5 4 3 2 1

# Preface

This workbook is designed to accompany *Mosby's EMT–Basic Textbook.* Many students find it helpful to use a workbook to enhance their knowledge and retention after reading a textbook chapter. The goal of this workbook is to provide questions in various testing formats that will challenge you to think and analyze the possible alternatives in providing care to your patients.

Some students will elect to study by themselves, whereas others will benefit more by working with groups of students to complete the materials. Pairs or small study groups may use this workbook to challenge each other's knowledge about the material in each chapter. You may want to complete some portions of the text alone and use the examinations at the end of each division with groups of fellow students.

Your instructor may ask you to complete certain sections of the workbook as classroom assignments. This is an excellent way to test your knowledge of the material that is being presented.

Two categories can be found in this workbook—recall and recognition. Questions of recognition are true/false, matching, and multiple choice. Recognition questions are designed to allow you to see the correct answer with distracting answers.

Questions of recall are completion, short answer, and fill-in-the-blank exercises. These types of questions require that you to know the answer. These are higher-end educational questions that truly challenge your knowledge. This workbook provides both recall and recognition questions for your educational enhancement.

Case studies are also included, which allow you to integrate knowledge from the current chapter and previous chapters to make patient care decisions. These types of exercises will challenge your ability to synthesize materials.

The workbook chapters correspond to the chapters of the textbook. The following elements are found in most workbook chapters:

- Textbook chapter outlines to facilitate note taking
- Key term–matching exercises
- True or false questions
- Short answer and fill-in-the-blank questions
- Multiple-choice questions
- Case studies

Multiple-choice examinations are provided at the end of each division to simulate examinations you may take for certification.

In Section II of the workbook, you will find the answers to each question with a rationale explaining the critical points of knowledge.

# Publisher's Acknowledgments

The editors wish to acknowledge and thank the reviewers of this workbook. Their comments were invaluable in helping develop and fine-tune this manuscript.

**John Gosford,** AS
Training Coordinator
State of Florida
Tallahassee, Florida

**Robert C. Hecker,** NREMT-P
Fire Captain
St. Tammany Fire District #4
Mandeville, Louisiana

**Douglas R. Smith,** MAT, EMT-P, I/C
Chief Operational Officer
Platinum Educational Group
Jenison, Michigan

# Contents

DIVISION **ONE:** Preparatory

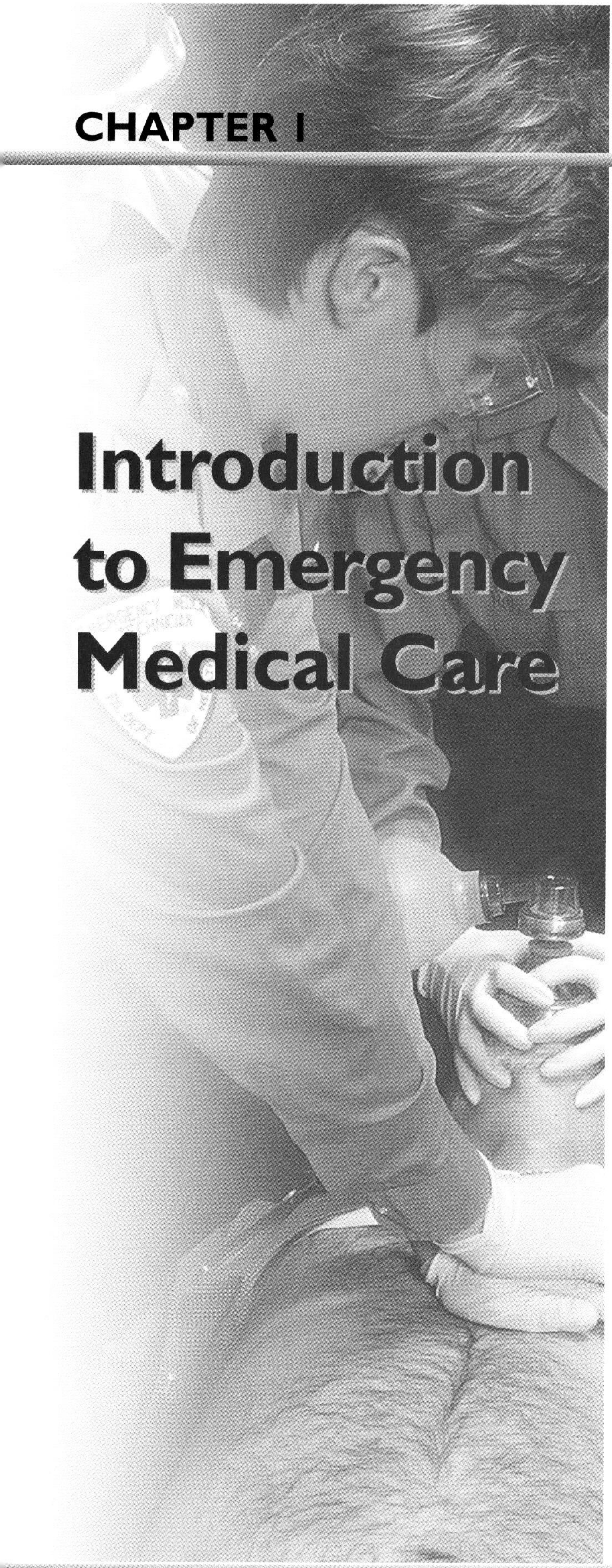

## CHAPTER 1

# Introduction to Emergency Medical Care

### CHAPTER OUTLINE

I. Emergency Medical Services System
   A. National Highway Traffic Safety Administration Technical Assistance Program
   B. Access to the Emergency Medical Services System
   C. Levels of Education
   D. Health Care System
   E. Liaison With Other Public Safety Workers
II. Emergency Medical Technician–Basic
   A. Roles and Responsibilities
      1. Personal safety
      2. Safety of the crew, patient, and bystanders
      3. Patient assessment and care
      4. Lifting and moving patients
      5. Transport and transfer of care
      6. Patient advocacy
   B. Professional Attributes
III. Quality Care
   A. Quality Improvement
   B. Medical Direction

## MATCHING 1

*Match the terms in Column 1 with the correct definition in Column 2.*

**Column 1**

1. ______ Direct medical direction
2. ______ Emergency medical services (EMS) system
3. ______ Indirect medical direction
4. ______ Medical direction
5. ______ National EMS Education and Practice Blueprint
6. ______ Quality improvement

**Column 2**

a. A method for planning, providing, and monitoring emergency care
b. The process of ensuring that care is medically appropriate
c. A method for evaluating and improving care
d. Offline activities such as system design, education, developing protocols, and standing orders
e. Physicians speaking directly with personnel in the field
f. Core content for scope of practice for EMS providers

## MATCHING 2

*Match the terms in Column 1 with the correct definition in Column 2.*

**Column 1**

7. ______ Emergency medical dispatcher
8. ______ Emergency medical technician (EMT)
9. ______ EMT–Basic
10. ______ EMT–Intermediate
11. ______ EMT–Paramedic
12. ______ First Responder

**Column 2**

a. General term for a prehospital care provider
b. Gives instructions over the telephone until EMS personnel arrive
c. Highest level of EMT, with full advanced life-support capabilities
d. Provides initial emergency care until the ambulance arrives
e. EMTs with additional education such as vascular access but not full advanced life support
f. EMT who provides primary care before the patient reaches the hospital

## REVIEW QUESTIONS

1. ______ Public information and education and resource management are part of the National Highway Traffic Safety Administration's (NHTSA) 10 standards for EMS. True (T) or false (F)?

2. ______ Which of NHTSA's 10 standards for EMS ensures adequate funding for EMS?
   a. Regulation and policy
   b. Resource management
   c. Facilities
   d. Evaluation

3. ______ NHTSA's facilities standard helps ensure that patients are transported to the closest appropriate hospital. True (T) or false (F)?

4. ______ 911 is the universal access code to EMS that can be used anywhere in the United States. True (T) or false (F)?

5. ______ The role of a First Responder is to:
   a. Stabilize and transport an ill or injured person
   b. Provide advanced care to an ill or injured person
   c. Provide advanced care without transporting an ill or injured person
   d. Provide initial stabilization until more advanced EMS personnel arrive

6. ______ The EMT–Basic course prepares people to:
   a. Provide advanced care for trauma patients
   b. Establish intravenous access and administer medications
   c. Manage life-threatening illnesses and injuries
   d. Stabilize a patient's injury until further help arrives

7. List three ways to help ensure personal safety.

   a. ______________________________

   b. ______________________________

   c. ______________________________

8. ______ EMT–Basics are responsible for the safety of their crew and the patient, and police and other emergency workers are responsible for the safety of bystanders. True (T) or false (F)?

9. List three roles and responsibilities of the EMT–Basic.

   a. ______________________________

   b. ______________________________

   c. ______________________________

10. ______ Which of the following terms is used to describe the physician who monitors the activities of an EMS system?
    a. Physician in charge
    b. Trauma physician
    c. Medical director
    d. EMS physician

11. ______ Direct medical direction and online medical direction refer to face-to-face, telephone, or radio communication between the physician and the EMS provider. True (T) or false (F)?

12. Define quality improvement.

    ______________________________

    ______________________________

    ______________________________

13. ______ Which of the following is *true* of medical direction?
    a. Requires direct communication between the physician and the EMT
    b. Is not recommended at the EMT–Basic level
    c. Is a physician monitoring the care of EMT–Basics
    d. Includes only education or protocol development before an EMS call

14. You have been asked to speak at an elementary school during Health Awareness Week. The school principal wants you to describe your job and to explain how students can access health care during an emergency.

    a. What are the roles and responsibilities of the EMT–Basic?

    ______________________________

    ______________________________

    b. What are the components of an EMS response?

    ______________________________

    ______________________________

    c. How can citizens access the EMS system?

    ______________________________

    ______________________________

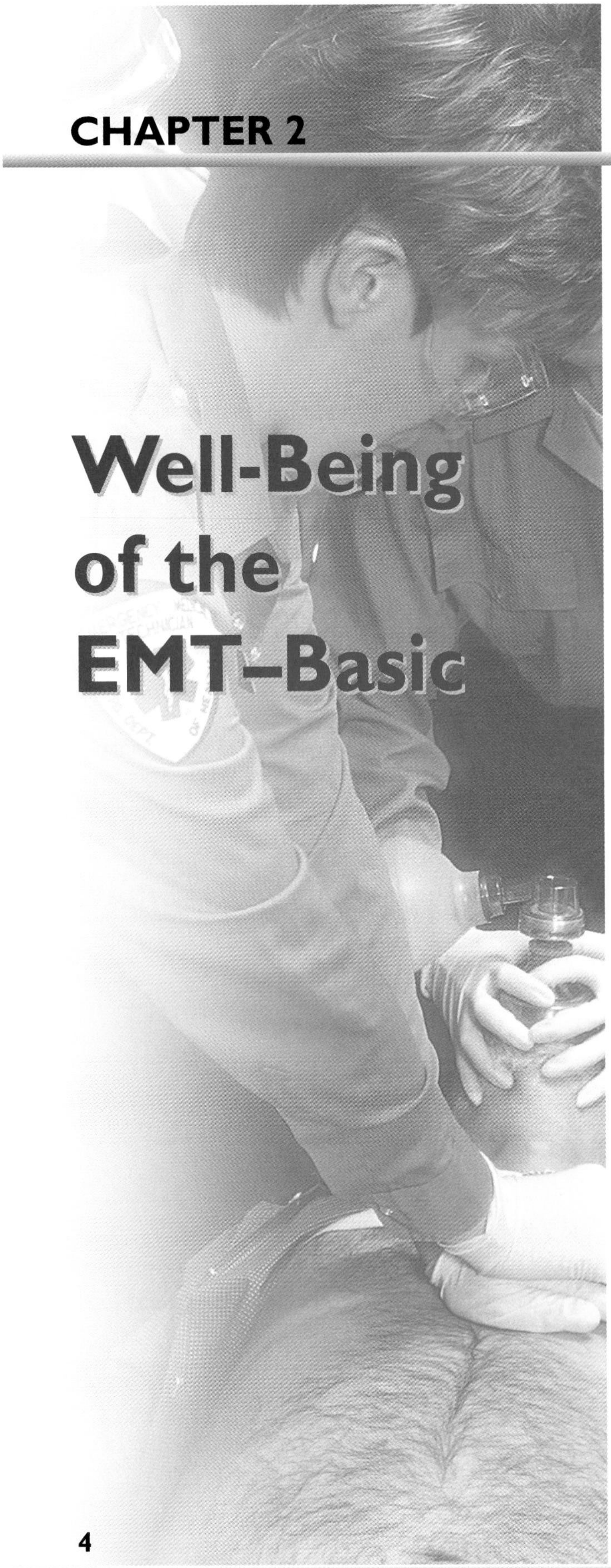

## CHAPTER 2

# Well-Being of the EMT–Basic

### CHAPTER OUTLINE

I. Emotional Aspects of Emergency Care
   A. Death and Dying
   B. Stressful Situations
   C. Stress Management
   D. Critical Incident Stress Debriefing
   E. Comprehensive Critical Incident Stress Management
II. Scene Safety
   A. Body Substance Isolation Precautions
      1. Hand washing
      2. Eye protection
      3. Gloves
      4. Gowns
      5. Masks
      6. Reporting an exposure
   B. Advance Safety Precautions
   C. Personal Protection
      1. Hazardous materials
      2. Rescue
      3. Violence

## MATCHING

*Match the terms in Column 1 with the correct definition in Column 2.*

**Column 1**

1. ______ Body substance isolation (BSI) precautions
2. ______ Critical incident
3. ______ Critical incident stress debriefing
4. ______ Hazardous material
5. ______ Stress

**Column 2**

a. Tension resulting from physical, chemical, or emotional factors
b. Causes unusually strong reactions and interferes with work
c. Process to help emergency workers deal with emotions and feelings
d. Steps taken to prevent exposure to blood or other body fluids
e. Substance that poses an unreasonable risk on release

## REVIEW QUESTIONS

1. Number the five stages in the death and dying process, with 1 as the first stage and 5 as the last.

   ______ Anger
   ______ Acceptance
   ______ Bargaining
   ______ Depression
   ______ Denial

2. Indicate the order of the scene responsibilities of the EMT–Basic, with 1 as the first priority and 4 as the last.

   ______ The patient's safety
   ______ Personal safety
   ______ Bystander safety
   ______ Other crew members' safety

3. ______ People generally move through Kübler-Ross's stages of death and dying in order and in a standard time frame. True (T) or false (F)?

4. List two actions the EMT–Basic may take to help a patient who is dying or the family members of a patient who is dying deal with their emotions.

   a. ______________________________
   b. ______________________________

5. ______ Which of the following is a stress-reduction technique?
   a. Quitting smoking
   b. Volunteering as an EMT–Basic outside of your job
   c. Decreasing exercise programs
   d. Maintaining a constant work schedule

6. List three situations that may cause stress for the EMT–Basic.

   a. ______________________________
   b. ______________________________
   c. ______________________________

7. Stress can be caused by ______________________________, ______________________________, or ______________________________ factors.

8. List three warning signs of stress.

   a. ______________________________
   b. ______________________________
   c. ______________________________

9. ______ A critical level of stress can be the result of one incident or a slow build-up over time. True (T) or false (F)?

10. ______ The purpose of critical incident stress debriefing (CISD) is to help the EMT–Basic speed up the normal recovery process. True (T) or false (F)?

11. ______ Families of EMT–Basics seldom face stresses related to their outside involvement in the profession of EMS. True (T) or false (F)?

12. ______ EMT–Basics are experiencing critical incident stress when:
    a. Their emotional reactions interfere with their ability to function.
    b. They feel guilty about the death of a patient.
    c. They doubt that they treated a patient appropriately.
    d. They are unable to relate their feelings to their family.

13. ______ Which of the following is *true* of CISD?
    a. Debriefings should be held approximately 1 week after the event.
    b. Debriefings should be one on one between the EMT and a mental health professional.
    c. Debriefings should be an opportunity to find out what went wrong.
    d. Debriefings should be followed with referrals for additional help.

14. What is comprehensive critical incident stress management?

______________________________________________

______________________________________________

15. ______ EMT–Basics should determine scene safety immediately after assessing the patient's airway, breathing, and circulation. True (T) or false (F)?

16. ______ What is the single most important measure to take to help prevent the spread of disease?
    a. Wearing gloves
    b. Disinfecting the ambulance between patient encounters
    c. Hand washing
    d. Having the patient wear a mask

17. ______ Which of the following combinations of BSI precautions should be worn when caring for an injury with minimal bleeding?
    a. Gloves only
    b. Gloves and protective eyewear
    c. Gloves and mask
    d. Mask only

18. ______ Eye protection and masks should be worn in addition to gloves when a possibility exists that blood or body fluids might splash during patient care. True (T) or false (F)?

19. ______ EMT–Basics responding to a hazardous materials incident should:
    a. Assume command of the scene.
    b. Begin treatment and transport of all ill or injured persons.
    c. Wait until a specialized hazardous materials team secures the scene.
    d. Begin to decontaminate the scene.

20. ______ Turnout gear, puncture-proof gloves, steel-toed boots, and a helmet are the type of equipment necessary for:
    a. Most hazardous materials
    b. Most rescue situations
    c. Routine emergencies
    d. Firefighting only

21. You have been dispatched to the home of a terminally ill patient who has been involved in a hospice program. The patient's wife is distraught, and her daughter has requested EMS assistance.

    a. Describe, in order, the stages through which most patients and family members go when they discover that death is imminent.

    ________________________________________

    ________________________________________

    b. When you arrive at the scene, the wife pleads, "Please do something to make him live another day." This is an example of which stage?

    ________________________________________

    ________________________________________

    c. How should you deal with the family members in this situation?

    ________________________________________

    ________________________________________

22. Over the last several weeks, your partner is having problems getting along with you. She has been very quiet and withdrawn and does not talk much to anybody.

    a. You know that your partner is showing warning signs of stress. What are other stress warning signs?

    ________________________________________

    ________________________________________

    b. List seven techniques that can reduce stress and help avoid burnout.

    ________________________________________

    ________________________________________

    ________________________________________

    ________________________________________

    ________________________________________

    ________________________________________

    ________________________________________

    c. Describe situations that can cause stress in EMS.

    ________________________________________

    ________________________________________

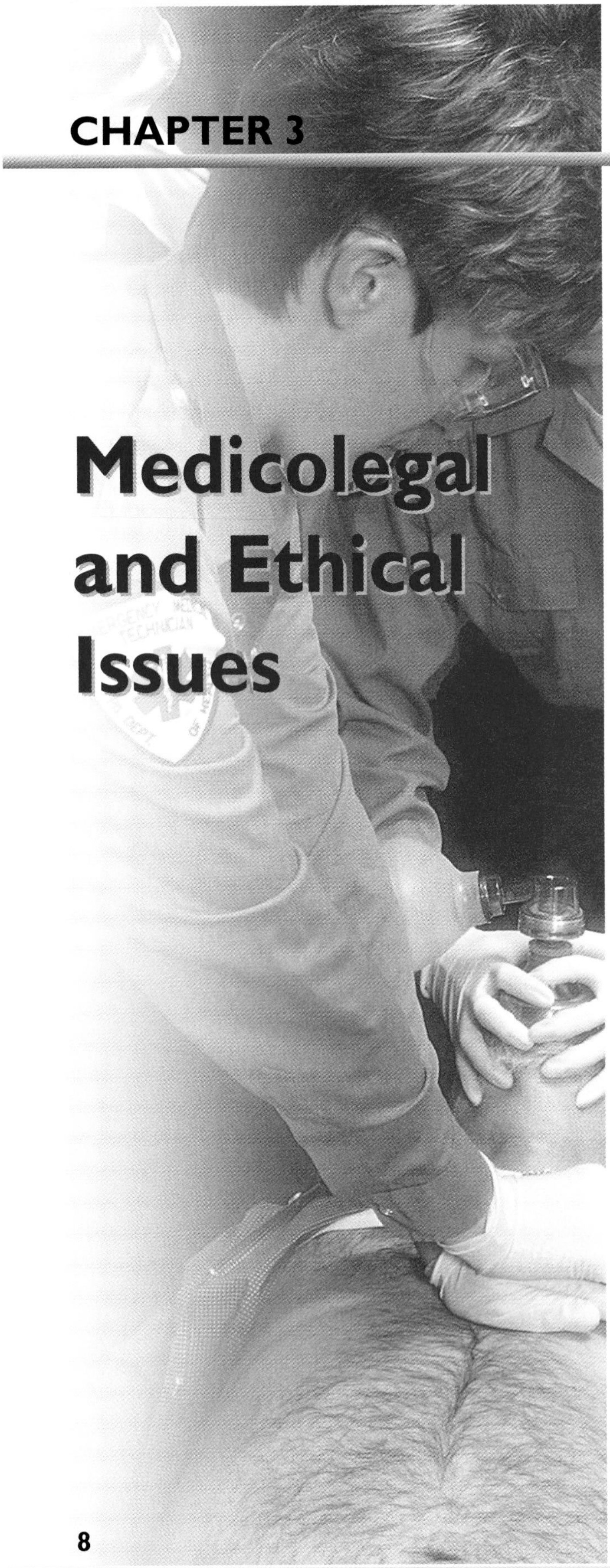

# CHAPTER 3

# Medicolegal and Ethical Issues

## CHAPTER OUTLINE

I. Scope of Practice
   A. Legal Duties to the Patient, Medical Director, and Public
   B. Ethical Responsibilities
   C. Duty to Act
      1. Legal considerations
         a. Negligence
         b. Abandonment
      2. Ethical considerations

II. Consent for Treatment and Transport
   A. Expressed Consent
   B. Implied Consent
   C. Children and Mentally Incompetent Adults
   D. Refusal of Treatment and Transport
   E. Assault and Battery
   F. Advance Directives
      1. Living wills
      2. Durable power of attorney
      3. Do not resuscitate orders

III. Patient Confidentiality
   A. Confidential Information
   B. Releasing Confidential Information
   C. Situations Requiring Special Reporting
   D. Health Insurance Portability and Accountability Act (HIPAA)

IV. Special Situations
   A. Potential Organ Donors
   B. Medical Condition Identification Insignia
   C. Considerations at Possible Crime Scenes

## MATCHING 1

*Match the terms in Column 1 with the correct definition in Column 2.*

**Column 1**

1. ______ Abandonment
2. ______ Advance directives
3. ______ Assault
4. ______ Battery
5. ______ Duty to act
6. ______ Durable power of attorney

**Column 2**

a. Legal obligation to provide care when opportunity exists
b. Termination of care without consent or transfer to an equal or higher level of provider
c. Threatening or attempting to inflict offensive physical contact
d. Orders regarding care to be given in certain emergency situations
e. Offensive touching of a person without his or her consent
f. Document identifying a guardian who can make medical decisions for a patient

## MATCHING 2

*Match the terms in Column 1 with the correct definition in Column 2.*

**Column 1**

7. ______ Expressed consent
8. ______ HIPAA
9. ______ Implied consent
10 ______ Negligence
11. ______ Scope of practice
12. ______ Standard of care

**Column 2**

a. Minimum acceptable level of treatment within a community
b. Duties and skills that can be performed by an EMT–Basic
c. Failure to act in a reasonable and prudent manner
d. Condition to provide care when a patient is physically, mentally, or emotionally unable to consent
e. Condition in which the patient agrees and gives permission for treatment
f. A federal law with provisions for patient privacy

## REVIEW QUESTIONS

1. ______ In most states, the EMT–Basic's scope of practice is based on which of the following?
   a. The U.S. Department of Transportation National Highway Traffic Safety Administration's National Standard Curriculum
   b. The individual medical director for each agency
   c. Each individual EMT–Basic
   d. The service or agency to which the EMT–Basic belongs

2. ______ Protocols and standing orders are used to narrow the scope of practice for EMT–Basics. True (T) or false (F)?

3. What conditions would cause an EMT–Basic to have a "duty to act?"

______________________________________

______________________________________

______________________________________

4. List the four criteria necessary for an EMT–Basic to be accused of negligence.

   a. ______________________________

   b. ______________________________

   c. ______________________________

   d. ______________________________

5. ______ In which of these situations can you release the patient for continued care and not be accused of abandonment?
   a. EMT–Basic to a bystander
   b. EMT–Basic to the hospital staff
   c. EMT–Basic to First Responder
   d. EMT–Paramedic to EMT–Basic

6. The term that describes permission to be treated is called ______________________________.

7. What conditions must exist for the patient to be able to give expressed consent?

   ______________________________

   ______________________________

8. ______ Children have the right to refuse care, even if their parents consent for them to be treated. True (T) or false (F)?

9. Under what conditions is a child considered to be an emancipated minor?

   ______________________________

   ______________________________

10. What steps should the EMT–Basic take when a patient refuses treatment or transport?

    ______________________________

    ______________________________

11. ______ Threatening to touch someone without his or her permission is called:
    a. Aggression
    b. Battery
    c. Assault
    d. Negligence

12. ______ Advance directives are written documents used to express patients' wishes for the type of care they want or do not want in the future. True (T) or false (F)?

13. ______ If the family members of a patient in cardiac arrest state the patient has a do not resuscitate (DNR) order, but they do not or cannot produce a copy of the DNR order, you should:
    a. Withhold care while the family locates the DNR order.
    b. Begin resuscitation.
    c. Contact the patient's physician and ask him or her what should be done.
    d. Provide cardiopulmonary resuscitation (CPR), but do not request additional advanced life support.

14. List three situations when an EMT–Basic can release confidential information.

    a. ______________________________

    b. ______________________________

    c. ______________________________

15. ______ Which of the following is a reportable case in most states?
    a. Gunshot wounds
    b. Alcohol intoxication
    c. Motor vehicle crashes
    d. Human bite

16. What is the purpose of HIPAA?

    ______________________________

    ______________________________

17. ______ Patients who are dying can become organ donors by making their wishes known to an EMT–Basic when they are dying. True (T) or false (F)?

18. ______ When treating a victim of a violent crime, the EMT–Basic should never disturb the crime scene. True (T) or false (F)?

19. Last year, you worked a call involving a motor vehicle crash. At the scene were two patients with serious injuries and one fatality. One of the survivors now claims that you did not perform to the standard of care and were negligent in your delivery of emergency care.

    a. Define standard of care.

    ______________________________

    ______________________________

    b. Define negligence.

    ______________________________

    ______________________________

    c. List the four criteria that must be met before negligence can be proven.

    ______________________________

    ______________________________

    ______________________________

    ______________________________

20. You are caring for a patient who has fallen and struck his head. He is unresponsive and has a notable amount of bleeding from a scalp laceration.

    a. How would you obtain permission to treat this patient?

    ______________________________

    ______________________________

    b. What is the legal basis that allows you to initiate emergency care?

    ______________________________

    ______________________________

    c. Define expressed consent.

    ______________________________

    ______________________________

21. You are caring for a 68-year-old man who collapsed at his neighbor's home from cardiac arrest. The automated external defibrillator is applied, CPR is in progress, and the patient's airway is being managed. The patient's son arrives on the scene and advises you that he has durable power of attorney for his father's health care. His father is terminally ill and has signed a living will that requests that he not be resuscitated. He demands that you stop CPR and allow his father to "die in peace."

    a. What is a living will?

    ______________________________

    ______________________________

    b. What is durable power of attorney?

    ______________________________

    ______________________________

    c. How will you handle this situation?

    ______________________________

    ______________________________

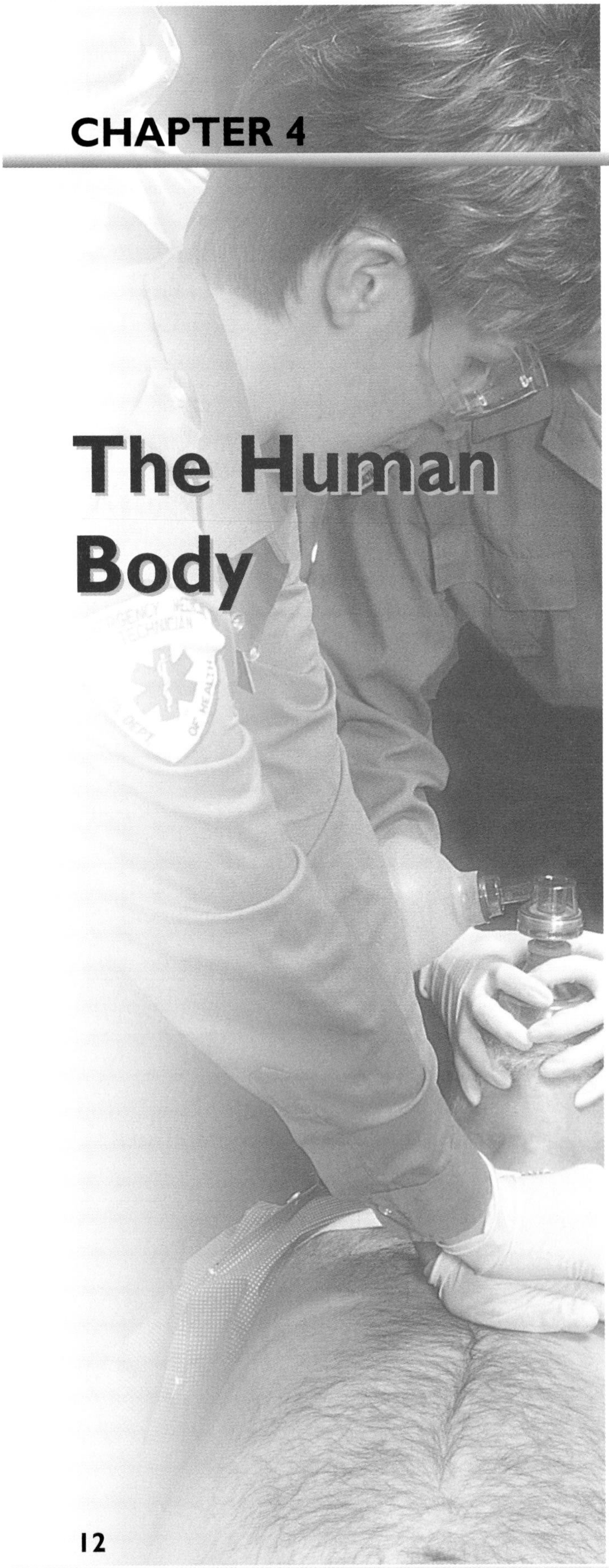

## CHAPTER 4

# The Human Body

**CHAPTER OUTLINE**

- I. Anatomic Terms
  - A. Anatomic Position
  - B. Descriptive Anatomic Terms
- II. Body Systems
  - A. Respiratory System
    - 1. Airway
    - 2. Lungs
      - a. Gas exchange
    - 3. Normal breathing
    - 4. Respiratory system of infants and children
  - B. Circulatory System
    - 1. Heart
    - 2. Blood vessels
    - 3. Blood
    - 4. Circulation of blood
  - C. Musculoskeletal System
    - 1. Skeleton
      - a. Skull
      - b. Spinal column and rib cage
      - c. Pelvis and lower extremities
      - d. Upper extremities
    - 2. Joints
    - 3. Muscles
      - a. Skeletal muscles
      - b. Smooth muscles
      - c. Cardiac muscles
  - D. Nervous System
  - E. Skin
  - F. Digestive System
  - G. Endocrine System

## MATCHING 1

*Match the terms in Column 1 with the correct definition in Column 2.*

**Column 1**

1. ______ Accessory muscles
2. ______ Breath sounds
3. ______ Intercostal muscles
4. ______ Thorax
5. ______ Tidal volume

**Column 2**

a. Sound made by air moving in and out of the lungs
b. Used in respiratory distress to draw more air into the lungs
c. The volume of air per breath
d. Bone structure composed of 12 pairs of ribs and the sternum
e. Muscles between each rib that move with breathing

## MATCHING 2

*Match the terms in Column 1 with the correct definition in Column 2.*

**Column 1**

6. ______ Adrenaline
7. ______ Hemoglobin
8. ______ Hormones
9. ______ Insulin
10. ______ Platelets
11. ______ Red blood cells
12. ______ White blood cells

**Column 2**

a. Body defense against infection
b. Regulate body activities and functions in many body systems
c. Hormone that helps prepare the body for emergencies
d. Blood cells containing hemoglobin
e. Blood component that plays a role in clotting
f. Carries oxygen in blood and releases it when it reaches the tissue
g. Hormone that is crucial for the body's use of sugar

## MATCHING 3

*Match the terms in Column 1 with the correct definition in Column 2.*

**Column 1**

13. ______ Anatomic position
14. ______ Bilateral
15. ______ Midaxillary line
16. ______ Midclavicular line
17. ______ Midline

**Column 2**

a. Standing upright with feet, palms, eyes facing forward
b. Two lines dividing the collarbone in two, extending through the nipples
c. Line from the armpits to the ankles, dividing the body in halves
d. The right and left sides of the body relative to each other
e. Line through the middle of the body through nose and umbilicus

## MATCHING 4

*Match the terms in Column 1 with the correct definition in Column 2.*

**Column 1**

18. ______ Blood pressure
19. ______ Central pulse
20. ______ Heart rate
21. ______ Perfusion
22. ______ Peripheral pulse
23. ______ Sutures

**Column 2**

a. A measure of the force exerted against the arterial walls
b. Number of heartbeats in 1 minute
c. A pulse point in an extremity
d. A pulse point in or near the trunk
e. The process of circulating blood, delivering oxygen, and removing waste
f. Joints between the skull bones

## LABELING

1. Label the figure below with the following directional terms:

| | | |
|---|---|---|
| Anterior | Medial | Posterior |
| Inferior | Midaxillary line | Superior |
| Lateral | Midline | |

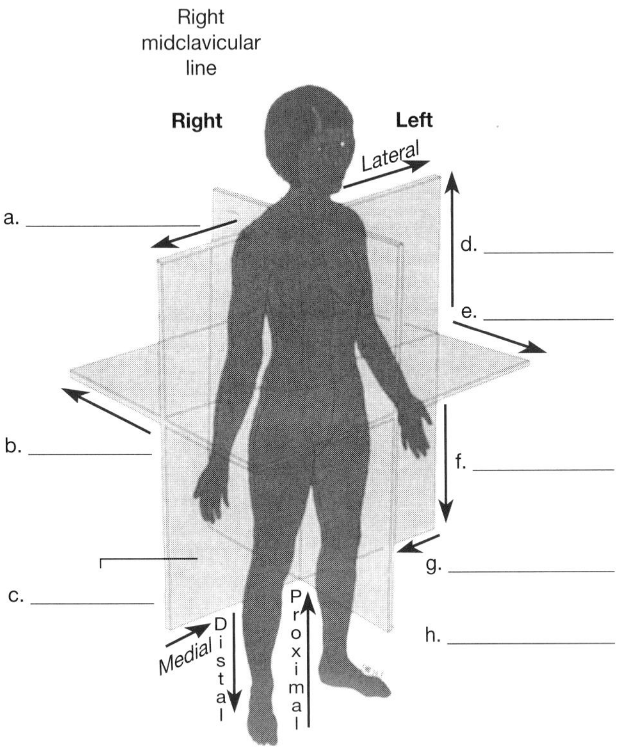


2. Label the figure below with the following skeletal structures:

| | | |
|---|---|---|
| Clavicle | Patella | Skull |
| Femur | Pelvis | Sternum |
| Humerus | Radius | Tibia |
| Mandible | Ribs | Vertebral column |

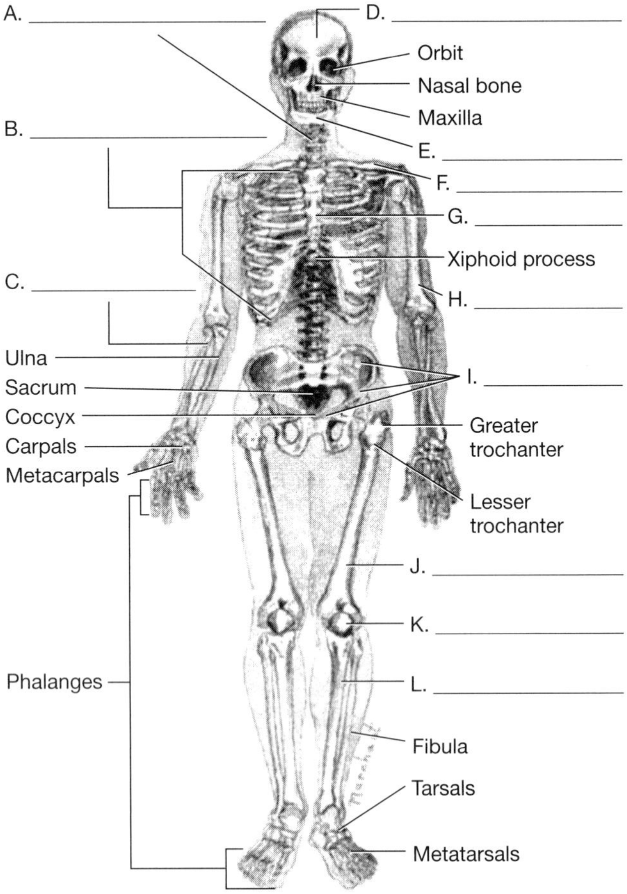

## REVIEW QUESTIONS

1. ______ The midaxillary line divides the body into the ________ and ________ planes.
   a. Anterior, posterior
   b. Superior, inferior
   c. Posterior, medial
   d. Anterior, inferior

2. The sole of the foot is called the

   ________________________________ surface.

3. ______ Supine patients are lying:
   a. On their back
   b. With their head elevated
   c. With their legs elevated
   d. Face down

4. ______ Which of the following terms is used to describe the portion of the throat directly behind the mouth?
   a. Nasopharynx
   b. Epiglottis
   c. Larynx
   d. Oropharynx

5. ______ The trachea is the anatomic term for the:
   a. Windpipe
   b. Throat
   c. Lungs
   d. Mouth

6. ______ The two main sets of muscles used during the normal breathing process are the ________ and the __________________.
   a. Diaphragm, intervertebral muscles
   b. Intercostal muscles, bronchi
   c. Diaphragm, intercostal muscles
   d. None of the above

7. ______ Which of the following best describes the action of the diaphragm during inspiration?
   a. The muscle fibers relax, and the dome flattens and lowers.
   b. The muscle fibers contract, and the dome flattens and lowers.
   c. The muscle fibers relax, and the dome flattens and raises.
   d. The muscle fibers contract, and the dome flattens and raises.

8. ______ Blood returned from the body to the lungs is:
   a. High in carbon dioxide and oxygen
   b. High in carbon dioxide and low in oxygen
   c. Low in carbon dioxide and oxygen
   d. Low in carbon dioxide and high in oxygen

9. ______ The normal respiratory rate for an adult is between __ and __ breaths per minute.
   a. 6, 30
   b. 12, 20
   c. 15, 25
   d. 20, 30

10. ______ The trachea of a small child is:
    a. Well formed but easily obstructed
    b. Soft and easily obstructed
    c. Rigid and not easily obstructed
    d. Rigid and easily obstructed

11. ______ The heart is a pump and consists of _____ chambers.
    a. Two
    b. Four
    c. Six
    d. Eight

12. ______ Which of the following best describes the flow of blood through the heart?
    a. Right ventricle, right atrium, lungs, left atrium, left ventricle, body
    b. Right atrium, right ventricle, lungs, left atrium, left ventricle, body
    c. Left atrium, left ventricle, lungs, right atrium, right ventricle, body
    d. Right ventricle, right atrium, lungs, left ventricle, left atrium, body

13. ______ ________ carry the blood away from the heart, and _____ carry blood to the heart.
    a. Veins, arteries
    b. Veins, capillaries
    c. Arteries, capillaries
    d. Arteries, veins

14. ______ How many liters of blood does the average-sized adult man have in his body?
   a. 3 to 4
   b. 5 to 6
   c. 2 to 4
   d. 7 to 8

15. ______ Plasma is the:
   a. Red blood cell
   b. White blood cell
   c. Fluid of blood
   d. Clotting factor

16. ______ The first number recorded in the blood pressure is the:
   a. Systolic pressure
   b. Diastolic pressure
   c. Aortic pressure
   d. Venous pressure

17. ______ The zygomatic bones form the:
   a. Orbits of the eye
   b. Bridge of the nose
   c. Jaw
   d. Cheekbones

18. ______ The vertebrae of the neck are called the:
   a. Cervical vertebrae
   b. Thoracic vertebrae
   c. Lumbar vertebrae
   d. Sacral vertebrae

19. ______ The superior portion of the breastbone is called the:
   a. Sternum
   b. Xiphoid process
   c. Thorax
   d. Manubrium

20. ______ Which of the following is an example of a ball-and-socket joint?
   a. Shoulder
   b. Neck
   c. Elbow
   d. Ankle

21. ______ The central nervous system consists of the:
   a. Brain and spinal cord
   b. Brain and peripheral nerves
   c. Spinal cord and peripheral nerves
   d. Brain and sensory nerves

22. ______ The peripheral nerves carry information between the spinal column and the other parts of the body. True (T) or false (F)?

23. ______ Signals to the motor nerves cause contractions in the skeletal muscles. True (T) or false (F)?

24. ______ Which layer of the skin contains the blood vessels and nerves?
   a. Epidermis
   b. Dermis
   c. Subcutaneous layer
   d. Connective tissue

25. What is the role of the digestive system?

______________________________________________

______________________________________________

26. Chemicals released from glands within the body are called ______________________________.

27. You are observing an autopsy as part of a continuing education program. After exposing the thoracic cavity, the medical examiner performing the autopsy asks you the following questions:

   a. Where do the bronchi begin and end?

   ______________________________________________

   ______________________________________________

   b. What muscles are involved in the process of ventilation and how do they work during inhalation and exhalation?

   ______________________________________________

   ______________________________________________

   c. How does gas exchange occur in the alveoli?

   ______________________________________________

   ______________________________________________

28. You are working at a local health fair to assist with blood pressure screenings. A middle-aged woman asks you to take her blood pressure and to explain to her the meaning of the two numbers in the measurement. The reading you obtain is 184/96 mm Hg.

    a. How would you explain blood pressure measurement to her?

    ______________________________

    ______________________________

    b. How would you explain the meaning of the two measurement numbers?

    ______________________________

    ______________________________

    c. What else should you tell this woman about her blood pressure reading?

    ______________________________

    ______________________________

29. You are hosting an EMT–Basic study group for your classmates at your home. The group decides to take a break from studying and to play "EMS Jeopardy." What are the questions to the following answers?

    a. They are muscles that are attached to bones.

    ______________________________

    ______________________________

    b. This system consists of sensory and motor nerves found outside the skull or spinal cord.

    ______________________________

    ______________________________

    c. This is the layer of skin that contains sweat glands, hair follicles, blood vessels, and nerve endings.

    ______________________________

    ______________________________

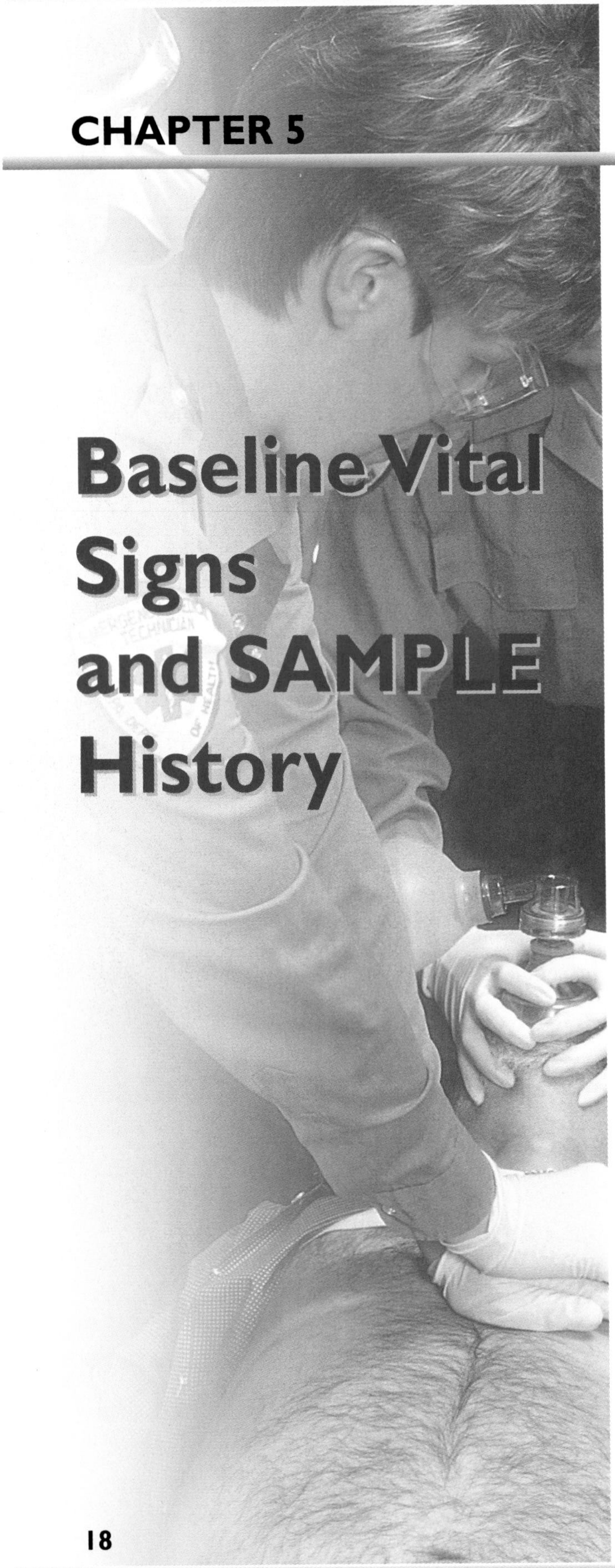

## CHAPTER 5

# Baseline Vital Signs and SAMPLE History

## CHAPTER OUTLINE

- I. Baseline Vital Signs
  - A. Breathing
    - 1. Rate
    - 2. Quality
  - B. Pulse
    - 1. Rate
    - 2. Quality
  - C. Skin
    - 1. Color
    - 2. Temperature
    - 3. Condition
    - 4. Capillary refill
  - D. Pupils
  - E. Blood Pressure
  - F. Vital Sign Reassessment
- II. SAMPLE History

## MATCHING 1

*Match the terms in Column 1 with the correct definition in Column 2.*

**Column 1**

1. ______ Accessory muscles
2. ______ Capillary refill
3. ______ Diastolic blood pressure
4. ______ History
5. ______ Reactive to light
6. ______ Sign
7. ______ Symptom
8. ______ Systolic blood pressure
9. ______ Trending

**Column 2**

a. Amount of time required for blood to return to vessels after applying pressure
b. Referring to pupil constriction when exposed to light
c. A condition that can be observed and identified in the patient
d. Additional muscles used to breathe by patients in respiratory distress
e. Measurement of pressure against the arteries when the heart contracts
f. A nonobservable condition that the patient describes
g. Comparing sets of vital signs over time
h. A concise and inclusive set of information the EMT–Basic gathers about the patient
i. Measurement of pressure against the arteries when the heart is at rest

## MATCHING 2

*Match the terms in Column 1 with the correct definition in Column 2.*

**Column 1**

10. ______ Crowing
11. ______ Grunting
12. ______ Gurgling
13. ______ Snoring
14. ______ Stridor
15. ______ Wheezing

**Column 2**

a. A long, high-pitched sound when breathing in
b. A loud, high-pitched airway noise that usually occurs during inspiration; can indicate obstruction
c. Sound made when liquid is present in the airway
d. Sound made because of the tongue falling back and partially obstructing the airway
e. Sound made when exhaling forcefully against a closed glottis
f. High-pitched whistling sound caused by constriction of the smaller airways

## MATCHING 3

*Match the terms in Column 1 with the correct definition in Column 2.*

**Column 1**

16. ______ Labored respirations
17. ______ Noisy respirations
18. ______ Normal respirations
19. ______ Shallow respirations

**Column 2**

a. An increase in the effort expended to breathe
b. Any sound coming from the patient's airway; indicates a problem
c. Low volumes of air on inspiration and expiration
d. Respirations without noise or effort; occur at a rate of 12 to 20 per minute in adult patients

## REVIEW QUESTIONS

1. When assessing breathing, assess the ______________________ and ______________ of the respirations.

2. ______ The average respiratory rate for an adult at rest is ________ breaths per minute.
   a. 10 to 15
   b. 12 to 26
   c. 10 to 20
   d. 12 to 20

3. How would you assess a patient's respiratory rate?

   ______________________________

   ______________________________

4. ______ The noise made by the tongue partially blocking the airway is called crowing. True (T) or false (F)?

5. ______ The sound that indicates narrowing of smaller airways is called:
   a. Gurgling
   b. Grunting
   c. Snoring
   d. Wheezing

6. ______ The pulse can be felt where a vein passes over a bone near the surface of the skin. True (T) or false (F)?

7. When assessing a patient's pulse, note the ______________________________ and ______________________________.

8. ______ The average resting pulse rate in adults is
   a. 60 to 80 beats per minute
   b. 50 to 100 beats per minute
   c. 60 to 100 beats per minute
   d. 50 to 80 beats per minute

9. Define the following terms:

   Regular pulse:

   ______________________________

   ______________________________

   Irregular pulse:

   ______________________________

   ______________________________

   Weak pulse:

   ______________________________

   ______________________________

10. ______ Which of the following are the components of the assessment of the skin?
    a. Quality, color, and motor function
    b. Temperature, motor and sensory function
    c. Color, temperature, and condition
    d. Quality, color, and motor function

11. Why is the skin color assessed in the nail beds, oral mucosa, or conjunctiva?

    ______________________________

    ______________________________

12. Abnormal skin colors include ______________ or red, blue-gray, ______________________, ______________________, or yellow, and pale.

13. To identify skin temperature, the skin of the ______________________ is more reliable compared with the skin of the extremities.

14. List three abnormal skin temperatures and the conditions that may cause them.

 a. ______________________________

 b. ______________________________

 c. ______________________________

15. The normal skin condition is

______________________________.

16. ______ Normal capillary refill in an infant or child should take less than _____ seconds.
 a. 1
 b. 2
 c. 3
 d. 4

17. ______________________ pupils are big and

______________________ pupils are small.

18. Define the terms equal and reactive to light in relation to the pupil of the eye.

______________________________

______________________________

19. ______ When pupils react normally to light, they ______________.
 a. Dilate
 b. Remain unchanged
 c. Constrict
 d. One constricts, one dilates

20. How would you assess a patient's pupils in bright sunlight?

______________________________

______________________________

______________________________

______________________________

21. ______ Blood pressure is a measure of the amount of force exerted on the blood vessel walls during each heartbeat. True (T) or false (F)?

22. Blood pressure can be measured by listening with

a stethoscope, called ______________________,

or by feeling for the return of a pulse, called

______________________________.

23. ______ Reassess stable patients every __________ minutes and unstable patients every __________ minutes.
 a. 5, 15
 b. 6, 10
 c. 15, 10
 d. 15, 5

24. ______ The "A" in the SAMPLE history stands for allergies. True (T) or false (F)?

25. ______ The medical history should include a detailed account of any medical condition the patient may have experienced. True (T) or false (F)?

26. ______ Medical identification tags generally do not provide any information that is pertinent in the prehospital setting. True (T) or false (F)?

27. List two reasons why accurately recording a patient's history and vital signs is important.

 a. ______________________________

 b. ______________________________

28. What are pertinent negatives?

 a. ______________________________

 b. ______________________________

29. You are participating in a clinical rotation at a local pediatrician's office. You have been asked to take a complete set of vital signs on three patients.
    a. What is a normal respiratory rate range for a 1-year-old child?

    ______________________________________

    ______________________________________

    b. What is a normal pulse rate range for a 3-year-old child?

    ______________________________________

    ______________________________________

    c. What is a normal blood pressure range for a 7-year-old child?

    ______________________________________

    ______________________________________

30. ______ You have been dispatched to care for a patient with difficulty breathing. On arrival, you find a 28-year-old man with labored respirations and audible wheezing. His wife tells you that he has a history of asthma.
    a. What two components do you evaluate in a respiratory assessment?

    ______________________________________

    ______________________________________

    b. If the patient is in respiratory distress, what accessory muscles might he use to assist with breathing?

    ______________________________________

    ______________________________________

    c. How would you describe "wheezing"?

    ______________________________________

    ______________________________________

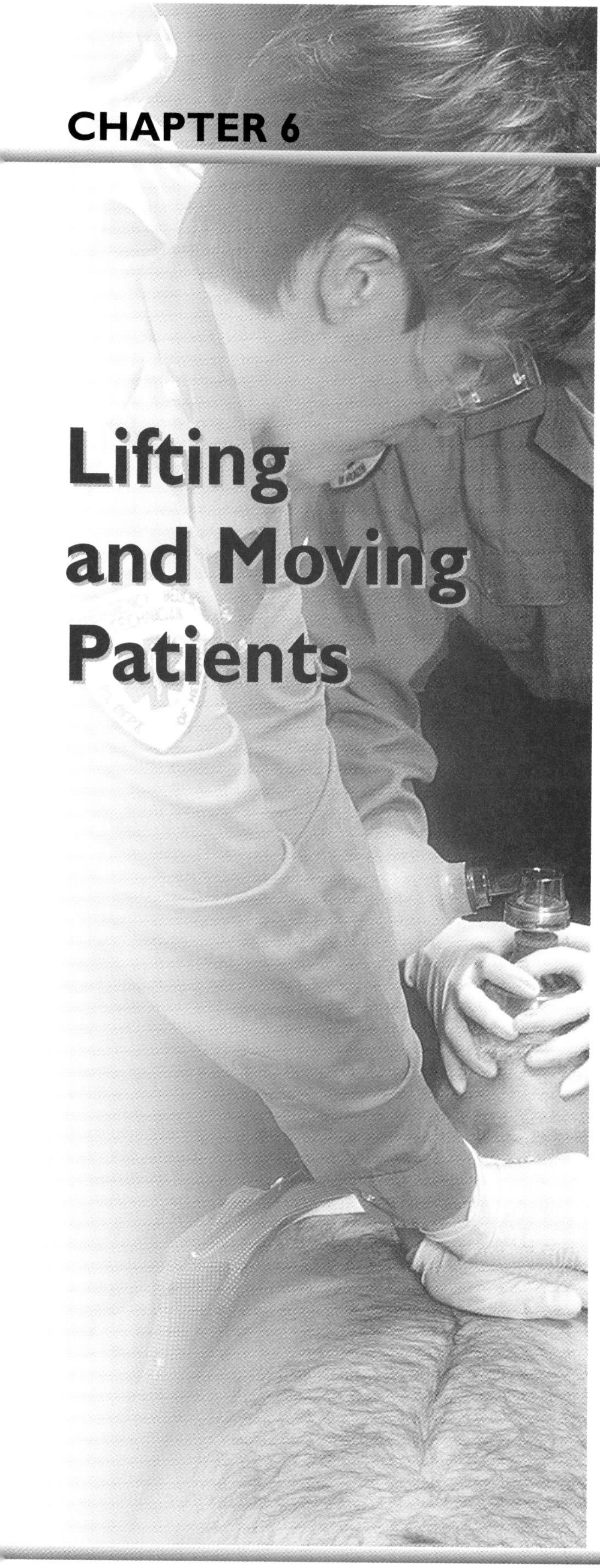

## CHAPTER 6

# Lifting and Moving Patients

### CHAPTER OUTLINE

I. Body Mechanics
  - A. Lifting
  - B. Carrying
  - C. Reaching
  - D. Pushing and Pulling

II. Principles of Moving Patients
  - A. Emergency Moves
  - B. Urgent Moves
  - C. Nonurgent Moves

III. Equipment
  - A. Stretchers and Cots
    1. Wheeled stretcher
    2. Portable stretcher
    3. Scoop stretcher
    4. Flexible stretcher
    5. Basket stretcher
    6. Stair chair
    7. Backboards
  - B. Patient Positioning

## MATCHING 1

*Match the terms in Column 1 with the correct definition in Column 2.*

**Column 1**

1. ______ Body mechanics
2. ______ Emergency move
3. ______ Nonurgent move
4. ______ Power grip
5. ______ Recovery position
6. ______ Urgent move

**Column 2**

a. A move required when danger to the crew or patient exists if the patient is not moved
b. Left lateral recumbent position, used for unresponsive, nontrauma patients
c. A move used when no immediate threats exist
d. Principles of movement used during lifting and moving
e. A patient move used when the patient's condition may become life threatening
f. Hand position providing maximum force to the object being lifted

## MATCHING 2

*Match the following pieces of equipment in Column 1 with the correct applications in Column 2.*

**Column 1**

7. ______ Long backboard
8. ______ Scoop stretcher
9. ______ Stair chair
10. ______ Basket stretcher
11. ______ Short backboard

**Column 2**

a. Lifting from a supine position to a stretcher
b. Immobilizing an entire patient
c. Moving patient through narrow halls
d. Immobilization during extrication when the patient is in a seated position
e. Can be attached to ropes and other lifting devices for rescue situations

## REVIEW QUESTIONS

1. ______ You and your partner should be able and prepared to lift and move every patient for whom you care. True (T) or false (F)?

2. List two components of safe lifting or carrying.

   a. ________________________________

   b. ________________________________

3. ______ Carrying a patient should always be avoided. True (T) or false (F)?

4. ______ One-handed carrying techniques are dangerous. EMTs should always use two hands when lifting. True (T) or false (F)?

5. What is the safest way to transport a patient down a flight of stairs?

   ________________________________

   ________________________________

6. ______ Avoid lifting situations when you must reach more than ______________ in front of you and when you must reach for more than ______________.
   a. 20 inches, 30 seconds
   b. 20 inches, 1 minute
   c. 25 inches, 30 seconds
   d. 25 inches, 1 minute

7. Describe how to reach safely when performing a log roll.

_______________________________________________

_______________________________________________

8. ______ __________ rather than __________ any object is always preferable.
   a. Pushing, pulling
   b. Pulling, pushing
   c. Carrying, pulling
   d. Pushing, dragging

9. Although you will not take time to immobilize a patient during an emergency move, consideration should be given to protecting the

_______________________________________________.

10. ______ If an immediate danger exists for the patient, such as fire, explosives, or other hazards, how should the patient be moved?
    a. Urgent move
    b. Emergency move
    c. Nonurgent move
    d. Rapid extrication move

11. ______ Spinal stabilization techniques can be implemented with an urgent move. True (T) or false (F)?

12. ______ When transporting a pregnant patient in the ambulance, she usually should be placed on her:
    a. Left side
    b. Right side
    c. Back
    d. Abdomen

13. ______ An unresponsive patient with a suspected spinal injury should be placed in the recovery position. True (T) or false (F)?

14. ______ How should a patient with signs and symptoms of shock (hypoperfusion) be transported?
    a. Flat on the back
    b. Head up 30 degrees
    c. Flat on the back, legs elevated 8 to 12 inches
    d. Head down 30 degrees

15. ______ How should a responsive patient who is nauseated or vomiting and has no suspected trauma be positioned for transport?
    a. In the position of comfort
    b. Supine
    c. On left side
    d. Head up 15 degrees

16. You have been dispatched to a patient with a possible allergic reaction. When you arrive at the scene, you are directed up a steep flight of stairs to the attic in an older home. There you find a 56-year-old man who was replacing fiberglass insulation when he became short of breath. You apply high-concentration oxygen and assess his vital signs. He is responsive and alert but says he is too weak to walk down the steps.

    a. What would be the best method of moving this patient to the main level of the house?

    _______________________________________________

    _______________________________________________

    b. When would use of this moving device be contraindicated?

    _______________________________________________

    _______________________________________________

    c. If this patient had also fallen, how should he be transported?

    _______________________________________________

    _______________________________________________

17. You have responded to a motor vehicle crash where fire and rescue personnel are on the scene. On arrival, you find the driver of the car trapped behind the steering column. The fire department has provided access through the driver's door. The patient is unresponsive and has gurgling respirations and an open chest injury. Is this patient a candidate for rapid extrication? If so, why?

_______________________________________________

_______________________________________________

_______________________________________________

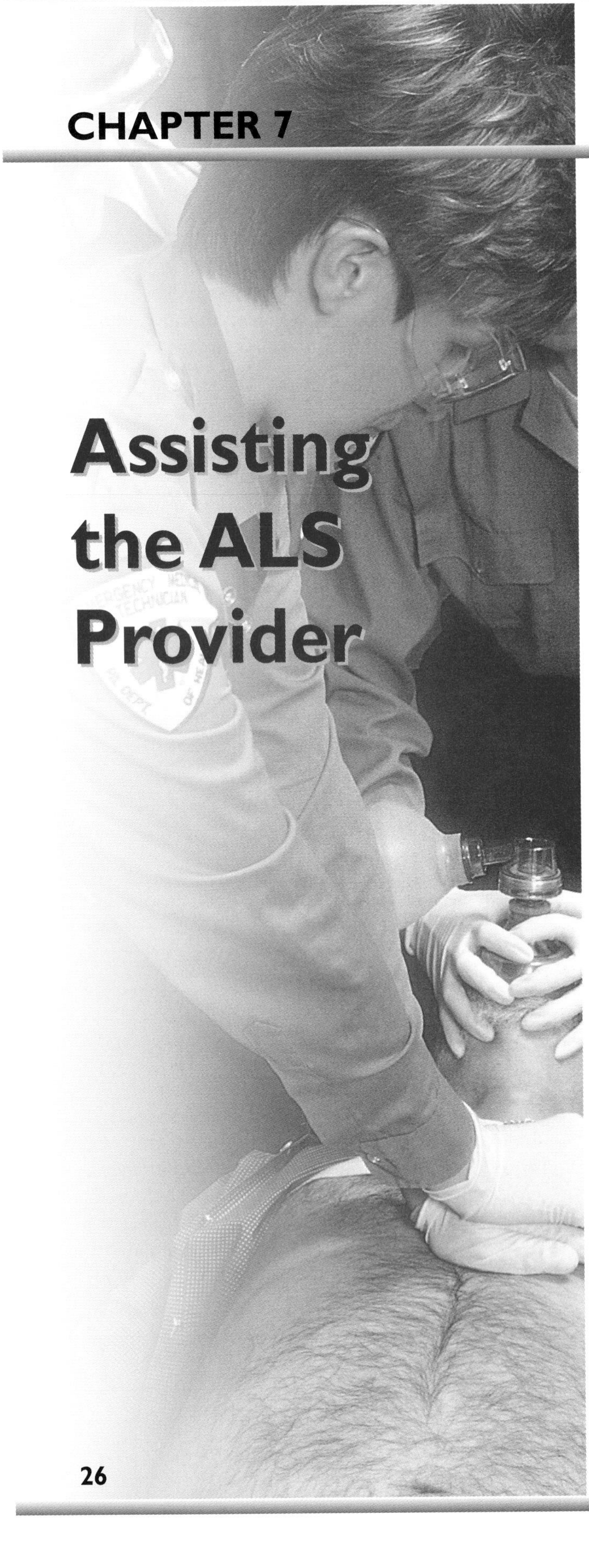

## CHAPTER 7

# Assisting the ALS Provider

## CHAPTER OUTLINE

I. Team Concept
II. ALS Procedures and Equipment
   A. Electrocardiogram (ECG) Monitoring
      1. Rationale
      2. Monitors and patient preparation
      3. Electrode placement
   B. Intravenous Therapy
      1. Rationale
      2. Preparation
         a. Assembly of equipment
         b. Patient preparation
      3. Securing and monitoring
   C. Endotracheal Intubation
      1. Rationale
      2. Equipment and patient preparation
      3. Assisting with the procedure
      4. Confirmation of endotracheal tube placement
      5. Securing and ventilating

## MATCHING

*Match the terms in Column 1 with the correct definition in Column 2.*

**Column I**

1. ______ ALS provider
2. ______ Capnometry
3. ______ Cardiac monitoring
4. ______ Direct laryngoscopy
5. ______ Endotracheal intubation
6. ______ End-tidal $CO_2$ detector
7. ______ Intravenous
8. ______ Microdrip
9. ______ Macrodrip
10. ______ Preoxygenate
11. ______ Pulse oximetry

**Column 2**

a. Fluid administration set producing large drops
b. Fluid administration set producing small drops
c. A device used to measure oxyhemoglobin in the blood
d. The placement of a tube into the trachea
e. A paramedic, nurse, or physician who performs advanced skills
f. Evaluation of the electrical activity of the heart
g. Within the vein
h. Detects the presence of carbon dioxide in exhaled air
i. Ventilatory assistance before procedures such as intubation and suctioning
j. A device that displays the proportion of carbon dioxide in exhaled air
k. The use of a laryngoscope to view the larynx

## REVIEW QUESTIONS

1. On three-lead electrocardiograms (ECGs), the right arm lead is ______________________, the left arm lead is ______________________, and the left leg lead is ______________________.

2. Describe steps that might be necessary to prepare the patient's skin before placing ECG electrodes.

   a. ______________________

   b. ______________________

3. List three reasons why a bag of intravenous (IV) fluid might be discarded.

   a. ______________________

   b. ______________________

   c. ______________________

4. ______ A macrodrip administration delivers _____ drops of fluid per ml.
   a. 10
   b. 20
   c. 30
   d. 40

5. ______ Which of the following steps comes first when preparing an administration set?
   a. Squeeze the drip chamber.
   b. Insert the spike into the bag of fluid.
   c. Unclamp the tubing.
   d. Clear air from the line.

6. Why is a small loop of IV tubing taped onto the patient's skin while securing the IV site?

   ______________________

   ______________________

7. ______ The most common method of endotracheal intubation is by:
   a. Direct laryngoscopy
   b. Nasal intubation
   c. Digital intubation
   d. Retrograde intubation

8. A straight laryngoscope blade is called a ______________________ blade. A curved laryngoscope blade is called a ______________________ blade.

9. What three steps might the EMT take to assist the ALS provider in preparing the endotracheal tube?

   a. ______________________________

   b. ______________________________

   c. ______________________________

10. List three ways to confirm proper endotracheal tube placement.

   a. ______________________________

   b. ______________________________

   c. ______________________________

# DIVISION **ONE**

## Preparatory



## DIVISION TEST

**Directions:** *Place the letter of the correct answer in the space provided.*

1. ______ EMT–Basics are best defined as:
   a. Responders who stabilize the patient until advanced help arrives
   b. Providers of definitive care for trauma patients
   c. Advanced level of prehospital care provider
   d. Providers of primary care before the patient reaches the hospital

2. ______ Which of the NHTSA standards for EMS ensures that everyone has access to basic emergency medical care?
   a. Regulation and policy
   b. Resource management
   c. Transportation
   d. Trauma systems

3. ______ The standard for the education of prehospital emergency care providers is set by:
   a. The National Registry of Emergency Medical Technicians
   b. The medical director
   c. The National EMS Education and Practice Blueprint
   d. NHTSA's 10 standards for EMS

4. ______ In most states, the minimum acceptable education level for ambulance staff is:
   a. First Responder
   b. EMT–Basic
   c. EMT–Intermediate
   d. EMT–Paramedic

5. ______ Which of the following statements is *true* concerning EMS?
   a. EMT–Basics rarely interact with other public safety workers.
   b. EMT–Basics should be concerned with the patient's rights.
   c. EMT–Basics should put the needs of the patient first, before their personal safety.
   d. EMT–Basics require little continuing education.

6. ______ Which of the following is a role or responsibility of the EMT–Basic?
   a. Patient assessment
   b. Providing medical direction
   c. Diagnosing a patient's medical problem
   d. Care based on diagnosis

7. ______ The first priority of the EMT–Basic at the scene of an emergency should always be:
   a. Scene and personal safety
   b. Communication with the patient
   c. Correct documentation
   d. Contacting medical direction

8. ______ Direct medical direction includes:
   a. Developing protocols
   b. Teaching continuing education courses
   c. Telephone communications during an EMS response
   d. Discussing problems following an EMS response

9. ______ Which of the following is included in the Kübler-Ross stages of death and dying?
   a. Anger
   b. Pity
   c. Disability
   d. Sympathy

10. ______ Which of the following statements is *true* when dealing with the dying patient and family members of the dying patient?
    a. Patient needs include dignity, respect, sharing, communications, privacy, and control.
    b. Separate the patient from the family members when possible.
    c. Provide false assurance if necessary to make the family feel better.
    d. Do not touch the patient unless medically necessary.

11. ______ What is CISD?
    a. Critical injury stabilization disorder
    b. Clinical incident stress disorder
    c. Clinical injury situation debriefing
    d. Critical incident stress debriefing

12. ______ Which of the following is a component of comprehensive critical incident stress management?
    a. Preincident stress education
    b. Financial compensation
    c. Debriefings 1 week after the incident
    d. Formal investigation into the cause of the problem

13. ______ Which of the following is associated with BSI precautions?
    a. Industrial-grade goggles
    b. Self-contained breathing apparatus
    c. Masks with eye shields
    d. Helmets with chin straps

14. ______ Negligence occurs when:
    a. A physician does not ensure a patient's continued care.
    b. A patient suffers damages or injury because an EMT–Basic fails to perform at the accepted level of care.
    c. The EMT–Basic treats the patient without consent.
    d. The EMT–Basic continues to treat the patient after he or she has refused treatment.

15. ______ If an EMT does not continue care after initiation of care, he or she is guilty of:
    a. Negligence
    b. Abandonment
    c. Assault
    d. Battery

16. ______ If EMTs have a formal contract with a municipality to provide care, they have a:
    a. Legal duty to act
    b. Moral duty to act
    c. Ethical duty to act
    d. Reasonable duty to act

17. ______ You are treating a seriously injured patient who is under the influence of alcohol. If he refuses care, you should:
    a. Have him sign a refusal and discontinue care.
    b. Have the patient's friend sign the refusal.
    c. Treat the patient under implied consent.
    d. Treat the patient under expressed consent.

18. ______ Which of the following statements regarding consent is *true?*
   a. Responsive and unresponsive patients can provide expressed consent.
   b. Use implied consent to treat the unresponsive patient.
   c. Use implied consent to treat children whose parents do not want them to be treated.
   d. The patient cannot withdraw his or her consent once it is given.

19. ______ Which of the following statements is *true* concerning refusals in patient care?
   a. Children can refuse care, even if their parents want them to be treated.
   b. The patient cannot withdraw from treatment after it has begun.
   c. Patients who do not want care must simply sign a release.
   d. When in doubt, if the patient is competent to refuse treatment, err in the favor of treatment.

20. ______ Which of the following statements is *true* regarding DNR orders?
   a. The patient has the right to refuse certain resuscitation efforts.
   b. In general, DNR orders do not require written orders from a physician.
   c. All states recognize DNR orders for prehospital personnel.
   d. The DNR order does not have to be seen by the EMT–Basic to be honored.

21. ______ In which of the following situations can an EMT–Basic release confidential information?
   a. In a case review for continuing education
   b. Any time law enforcement personnel request information
   c. When a reportable situation occurs
   d. All of the above

22. ______ Which of the following terms is associated with the respiratory system?
   a. Pharynx
   b. Mitral valve
   c. Olecranon process
   d. Adrenaline

23. ______ Gas exchange normally takes place in the:
   a. Oropharynx
   b. Trachea
   c. Bronchi
   d. Alveoli

24. ______ Which of the following statements is *true* of normal respiratory rates?
   a. Children breathe more quickly than adults.
   b. The oxygen needs of infants and children are less than adults.
   c. Adults normally breathe 10 to 30 times per minute.
   d. Children normally breathe 15 to 25 times per minute.

25. ______ Which of the following statements concerning anatomic considerations in infants and children is *true?*
   a. In general, all structures are smaller and less easily obstructed.
   b. The tongue is smaller proportionally and rarely causes problems.
   c. Swelling obstructs the trachea more easily.
   d. The trachea is less flexible because it is less developed.

26. ______ Which of the following statements about the circulatory system is *true?*
   a. Oxygenated blood is pumped from the lungs to the left atrium.
   b. The average man has approximately 5 gallons of blood.
   c. Platelets are important for fighting infection.
   d. The upper chambers of the heart are the ventricles.

27. ______ What is the medical terminology used to describe the bone in the thigh?
   a. Tibia
   b. Femur
   c. Fibula
   d. Patella

28. ______ Which of the following statements is *true?*
   a. The digestive system contains glands that release hormones.
   b. The motor nerves carry information to the brain from the body.
   c. The middle layer of the skin is the dermis.
   d. The central nervous system is composed of motor and sensory nerves.

29. ______ The average pulse rate range for an adult is ________ beats per minute.
   a. 12 to 20
   b. 60 to 80
   c. 70 to 100
   d. 50 to 70

30. ______ Which of the following signs is characteristic of normal breathing?
   a. Increased effort
   b. Grunting and stridor
   c. Using accessory muscles
   d. Bilateral chest expansion

31. ______ Which of the following terms is used to describe a patient's skin temperature?
   a. Hot
   b. Dry
   c. Clammy
   d. Pale

32. ______ Which of the following statements is *correct?*
   a. Pupils should dilate equally when exposed to light.
   b. Capillary refill should be assessed in patients younger than 6 years of age.
   c. The diastolic pressure is the measurement of force exerted when the heart is contracting.
   d. Vital signs should be reassessed every 15 minutes for unstable patients.

33. ______ Which of the following statements concerning the SAMPLE history is correct?
   a. The "A" in SAMPLE stands for allergies to medications only.
   b. A complete medical history should be assessed.
   c. A symptom is any medical condition that can be observed.
   d. The "E" in SAMPLE stands for events leading to the illness or injury.

34. ______ Which of the following statements is *true* concerning lifting and moving?
   a. Use legs, not back, to lift.
   b. Use back, not legs, to lift.
   c. Twist when needed to help move patients.
   d. Use no more than three people to move a patient.

35. ______ Which of the following is a dangerous way to lift a stretcher?
   a. Using the power-lift
   b. Using the power-grip
   c. Bending at the waist
   d. Lifting while keeping back in locked-in position

36. ______ Which of the following statements is *true* regarding moving patients?
   a. An emergency move is necessary if you cannot provide lifesaving care because of the patient's position.
   b. Use urgent moves when an immediate danger is present.
   c. No time exists for spinal protection during urgent moves.
   d. A patient with signs and symptoms of shock would require a nonurgent move.

37. ______ How should the unresponsive patient, without suspected spine injury, be transported?
   a. In the recovery position
   b. Supine
   c. Prone
   d. In the position of comfort

38. ______ How should a responsive patient with chest pain or difficulty breathing and no signs of trauma be transported?
   a. In the recovery position
   b. Supine
   c. Prone
   d. In the position of comfort

39. ______ Twelve-lead EKG systems use ________ electrodes placed on the chest wall and four electrodes placed on the ________.
   a. six; chest wall
   b. six; extremities
   c. eight; chest wall
   d. eight: extremities

40. ______ An administration set that delivers 10 or 15 drops per milliliter of fluid is called a:
   a. Large administration set
   b. Small administration set
   c. Macrodrip administration set
   d. Microdrip administration set

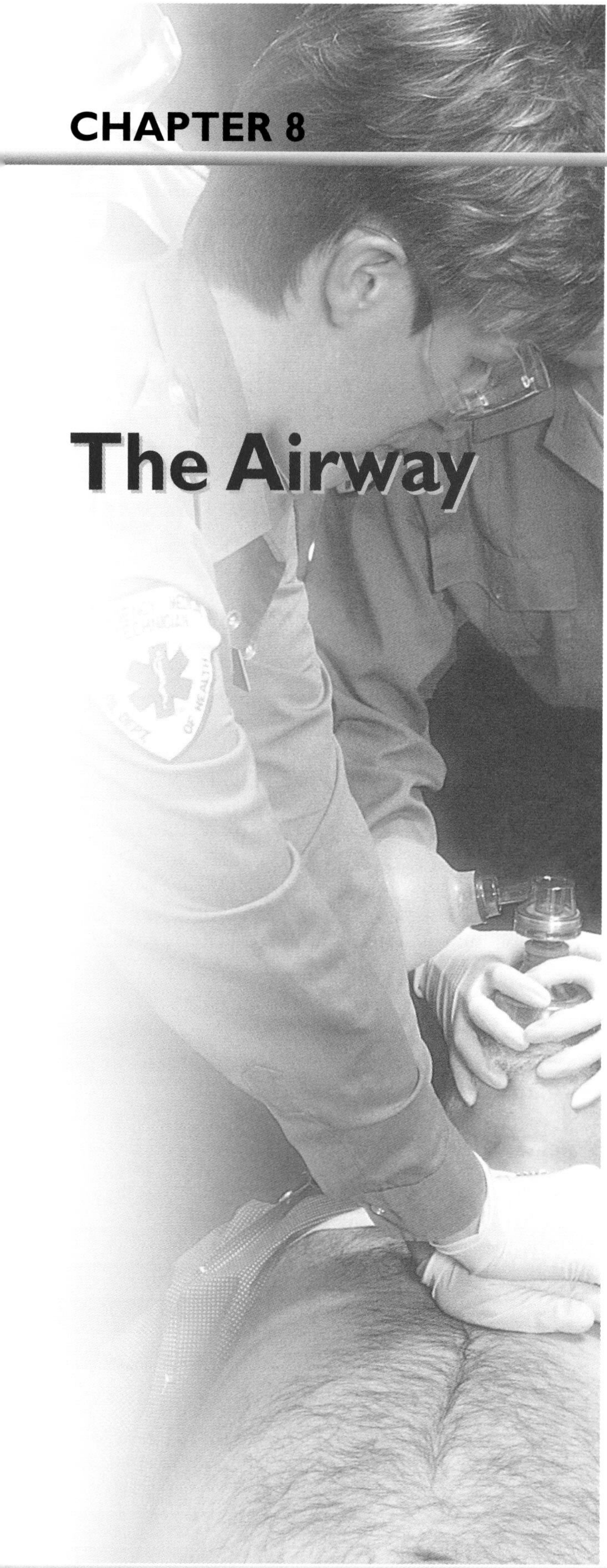

## CHAPTER 8

# The Airway

## CHAPTER OUTLINE

I. Respiratory System
   A. Respiratory Anatomy
   B. Respiratory Physiology
      1. Adequate breathing
      2. Inadequate breathing
      3. Considerations for infants and children
II. Oxygen
   A. Oxygen Sources
   B. Equipment for Oxygen Delivery
      1. Oxygen regulators
      2. Oxygen delivery devices
         a. Nonrebreather masks
         b. Nasal cannulas
III. Opening the Airway
   A. Manual Positioning
   B. Airway Adjuncts
      1. Oropharyngeal airway
      2. Nasopharyngeal airway
   C. Suction
IV. Artificial Ventilation
   A. Mouth-to-Mask With Supplemental Oxygen Technique
   B. Two-Person Bag-Valve-Mask Technique
   C. Flow-Restricted, Oxygen-Powered Ventilation Device
   D. One-Person Bag-Valve-Mask Technique
   E. Considerations for Trauma Patients
   F. Assessing the Adequacy of Artificial Ventilation
V. Special Situations in Airway Management
   A. Patients With Laryngectomies
   B. Ventilating Infants and Children
   C. Facial Injuries
   D. Obstructions
   E. Dental Appliances

## MATCHING 1

*Match the terms in Column 1 with the correct definition in Column 2.*

**Column 1**

1. ______ Airway
2. ______ Alveoli
3. ______ Bronchi
4. ______ Cricoid ring
5. ______ Glottis
6. ______ Tracheal stoma

**Column 2**

a. The passageway into the trachea from the pharynx
b. Respiratory system structures through which air passes
c. The two major branches of the trachea into each lung
d. The air sacs in the lungs where gas exchange takes place
e. A firm cartilage ring just inferior to the lower portion of the larynx
f. Permanent artificial opening in the trachea

## MATCHING 2

*Match the terms in Column 1 with the correct definition in Column 2.*

**Column 1**

7. ______ Bag-valve-mask (BVM)
8. ______ Nasal cannula
9. ______ Nasopharyngeal airway
10. ______ Nonrebreather mask
11. ______ Oropharyngeal airway
12. ______ Suction devices

**Column 2**

a. Devices that remove secretions and fluids from the airway
b. Device for delivering oxygen from tubing into nostrils
c. Inserted into mouth to lift the tongue out of the oropharynx
d. High-flow device for delivering oxygen to the patient
e. Ventilation device with a bag, a one-way valve, and a mask
f. Flexible tube inserted into the nostril to provide an air passage

## MATCHING 3

*Match the terms in Column 1 with the correct definition in Column 2.*

**Column 1**

13. ______ Cyanotic
14. ______ Diaphragm
15. ______ Gag reflex
16. ______ Intercostal muscles
17. ______ Jaw thrust
18. ______ Laryngectomy

**Column 2**

a. Causes the patient to retch when the throat is stimulated
b. Muscle separating the thoracic from the abdominal cavity
c. Color of mucous membranes caused by hypoperfusion
d. Muscles located between the ribs that move with breathing
e. Surgical procedure in which the larynx is removed
f. Opening the airway by displacing the mandible forward

## MATCHING 4

*Match the terms in Column 1 with the correct definition in Column 2.*

**Column 1**

19. ______ Epiglottis
20. ______ Larynx
21. ______ Nasopharynx
22. ______ Oropharynx
23. ______ Pharynx
24. ______ Trachea

**Column 2**

a. Prevents food and liquid from entering the trachea
b. Voice box; consists of cartilage that vibrates when speaking
c. Part of the airway behind the nose and mouth
d. Part of the pharynx behind the nose
e. Part of the airway behind the mouth
f. The windpipe

## LABELING

1. Label the following figure with these terms:
   Diaphragm, Left bronchus, Oropharynx, Larynx, Nasopharynx, Right bronchus, Epiglottis

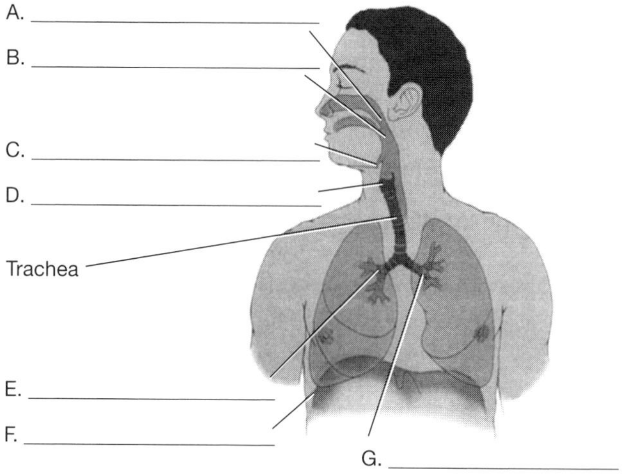


2. Label the following figure with these terms:
   Face mask, Oxygen reservoir valve, One-way valve, Oxygen supply, Oxygen reservoir, Self-inflating bag

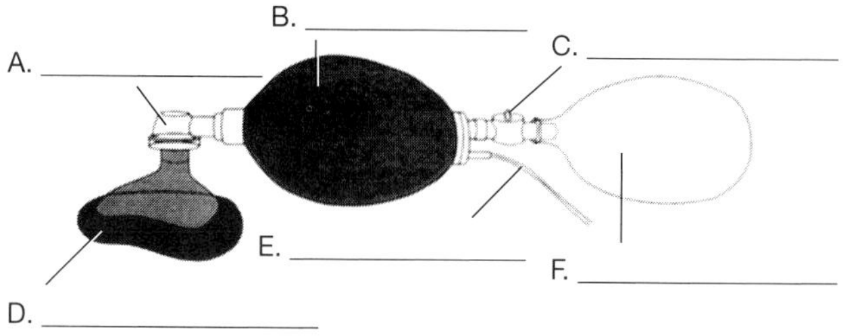


## REVIEW QUESTIONS

1. ______ Inspiration flattens the diaphragm, pulling air into the lungs through the nose and mouth. True (T) or false (F)?

2. ______ Exhalation and inhalation are considered active processes. True (T) or false (F)?

3. ______ The normal range of respiratory rates for an adult is:
   a. 10 to 12
   b. 12 to 30
   c. 12 to 20
   d. 15 to 18

4. ______ Indicate which of the following are signs and symptoms of inadequate breathing and which are signs of adequate breathing.
   a. Regular rhythm
   b. Equal chest expansion
   c. Shortness of breath
   d. Pale, cyanotic skin
   e. Decreased breath sounds
   f. Slow rate
   g. Quiet breathing

5. On what muscle or muscles do children rely most for respiration?

______________________________

______________________________

6. What equipment is necessary to deliver oxygen to a patient?

   a. ______________________________

   b. ______________________________

   c. ______________________________

7. What are the two types of oxygen delivery devices commonly used by EMT–Basics?

   a. ______________________________

   b. ______________________________

8. ______ Nonrebreather masks can deliver up to _____ oxygen at 15 L/min.
   a. 97%
   b. 92%
   c. 90%
   d. 100%

9. ______ When administering oxygen by non-rebreather mask, set the flow rate at:
   a. 2 L/min
   b. 4 L/min
   c. 6 to 8 L/min
   d. 15 L/min

10. ______ Similar to the nonrebreather mask, the nasal cannula delivers high oxygen concentrations to the patient and is therefore a good alternative to the nonrebreather mask. True (T) or false (F)?

11. ______ The flow rate of a nasal cannula can be set to a maximum of ____ L/minute.
    a. 2
    b. 4
    c. 6
    d. 8

12. What three actions can combine to prevent air from entering the lungs in an unresponsive patient?

    ______________________________

    ______________________________

13. ______ The most common method of opening the airway for a trauma patient is the head-tilt, chin-lift technique. True (T) or false (F)?

14. List the steps in performing the head-tilt, chin-lift technique and the jaw thrust maneuver.

    Head-tilt, chin-lift:

    ______________________________

    ______________________________

    Jaw thrust:

    ______________________________

    ______________________________

15. Oral airways are measured from the corner of the mouth to the ______________________________ or the ______________________________.

16. ______ How would you insert an oral airway for a child?
    a. Upside down, then gently rotate into place
    b. Right side up, using a tongue depressor
    c. Right side up, without a tongue depressor
    d. Oral airways are not recommended for children under 16 years of age.

17. ______ The nasal airway is preferred for patients who have a gag reflex. True (T) or false (F)?

18. The nasal airway is measured from the tip of the nose to the ______________________________.

    The airway is inserted with the bevel toward the ______________________________ of the nose.

19 If the EMT–Basic hears gurgling when assessing the patient's breathing, what should be done?

_______________________________________

_______________________________________

20. ______ Which statement about the rigid suction catheter is *true?*
   a. It is difficult to control.
   b. The tip should remain visible when inserted.
   c. It can be used only on unresponsive patients.
   d. It is also called a French catheter.

21. ______ Which of the following statements about bulb syringes is *true?*
   a. Used to suction the mouth and nose
   b. Inserted into the nostril and then compressed
   c. Dangerous to use for infants and children
   d. Can be used only for newborns up to 2 days of age

22. ______ Suctioning should never last more than ________ before applying more oxygen.
   a. 15 seconds
   b. 20 seconds
   c. 30 seconds
   d. 1 minute

23. List the steps in performing mouth-to-mouth ventilation.

_______________________________________

_______________________________________

24. ______ Mouth-to-mask is the preferred ventilation method because:
   a. Only one hand is used to form a mask seal.
   b. It requires two people to ventilate the patient.
   c. It provides excellent ventilatory volumes.
   d. Using an oxygen source with the mask is unnecessary.

25. ______ Which of the following statements is true regarding one- and two-person BVM techniques?
   a. With two people, one person maintains the mask seal and squeezes the bag, and the second person maintains an open airway.
   b. With two people, one person maintains the mask seal, and the second person squeezes the bag.
   c. The one-person technique is preferred when maintaining the mask seal is difficult.
   d. With the one- and two-person techniques, ventilate adult patients every second until the chest rises.

26. ______ The flow-restricted, oxygen-powered ventilation device:
   a. Can deliver oxygen at 65 L/minute
   b. Does not require the EMT–Basic to maintain a mask seal
   c. Is safe for infants and children
   d. Delivers 100% oxygen when the trigger is pushed

27. ______ Which of the following is a modification that must be made when ventilating a trauma patient?
   a. Use the head-tilt, chin-lift technique.
   b. The EMT–Basic maintaining the mask seal also performs the jaw thrust.
   c. Seal the mask over the bridge of the nose and well below the chin.
   d. The adult patient should be ventilated every 3 seconds.

28. Indicate with an "A" which of the following statements describes signs of adequate ventilation when using a BVM. Indicate with an "I" which of the statements describes inadequate ventilation when using a BVM.

______ The chest rises and falls with each ventilation.
______ The ventilatory rate is less than 12 times per minute.
______ Skin color is cyanotic.
______ Heart rate returns to normal.
______ The chest does not rise with each ventilation.
______ The stomach becomes distended.

29. Place in order the following steps in correcting poor chest rise during ventilation, with 1 as the first step and 4 as the last.
    ______ Check mask seal.
    ______ Reposition the jaw.
    ______ Try different technique.
    ______ Check for an obstruction.

30. How would you ventilate a patient who has a tracheal stoma?

    ______________________________________

    ______________________________________

31. ______ Oral airways should never be used on trauma patients. True (T) or false (F)?

32. ______ If at all possible, try to leave dentures and other dental appliances in place. They add shape and structure, making it easier to create a mask seal. True (T) or false (F)?

33. You have been dispatched to the home of a sick child. On arrival, the child's mother tells you that her 3-year-old daughter awoke from sleep with a barking cough. The patient is sitting in her father's lap and is leaning forward to breathe.
    a. What are important anatomic and physiologic considerations to keep in mind when caring for a pediatric patient with difficulty breathing?

    ______________________________________

    ______________________________________

    b. What are the signs and symptoms of inadequate breathing?

    ______________________________________

    ______________________________________

    c. What is tidal volume, and what is the easiest way to evaluate it?

    ______________________________________

    ______________________________________

34. You and your partner are using a two-person BVM technique to ventilate an unresponsive patient. During your assessment, you notice that the patient's skin color is not improving. You reposition the patient's jaw and check the mask seal, yet the patient's chest rise remains inadequate.
    a. What are the signs and symptoms of adequate ventilation that should be monitored while providing artificial ventilation?

    ______________________________________

    ______________________________________

    b. You decide to try an alternative method to ventilate this patient. What method would you choose?

    ______________________________________

    ______________________________________

    c. Alternative methods do not correct the patient's inadequate chest rise. What should you do next?

    ______________________________________

    ______________________________________

# DIVISION TWO

## Airway

Chapter 8 The Airway

## DIVISION TEST

**Directions:** *Place the letter of the correct answer in the space provided.*

1. ______ Which of the following occurs during inhalation?
   a. The diaphragm relaxes.
   b. The diaphragm rises.
   c. The chest expands.
   d. The ribs move downward and inward.

2. ______ Which of the following breathing rates is the average in children?
   a. 12 to 20 breaths per minute
   b. 15 to 30 breaths per minute
   c. 25 to 50 breaths per minute
   d. 12 to 50 breaths per minute

3. ______ Which of the following is characteristic of adequate breathing?
   a. Irregular rhythm
   b. Diminished or absent breath sounds
   c. Shallow respirations
   d. Equal chest expansion

4. ______ Which of the following statements is true of an infant or child's airway?
   a. The tongue takes up less room in the mouth than an adult's.
   b. The trachea is relatively wide.
   c. The cricoid ring is totally developed at birth.
   d. The airways are easily kinked with improper positioning.

5. ______ A patient presents with difficulty breathing, a respiratory rate of 20 breaths per minute, and cyanotic mucous membranes. The patient says that he is on oxygen at home via nasal cannula at 4 L/minute. How would you deliver oxygen to the patient?
   a. Nasal cannula at 2 to 4 L/minute
   b. Nasal cannula at 6 L/minute
   c. Nonrebreather mask at 6 L/minute
   d. Nonrebreather mask at 12 to 15 L/minute

6. ______ When administering oxygen by nasal cannula, the maximum oxygen flow rate is:
   a. 2 L/minute
   b. 6 L/minute
   c. 10 L/minute
   d. 15 L/minute

7. ______ How should the airway be opened on a patient with suspected cervical spine injury?
   a. Head-tilt
   b. Head-tilt, chin lift
   c. Jaw thrust
   d. Hyperextension of head

8. ______ Which of the following is appropriate when measuring or inserting an oral airway?
   a. Oral airways are used in unresponsive patients with a gag reflex.
   b. Oral airways are measured for size from the tip of the nose to the corner of the jaw.
   c. Oral airways are inserted upside down until the flange reaches the teeth then rotated.
   d. Oral airways may be inserted by using a tongue depressor.

9. ______ Nasal airways are inserted:
   a. After lubricating with water-soluble lubricant
   b. With the bevel facing the top of the nose
   c. In adult patients only
   d. In responsive patients who are managing their own airway

10. ______ How far should the suction catheter tip be inserted into the patient's mouth?
   a. Just to the front teeth
   b. To the central incisors
   c. To the molars
   d. Only as far as you can see

11. ______ What should be done if large amounts of emesis or secretions are present in the patient's airway?
   a. Log-roll the patient and clear the airway.
   b. Suction for up to 1 minute, then ventilate.
   c. Place the patient in the prone position.
   d. Ventilate the patient first, then suction.

12. ______ What is the maximum length of time to suction a patient between ventilations?
   a. 5 seconds
   b. 10 seconds
   c. 15 seconds
   d. 20 seconds

13. Place the four methods of ventilation in order of preference, with 1 as the most preferred method and 4 as the least.
   ______ One-person BVM
   ______ Mouth-to-mask
   ______ Flow-restricted, oxygen-powered ventilation device
   ______ Two-person BVM

14. ______ Which of the following statements is true of the BVM?
   a. The BVM has a self-inflating bag.
   b. The BVM has a pop-off valve set at 40 L/minute.
   c. BVMs come with a variety of adapters.
   d. Adult BVMs have 800 ml of air.

15. ______ Which of the following statements is *true* concerning a flow-restricted, oxygen-powered ventilation device?
   a. A peak flow rate of 80% oxygen occurs at 60 L/minute.
   b. Relief valve opens at approximately 100 ml of water.
   c. An alarm sounds when relief valve pressure is exceeded.
   d. The EMT–Basic should use only one hand to ventilate the patient.

16. ______ The one-person BVM technique is:
   a. Technically easy but very tiring
   b. The preferred method for ventilating infants or children
   c. Difficult to perform correctly and requires practice
   d. Easier to perform on large patients with receding chins

17. ______ When using a BVM on a trauma patient with suspected spinal injury, which of the following is an accepted technique of ventilation?
   a. Stabilize the head and neck before ventilation.
   b. Use the ring finger and little finger to bring jaw forward to the mask while tilting the head.
   c. A head-tilt, chin-lift maneuver should be performed to allow for best ventilation.
   d. Ventilate every 3 seconds for adults, children, and infants.

18. ______ If you are unable to ventilate a patient through their tracheal stoma, you should:
    a. Request advanced life support assistance for a surgical airway.
    b. Know that endotracheal intubation is required.
    c. Know that the patient cannot be ventilated.
    d. Cover the stoma and ventilate through the mouth and nose.

19. ______ Which of the following is a special consideration when ventilating infants and children?
    a. The head needs to be tilted further back for children and infants.
    b. Avoid excessive pressure when using the BVM.
    c. Gastric distention is less common in children.
    d. Use a BVM with a pop-off valve.

20. ______ What should you do if dentures become dislodged while you are ventilating a patient?
    a. Leave them in place.
    b. Take them out.
    c. Pull up on the jaw to hold them in place.
    d. Take out the upper teeth.

## CHAPTER 9

# Scene Size-Up

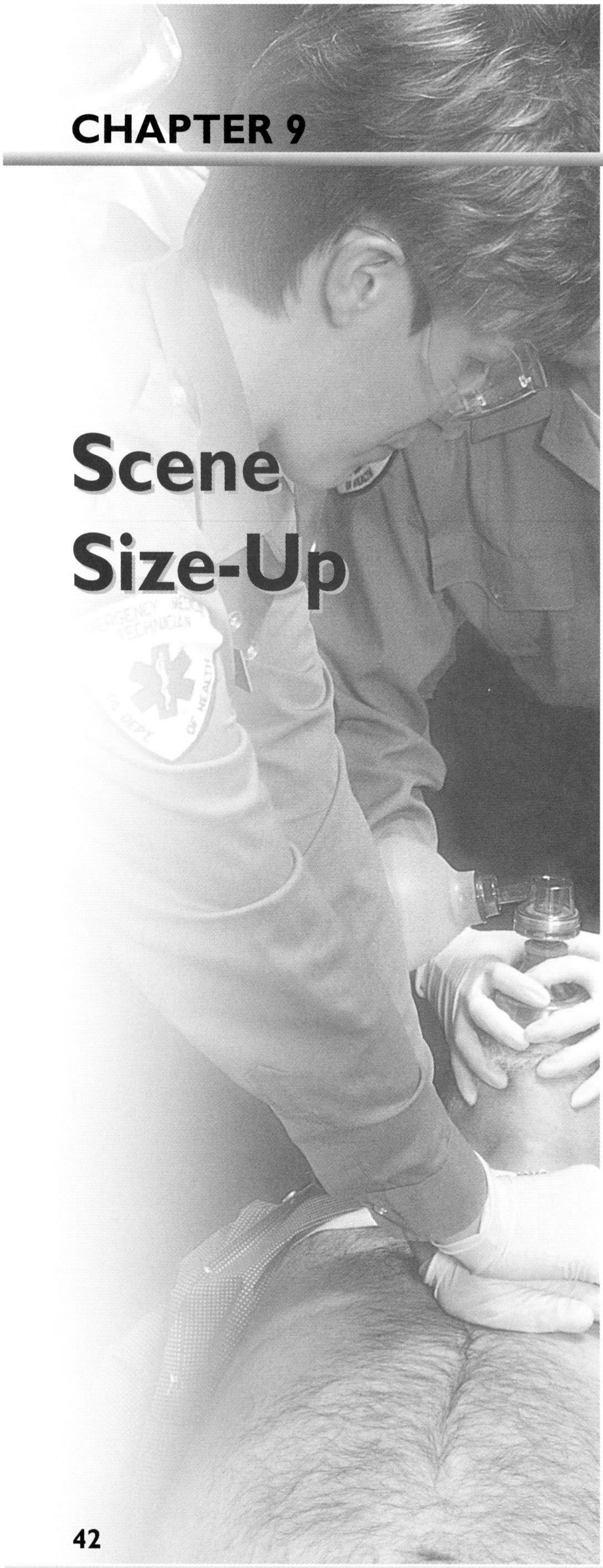

## CHAPTER OUTLINE

I. Body Substance Isolation Precautions
II. Scene Safety
  A. Personal Protection
  B. Protection of the Patient
  C. Protection of Bystanders
III. Nature of Illness and Mechanism of Injury
  A. Nature of Illness
  B. Mechanism of Injury
IV. Number of Patients and Need for Additional Help

## MATCHING

*Match the terms in Column 1 with the correct definition in Column 2.*

**Column 1**

1. ______ Body substance isolation
2. ______ Chief complaint
3. ______ Index of suspicion
4. ______ Mechanism of injury
5. ______ Nature of illness
6. ______ Scene size-up
7. ______ Tunnel vision

**Column 2**

a. The patient's description of the medical problem
b. Evaluation of the entire environment for possible risks
c. Event or forces that caused the damage to the patient
d. The reason EMS was called
e. Precautions from contact with blood and other body fluids
f. Focusing on a noncritical aspect of the situation
g. Anticipating injuries based on the forces causing trauma

## REVIEW QUESTIONS

1. ______ Personal protection includes BSI precautions and appropriate clothing for the environment and situation. True (T) or false (F)?

2. List the steps of the scene size-up.

______________________________

______________________________

3. ______ Scene safety includes which of the following?
   a. Bystander protection
   b. Primary evaluation of the patient
   c. Patient assessment
   d. Determining the number of patients

4. List three hazards that may be present at the scene of an automobile crash.

   a. ______________________________

   b. ______________________________

   c. ______________________________

5. What types of hazards may be present at the scene of a medical call?

______________________________

______________________________

6. How would you determine if the scene was safe to enter?

______________________________

______________________________

7. The most important statement to remember concerning scene safety is:

______________________________

______________________________

8. ______ The nature of illness is also called the:
   a. Chief complaint
   b. Medical history
   c. Mechanism of injury
   d. Patient assessment

9. ______ You can usually determine the mechanism of injury for a trauma patient by looking at the surroundings. True (T) or false (F)?

10. Why is identifying the mechanism of injury important for a trauma patient?

______________________________

______________________________

11. Why is determining the total number of patients at the scene important?

_______________________________________

_______________________________________

12. List three reasons to request additional help.

   a. _______________________________________

   b. _______________________________________

   c. _______________________________________

13. You have been dispatched to a domestic disturbance where "shots have been fired." En route, you are advised by dispatch that police have secured the scene and that it is safe to enter.
   a. Based on this information, what preparations should you make while responding to the scene?

   _______________________________________

   _______________________________________

   b. On arrival in the area, law enforcement personnel escort you to the scene. What are your priorities in managing this scene?

   _______________________________________

   _______________________________________

   c. While assessing a woman who has been shot in the abdomen, the perpetrator breaks away from police custody. What should you do?

   _______________________________________

   _______________________________________

14. You have responded to a motor vehicle crash involving three cars and multiple patients. Fire and rescue personnel are en route, but your crew is first to arrive at the scene.
   a. What are your responsibilities during the scene size-up?

   _______________________________________

   _______________________________________

   b. Using your senses of vision, smell, and sound, how would you evaluate this scene for safety?

   _______________________________________

   _______________________________________

   c. What are your responsibilities in protecting a patient from further injury during extrication?

   _______________________________________

   _______________________________________

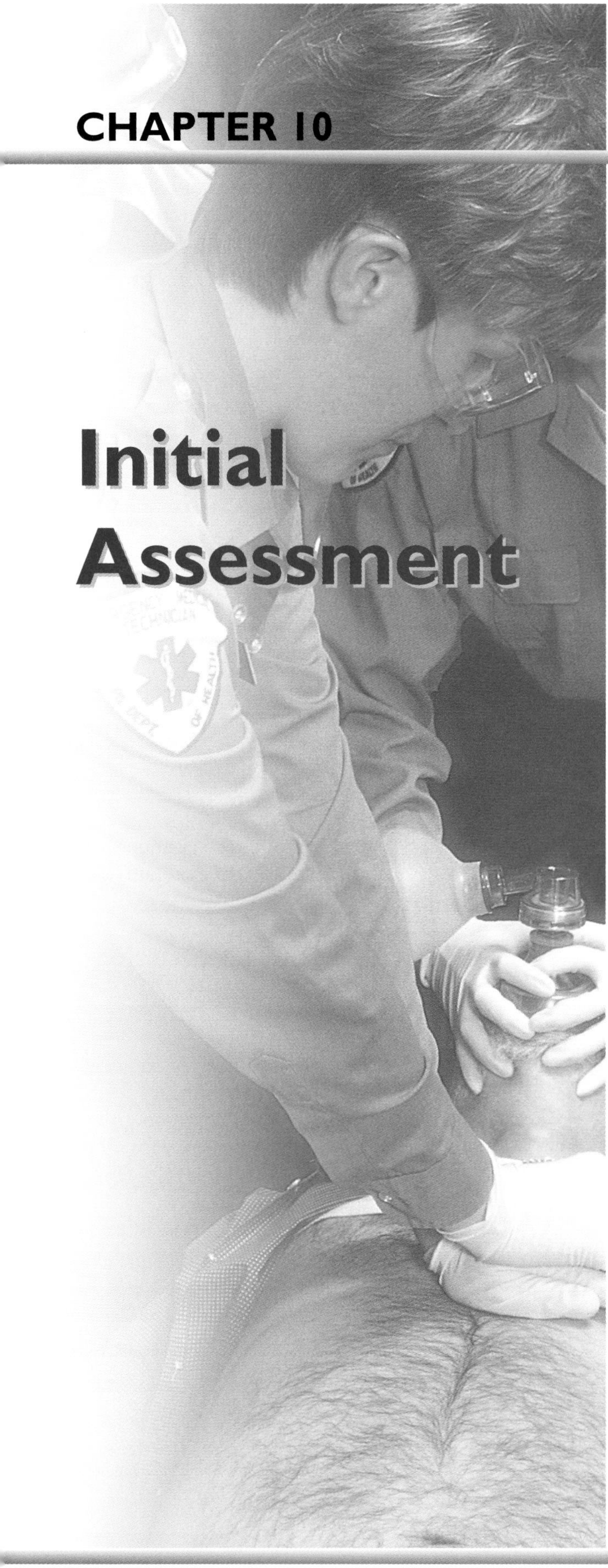

## CHAPTER 10

# Initial Assessment

## CHAPTER OUTLINE

## MATCHING

*Match the terms in column 1 with the correct definition in column 2.*

**Column 1**

1. ______ Capillary refill
2. ______ General impression
3. ______ Mechanism of injury (MOI)
4. ______ Nature of illness (NOI)

**Column 2**

a. The event or forces that caused the patient's injury
b. The patient's description of the chief complaint
c. Immediate assessment of the patient
d. An indicator of shock in patients younger than 6 years of age

## REVIEW QUESTIONS

1. List two reasons for forming a general impression of the patient.

   a. ________________________________

   b. ________________________________

2. ______ The general impression should include which of the following?
   a. Medical history
   b. Name
   c. Mechanism of injury
   d. Allergies

3. ______ Because young children cannot answer questions, the level of their mental status cannot be determined. True (T) or false (F)?

4. How would you assess if a patient is alert, responsive to verbal stimuli, responsive to painful stimuli, or unresponsive?

   ________________________________

   ________________________________

5. ______ Changes in mental status are a late indication of a change in patient condition. True (T) or false (F)?

6. ______ The head-tilt, chin-lift maneuver is used for ________ patients, and the jaw thrust is used for ______________ patients.
   a. Medical, unresponsive
   b. Trauma, medical
   c. Medical, trauma
   d. Unresponsive, uncooperative

7. Why is the head manually stabilized in the neutral position for trauma patients?

   ________________________________

   ________________________________

8. How should the EMT–Basic administer oxygen to an adult patient who is breathing fewer than eight times a minute?

   ________________________________

   ________________________________

9. How would you determine whether a patient was breathing, and how would you evaluate breathing efforts?

   ________________________________

   ________________________________

10. ______ When assessing the breathing of an infant, assessing the rate is of little importance compared with assessing the quality, and no care needs to be provided for changes in rate. True (T) or false (F)?

11. ______ Immediately after completing the initial assessment, EMT–Basics should care for any life-threatening injuries found. True (T) or false (F)?

12. ______ Assess the adult patient's pulse initially by palpating the __________ artery, the child's pulse by palpating the ________ artery, and an infant's pulse by palpating the __________ artery.
    a. Radial, radial, brachial
    b. Radial, brachial, brachial
    c. Carotid, carotid, radial
    d. Carotid, brachial, radial

13. The first time the EMT–Basic assesses for external bleeding is during the ____________________ and assesses for external bleeding again when evaluating the patient's ____________________.

14. List three abnormal skin colors, three abnormal skin temperatures, and three abnormal skin conditions.

    Color ______________________________

    ______________________________

    ______________________________

    Temperature ______________________________

    ______________________________

    ______________________________

    Condition ______________________________

    ______________________________

    ______________________________

15. ______ Capillary refill should be less than 2 seconds when evaluating infants and children. True (T) or false (F)?

16. ______ Which of the following situations constitutes a priority patient?
    a. Uncomplicated childbirth
    b. Severe abdominal pain
    c. Patient with a broken femur
    d. Chest pain and systolic blood pressure of 140 mm Hg

17. Why do EMT–Basics determine if a patient has a priority condition during the initial assessment?

    ______________________________

    ______________________________

18. You have been dispatched to a motorcycle crash. Police are on the scene, and the scene is safe. On arrival, you find a teenage boy lying in the road.
    a. What are seven elements of patient evaluation to consider during the initial assessment?

       ______________________________

       ______________________________

    b. The patient is lying on his left side. Blood, vomit, and broken teeth are in his mouth. How will you manage his airway?

       ______________________________

       ______________________________

    c. The patient is not responsive to verbal stimulus but withdraws appropriately from painful stimulus. How would you describe this patient's level of responsiveness?

       ______________________________

       ______________________________

19. Your EMS crew is caring for three patients who are victims of a drive-by shooting. The first patient is a 15-year-old girl who was grazed on the upper arm by a passing bullet. She is hysterical and is difficult to assess. The second patient is a 27-year-old man who was shot in the chest and has lost a large amount of blood. The third patient is a 54-year-old woman who has a wound to her lower back and is unable to feel or move her lower extremities.
    a. Based on your initial assessment, which of these patients is a "priority patient" who should be rapidly transported?

       ______________________________

       ______________________________

b. Because your ambulance is the only one on the scene, how would you arrange for rapid transport of the priority patient?

________________________________________

________________________________________

c. Define ways to identify priority patients.

________________________________________

________________________________________

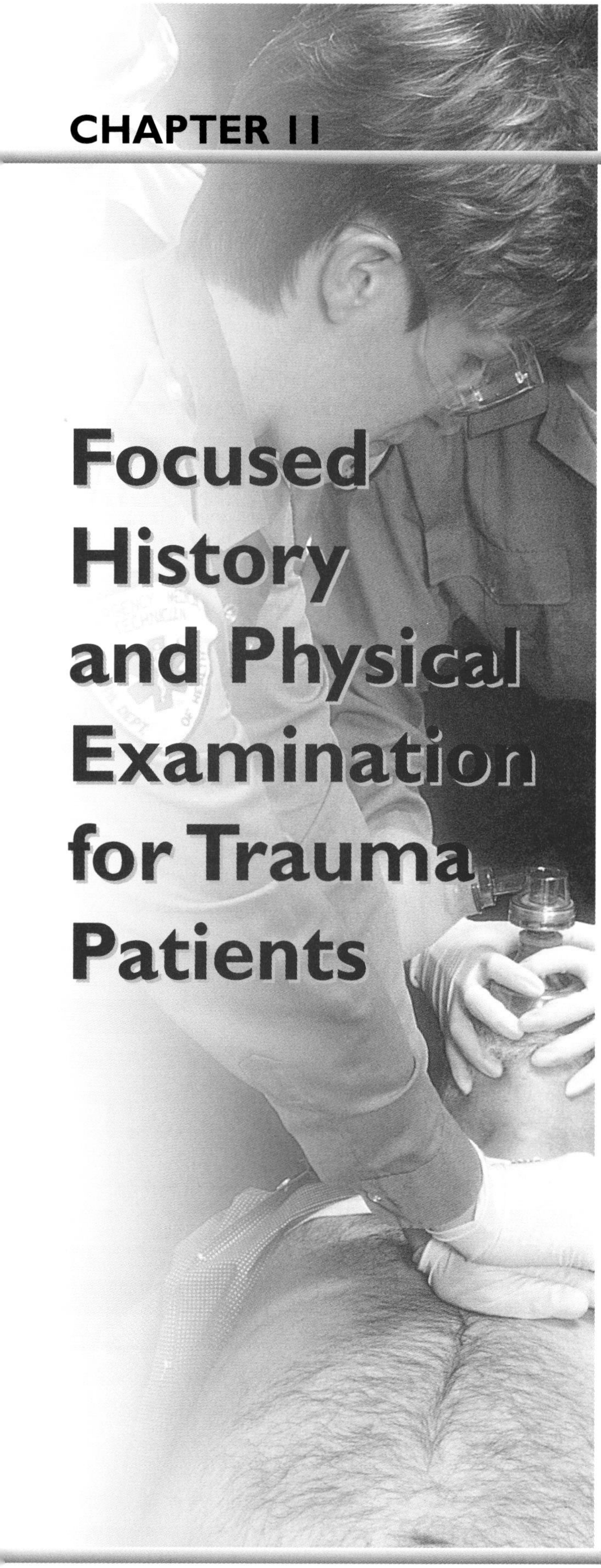

## CHAPTER 11

# Focused History and Physical Examination for Trauma Patients

**CHAPTER OUTLINE**

I. Mechanism of Injury
II. Evaluating Patients With Serious Injuries or Mechanisms of Injury
   A. Performing the Rapid Trauma Assessment
   B. Baseline Vital Signs and SAMPLE History
III. Evaluating Patients With No Significant Mechanism of Injury

## MATCHING

*Match the terms in Column 1 with the correct definition in Column 2.*

**Column 1**

1. ______ Crepitation
2. ______ DCAP-BTLS
3. ______ Distal pulse
4. ______ Iliac wings
5. ______ Jugular vein distention
6. ______ Motor function
7. ______ Multitiered response system
8. ______ Paradoxical motion
9. ______ Sensation

**Column 2**

a. System in which care is provided at basic and advanced levels
b. Testing the ability to move
c. Grating or crackling sound or sensation
d. Ability to feel a touch against the skin
e. Pulse taken away from the center of the body (e.g., wrist)
f. Anterosuperior tips of the pelvis
g. Acronym standing for the eight components of assessment
h. Abnormal enlargement of the blood vessels on the sides of the neck
i. Abnormal movement of the chest wall during inspiration and exhalation in which the affected portion moves opposite the unaffected portion

## REVIEW QUESTIONS

1. If you are unsure if a patient has a medical condition or a traumatic injury, which focused history and physical examination should you use?

______________________________

______________________________

2. Explain why identifying the mechanism of injury is important.

______________________________

______________________________

3. List three serious mechanisms of injury.

a. ______________________________

b. ______________________________

c. ______________________________

4. ______ Elderly patients, infants, and children can be more easily injured than healthy adults. True (T) or false (F)?

5. Fill in the blanks with the appropriate term from the DCAP-BTLS acronym.

D ______________________________

C ______________________________

A ______________________________

P ______________________________

B ______________________________

T ______________________________

L ______________________________

S ______________________________

6. The rapid trauma assessment should take approximately __________ seconds to complete.

7. What should you do if you discover any life-threatening conditions during the rapid trauma assessment?

_______________________________________________

_______________________________________________

8. ______ Breath sounds are auscultated at the ______________ at the midclavicular line and ____________ at the midaxillary line.
   a. Clavicles, ribs
   b. Apices, bases
   c. Upper quadrant, lower quadrant
   d. Lungs, intercostal space

9. ______ At rest, most patients will have a _______ abdomen.
   a. Soft
   b. Firm
   c. Rigid
   d. Tender

10. ______ Which of the following best describes the motions used in evaluation of the pelvis?
    a. Rock and tilt
    b. Squeeze and tilt
    c. Flex and compress
    d. Flex and squeeze

11. The extremities must be evaluated for DCAP-BTLS, as well as ________________. *(Place a check next to all that are appropriate.)*

______ Sensation
______ Motor function
______ Distal pulses
______ Extension
______ Flexion
______ Response to deep pain

12. ______ For patients who have sustained a serious mechanism of injury but who complain only of an isolated injury, the assessment should be focused on the isolated injury. True (T) or false (F)?

13. ______ Every trauma patient should receive a rapid trauma assessment. True (T) or false (F)?

14. ______ Patients generally know when they have a more serious underlying injury that is not apparent. True (T) or false (F)?

*For questions 15 through 17, indicate the patients who should receive a rapid trauma assessment (R) and who should receive a focused history and physical examination directed only toward the injury (F).*

15. ______ 10-year-old girl who was hit by her brother in the forearm with a rake

16. ______ 47-year-old woman who twisted her ankle when stepping off the curb

17. ______ 28-year-old man who fell off a roof while working and is up walking around at the scene, complaining of forearm pain

18. You and your crew have been dispatched to a construction site where a worker has fallen from the roof of a two-story building. On arrival, you find a 30-year-old man lying supine on the ground. He is responsive and alert and tells you, "I'm fine." His supervisor is trying to persuade him to go to the hospital.

    a. Would this patient be considered at high risk for hidden injury? Why or why not?

    _______________________________________________

    _______________________________________________

    b. What questions would you ask this patient as you obtain a focused history?

    _______________________________________________

    _______________________________________________

    c. Following your initial assessment, how would you prepare this patient for transport?

    _______________________________________________

    _______________________________________________

19. Your crew is one of three EMS units that have been dispatched to an explosion at a chemical plant. En route, you are advised that five patients have serious injuries. Police and fire and rescue personnel have secured the scene and made it safe. The patient under your care is an unresponsive 47-year-old woman. She has obvious soft-tissue injuries and is breathing with gurgling respirations.

    a. What is your first priority in managing this patient?

    ______________________________________

    ______________________________________

    b. Because you suspect a head injury, what steps would you take before initiating the rapid trauma assessment?

    ______________________________________

    ______________________________________

    c. Describe the head-to-toe assessment you would perform on this patient and how you would evaluate her for injury using DCAP-BTLS.

    ______________________________________

    ______________________________________

## CHAPTER 12

# Focused History and Physical Examination for Medical Patients

**CHAPTER OUTLINE**

I. Responsive Medical Patients
   A. The Patient's History
   B. Rapid Assessment
   C. Vital Signs
   D. Emergency Care
II. Unresponsive Medical Patients

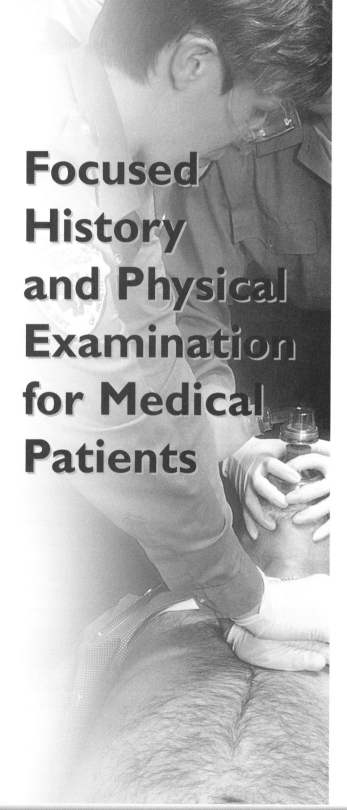

## MATCHING

*Match the terms in Column 1 with the correct definition in Column 2.*

**Column 1**

1. ______ Objective assessment
2. ______ OPQRST
3. ______ Palliative
4. ______ Provocation
5. ______ Rapid assessment
6. ______ SAMPLE history
7. ______ Subjective assessment

**Column 2**

a. Acronym for eliciting patient information about a particular condition
b. Quick evaluation of the patient, accomplished in 60 to 90 seconds
c. Term referring to something that induces a physical reaction
d. Acronym used to evaluate a patient's past medical condition and current events
e. Information obtained during physical assessment
f. What makes the patient's condition improve
g. Information about the patient obtained through questions

## REVIEW QUESTIONS

1. ______ Responsive and unresponsive medical patients receive the same focused history and physical examination. True (T) or false (F)?

2. Fill in the blanks with the correct terms of the OPQRST acronym.

O ______________________________

P ______________________________

Q ______________________________

R ______________________________

S ______________________________

T ______________________________

*Using the appropriate letter of the OPQRST acronym, indicate which component of the patient information is represented for questions 3 through 9.*

3. ______ What position makes you feel better?

4. ______ How long have you had cardiac problems?

5. ______ How long have you had this pain?

6. ______ Is this pain the worst you have ever had?

7. ______ What makes the pain worse?

8. ______ Does the pain spread or move?

9. ______ Can you describe the pain you are feeling?

10. ______ The OPQRST and SAMPLE assessments should be completed before care begins. True (T) or false (F)?

11. ______ A SAMPLE history should be assessed on every patient. True (T) or false (F)?

12. Fill in the blanks with the correct terms of the SAMPLE acronym.

S ______________________________

A ______________________________

M ______________________________

P ______________________________

L ______________________________

E ______________________________

13. The focused history and physical examination for the medical patient is guided by the patient's ____________ ____________.

14. Why is finding out if the patient has a known medical problem important during the focused history and physical examination of the medical patient? How might the history of a medical problem change the EMT–Basic's care for this patient?

____________________________________________

____________________________________________

15. ______ Unresponsive medical patients should be evaluated using the rapid trauma assessment. True (T) or false (F)?

16. When a medical patient is unresponsive and cannot provide a SAMPLE history, information can be obtained from ____________________.

17. ______ Which of the following is appropriate for the unresponsive medical patient without spinal trauma?
    a. Fowler's position
    b. Trendelenburg position
    c. Recovery position
    d. Supine position

18. You are caring for a 58-year-old man complaining of chest pain. He is alert and oriented and tells you that he thinks he is having a "heart attack." As your partner applies high-concentration oxygen and obtains vital signs, you begin to gather a patient history using the OPQRST acronym.

    a. What does the "O" signify, and what questions would be appropriate to ask this patient?

    ____________________________________________

    ____________________________________________

    b. What does the "Q" signify, and what questions would be appropriate to ask this patient?

    ____________________________________________

    ____________________________________________

    c. What does the "T" signify, and what questions would be appropriate to ask this patient?

    ____________________________________________

    ____________________________________________

19. You have been dispatched to a local shopping mall for an "unresponsive woman." On arrival, you find a young woman lying on the floor in a department store. Bystanders state that the woman "just collapsed." No other patient information is available.

    a. What are your first priorities in managing this patient?

    ____________________________________________

    ____________________________________________

    b. How would you assess this patient?

    ____________________________________________

    ____________________________________________

    c. If you could be certain no trauma is present, how would you transport this patient?

    ____________________________________________

    ____________________________________________

## CHAPTER 13

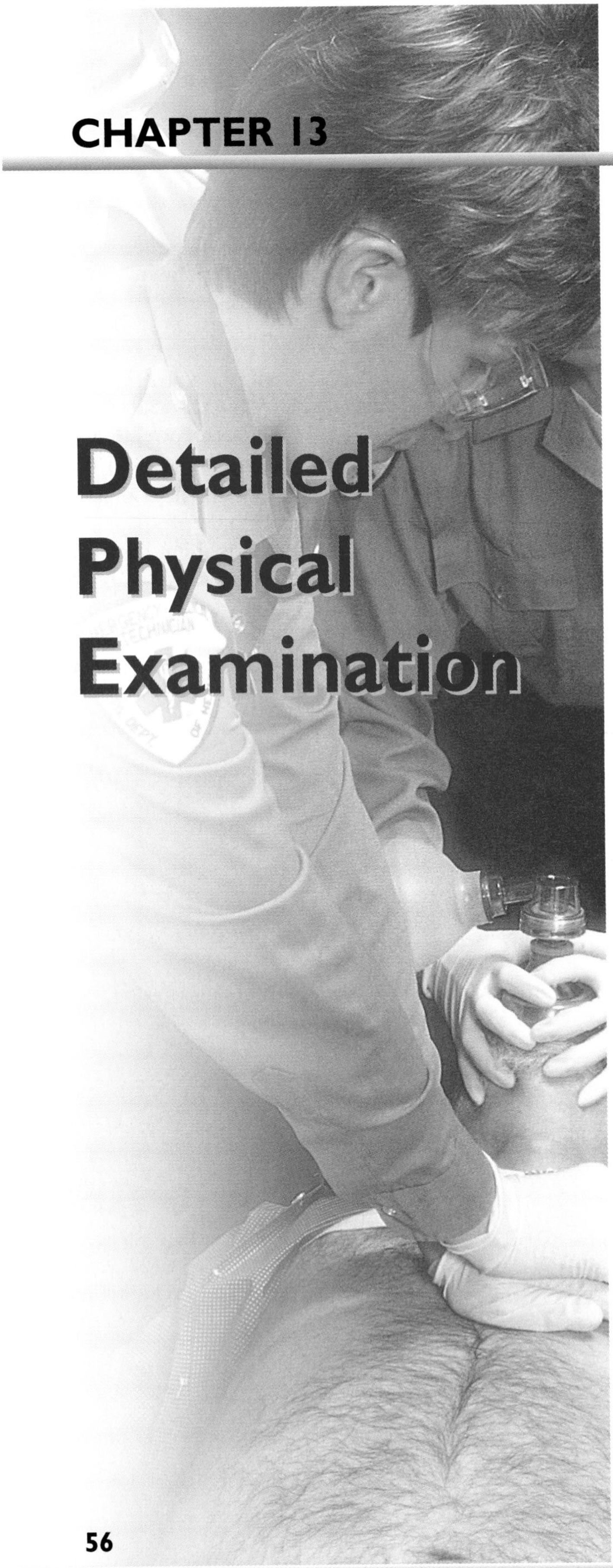

# Detailed Physical Examination

## CHAPTER OUTLINE

- I. Detailed Physical Examination
  - A. Patients Needing a Detailed Examination
  - B. Examination Procedure
- II. Assessing Vital Signs

## MATCHING

*Match the terms in column 1 with the correct definition in column 2.*

**Column 1**

1. ______ Bilaterally
2. ______ Crepitation
3. ______ Detailed physical examination
4. ______ DCAP-BTLS
5. ______ Mandible
6. ______ Maxilla
7. ______ Paradoxical motion
8. ______ Zygomatic arches

**Column 2**

a. Bone forming the lower jaw
b. Abnormal movement of the chest wall
c. Bones forming the cheek
d. Pertaining to both sides of the body
e. An acronym to remember the steps of the physical examination
f. A crackling or grating sound
g. Bones forming most of the upper face
h. In-depth assessment following the focused history and physical examination

## REVIEW QUESTIONS

1. ______ The purpose of the detailed physical examination is to gather details that may have been missed on the rapid trauma assessment. True (T) or false (F)?

2. ______ The detailed physical examination is a routine part of the assessment for all trauma patients. True (T) or false (F)?

3. ______ A patient involved in a rollover vehicle crash complains only of pain in her left lower leg and foot. This patient would still require a detailed physical examination. True (T) or false (F)?

4. When would a detailed physical examination be indicated for a medical patient?

______________________________________

______________________________________

5. Fill in the blanks with the appropriate terms of the DCAP-BTLS acronym.

D ______________________________________

C ______________________________________

A ______________________________________

P ______________________________________

B ______________________________________

T ______________________________________

L ______________________________________

S ______________________________________

6. ______ The light in the ambulance is adequate for evaluating the ears and nose for drainage and inspecting the mouth. True (T) or false (F)?

7. When evaluating the neck, you should assess for DCAP-BTLS and ______________________.

8. What conditions might lead an EMT–Basic to choose *not* to flex and compress a patient's pelvis?

______________________________________

______________________________________

9. ______ The best time to perform the detailed physical examination is:
   a. On scene, before transport
   b. In the back of the ambulance, before transport
   c. In the back of the ambulance, during transport
   d. At the receiving facility

10. You are caring for an 8-year-old girl who has fallen from a tree house. The child fell approximately 10 feet and landed on the grassy surface below the tree. She is alert and crying, and no apparent injuries are present.

    a. After completing the focused history and physical examination for a trauma patient, would this fall require a detailed physical examination?

    ______________________________

    ______________________________

    b. What are the eight components of the examination procedure that should be evaluated?

    ______________________________

    ______________________________

    c. Based on the mechanism of injury, during the focused history and physical examination, how would you evaluate the patient's neck?

    ______________________________

    ______________________________

11. You have been dispatched to a local restaurant where a waiter has been burned by hot coffee. Your initial assessment reveals superficial and partial-thickness burns to the patient's right hand and forearm. He is responsive, alert, and in extreme pain.

    a. Should this patient receive a detailed physical examination?

    ______________________________

    ______________________________

    b. How would you evaluate this patient's injury?

    ______________________________

    ______________________________

    c. Would you assess vital signs on this patient?

    ______________________________

    ______________________________

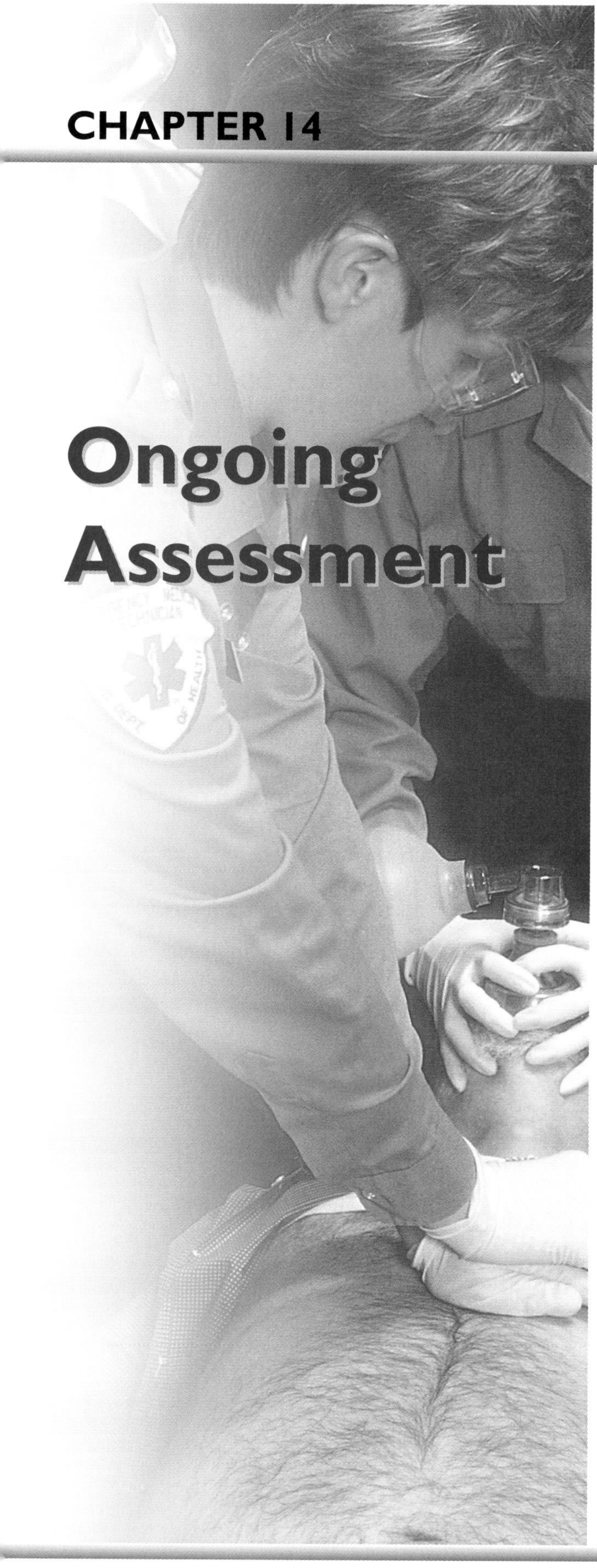

## CHAPTER 14

# Ongoing Assessment

### CHAPTER OUTLINE

I. Components of the Ongoing Assessment
II. Repeat the Initial Assessment
III. Repeat Vital Signs and Focused Assessment
IV. Check Interventions

## REVIEW QUESTIONS

1. List three purposes of the ongoing assessment.

   a. ______________________________

   b. ______________________________

   c. ______________________________

2. What are the components of the initial assessment that are repeated during the ongoing assessment?

   ______________________________

   ______________________________

3. How frequently do you reassess a stable patient?

   ______________________________

   ______________________________

4. Number the following steps in the ongoing assessment, with 1 as the first step and 6 as the last.

   ______ Assess skin color, temperature, condition, perfusion

   ______ Assess mental status

   ______ Assess pulse

   ______ Assess airway patency

   ______ Assess breathing rate and quality

   ______ Reassess patient priority

5. ______ The focused assessment of the chief complaint is not part of the ongoing assessment. True (T) or false (F)?

6. Why is documenting successive sets of vital signs over time important? What is this process called?

   ______________________________

   ______________________________

7. List three examples of interventions that the EMT–Basic should evaluate during the ongoing assessment.

   a. ______________________________

   b. ______________________________

   c. ______________________________

8. You are en route to the emergency department with a trauma patient who was a victim of a "hit-and-run" automobile-pedestrian collision. The patient is responsive to verbal stimulus, has multiple injuries, and is fully immobilized on a long spine board.

   a. How often should the ongoing assessment of this patient be performed?

   ______________________________

   ______________________________

   b. As part of your ongoing assessment, how will you reassess the patient's mental status?

   ______________________________

   ______________________________

   c. If the patient becomes unresponsive, how will you continue to assess his mental status?

   ______________________________

   ______________________________

9. You are caring for a 78-year-old woman who has difficulty breathing. She has a history of "heart failure" and is in moderate respiratory distress. You have applied high-concentration oxygen via a nonrebreather mask and allowed her to assume a position of comfort. Her vital signs are: blood pressure, 146/88 mm Hg; pulse, 134 beats per minute, strong and regular; respirations, 28 per minute, labored and noisy. En route to the emergency department, you check your interventions.

   a. How will you ensure the concentration of oxygen delivery?

   ______________________________________

   ______________________________________

   b. How can you check your method of oxygen delivery?

   ______________________________________

   ______________________________________

   c. What should you do if the patient cannot tolerate the facemask?

   ______________________________________

   ______________________________________

# CHAPTER 15

# Communications

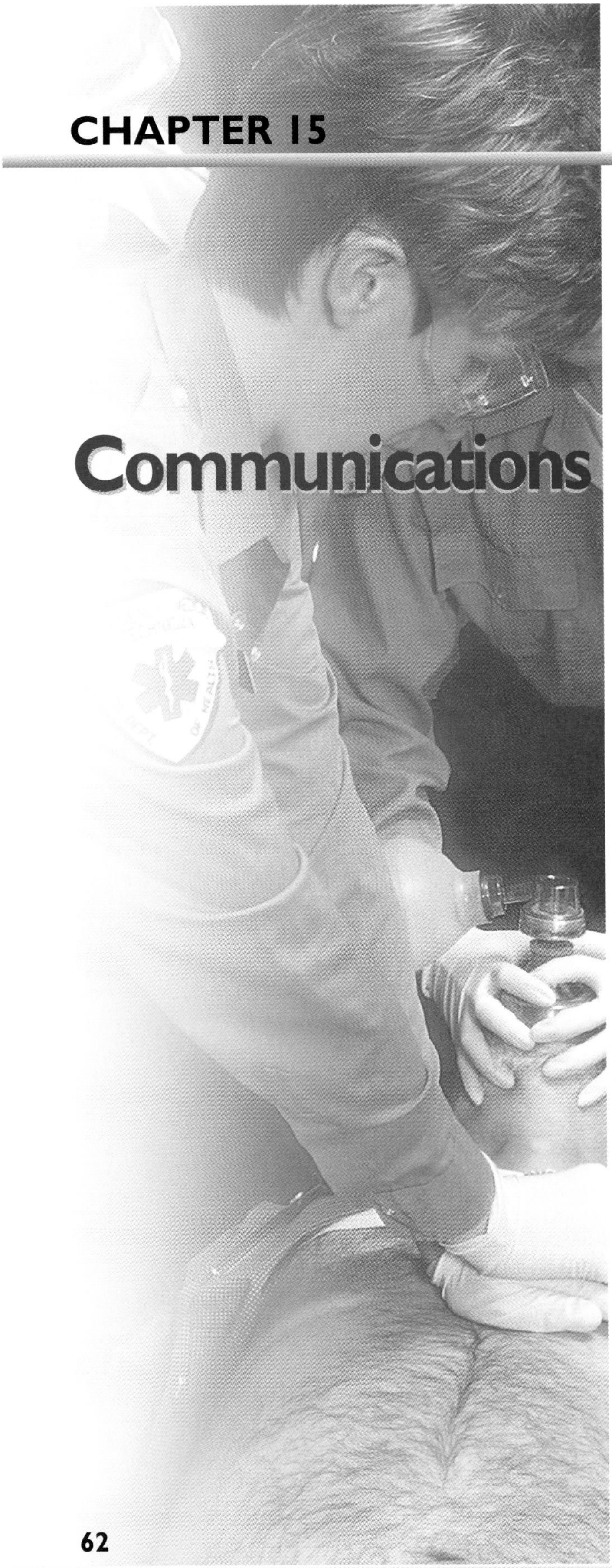

## CHAPTER OUTLINE

I. Communication Systems and Components
   A. Communication Components
   B. System Maintenance
II. Procedures for Radio Communications
   A. Communication with Dispatch
   B. Communication with Medical Direction
   C. Verbal Communication
III. Interpersonal Communication
   A. General Principles
   B. Tips for Effective Communication
   C. Special Populations

## MATCHING

*Match the terms in Column 1 with the correct definition in Column 2.*

**Column 1**

1. ______ Base station
2. ______ Communication
3. ______ Encoders and decoders
4. ______ Repeater

**Column 2**

a. Transmission or exchange of information, ideas, and skills through language and body movements
b. Digital radio equipment that allows the user to block out radio transmissions that are not intended for that unit
c. Radio transceiver located at a stationary site, such as a hospital, mountain top, or dispatch center
d. Remote receiver that receives a transmission from a low-power portable or mobile radio on one frequency and then transmits the signal at a higher power, often on another frequency

## REVIEW QUESTIONS

1. ______ A radio at a stationary site with superior transmission and receiving capabilities is called a:
   a. Repeater
   b. Base station
   c. Transceiver
   d. Encoder

2. The agency that regulates and monitors radio transmissions is called the ______________________.

3. You should monitor the radio frequency for __________ seconds before transmitting to ensure that the frequency is clear.

4. ______ How long should you wait to begin speaking after pushing the push-to-talk button?
   a. 1 second
   b. 3 seconds
   c. 5 seconds
   d. 10 seconds

5. The phrase ______________________ means to wait before continuing with the transmission.

6. ______ Use everyday language during radio communication to reduce confusion. True (T) or false (F)?

7. ______ Courtesy is an important part of radio communications, so be sure to use "please" and "thank you" on a regular basis. True (T) or false (F)?

8. ______ Which of the following is *true* of EMS radio channels?
   a. EMS channels are dedicated to their use and can be heard only by EMS providers.
   b. Operators outside of the EMS system can use EMS channels.
   c. EMS channels are considered to be public channels.
   d. Dispatch cannot legally record EMS channels.

9. ______ Which of the following actions is a routine part of communications with dispatch?
   a. Calling medical direction
   b. Arriving at the receiving facility
   c. Loading the patient at the scene
   d. Administering oxygen

10. ______ If the orders from a medical direction physician are unclear, you should:
    a. Ask dispatch to connect you with a different medical director.
    b. Withhold intervention until you arrive at the receiving hospital.
    c. Ask the medical direction physician to clarify the order.
    d. Complete the intervention you think was ordered.

11. ______ An effective radio report should be:
    a. Comprehensive
    b. Concise
    c. Coded
    d. Lengthy

12. List the 12 components included in the standard medical reporting format in order.

    a. ______________________________
    b. ______________________________
    c. ______________________________
    d. ______________________________
    e. ______________________________
    f. ______________________________
    g. ______________________________
    h. ______________________________
    i. ______________________________
    j. ______________________________
    k. ______________________________
    l. ______________________________

13. List three tips for effective interpersonal communication.

    a. ______________________________
    b. ______________________________
    c. ______________________________

14. ______ Body language consists of factors such as posture, facial expressions, and tone of voice. True (T) or false (F)?

15. You have been dispatched to a local bowling alley for a "possible heart attack." On arrival, you find an unresponsive woman in her middle 40s lying on the floor of the bathroom. She is breathing and has a pulse of 124 beats per minute. Her blood pressure is 108/64 mm Hg. No other information is available. As your partner monitors her airway, you contact medical direction via a cellular telephone.

    a. What information should you include about this patient in your initial report to the hospital?

    ______________________________

    ______________________________

    b. At the end of your radio report, what should you do before you end your transmission?

    ______________________________

    ______________________________

    c. The medical direction physician recommended an intervention that was unclear to you and your partner. What should you do?

    ______________________________

    ______________________________

16. You have responded to a crash scene involving a school bus and a city transportation vehicle for the elderly. The students on the bus are from a private school for the physically challenged. No major injuries are apparent, but the students and older passengers are frightened, and some are hysterical.

    a. What are some general considerations to keep in mind when dealing with ill or injured children?

    ______________________________________

    ______________________________________

    b. What are some general considerations to keep in mind when dealing with older patients?

    ______________________________________

    ______________________________________

    c. Several of the children are hearing impaired. What are ways to communicate with these patients?

    ______________________________________

    ______________________________________

## CHAPTER 16

# Documentation

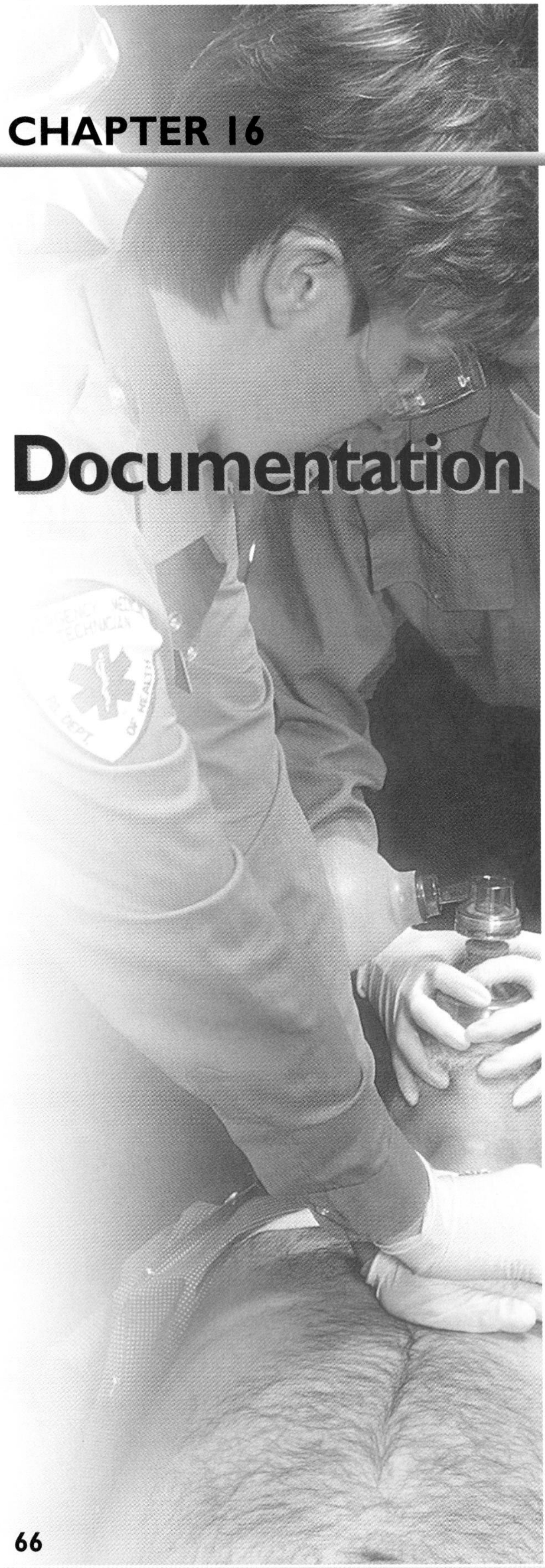

## CHAPTER OUTLINE

I. Minimum Data Set
II. The Prehospital Care Report
  A. Functions of the Prehospital Care Report
  B. Traditional Format
  C. Other Formats
  D. Distribution
  E. Documentation of Patient Care Errors
  F. Correction of Documentation Errors
III. Documentation of Patient Refusal
IV. Special Situations
  A. Multiple Casualty Incidents
  B. Special Situations

## MATCHING

*Match the terms in Column 1 with the correct definition in Column 2.*

**Column 1**

1. ______ Minimum data set
2. ______ Patient narrative
3. ______ Prehospital care report
4. ______ Trending

**Column 2**

a. Essential elements of patient and administrative data required for accurate and complete prehospital data collection
b. Section of a prehospital care report that allows EMT–Basics to document information using a standard medical reporting format
c. Process of comparing serial recordings of a patient's vital signs or other assessments to note changes
d. Form used to document the events occurring during a patient encounter

## REVIEW QUESTIONS

1. ______ Trending information requires that the same sets of information be collected and recorded over time. True (T) or false (F)?

2. ______ All of the following are elements of the patient information data set *except:*
   a. Injury description
   b. Skin color, temperature, and condition
   c. Chief complaint
   d. Time of arrival of patient

3. Write the following times in a 24-hour format.

   1:00 AM ______________________

   6:30 PM ______________________

   12:00 noon ______________________

   4:20 AM ______________________

   10:30 PM ______________________

   8:25 PM ______________________

   2:40 AM ______________________

   12:30 AM ______________________

4. ______ The prehospital care report is both a legal and a medical document. True (T) or false (F)?

5. Place an "S" next to statements that are subjective and an "O" next to statements that are objective.

   ______ I saw him drinking at that bar.

   ______ The patient was drunk.

   ______ It looked as if the car was going over the speed limit.

   ______ Her blood pressure was 120/80 and the pulse was 72.

   ______ The patient's skin is cool, clammy, and moist to the touch.

6. Name three things, other than documenting patient care, for which the prehospital care report can be used.

   ______________________________

   ______________________________

   ______________________________

7. Most prehospital care report forms have a section for writing a patient ______________________, allowing EMT–Basics to write about the events in the standard medical reporting format.

8. Write the common abbreviations for the following terms.

   Chief complaint ______________________________

   Gunshot wound ______________________________

   Every ______________________________

   Shortness of breath ______________________________

   History ______________________________

   Immediately ______________________________

   Treatment ______________________________

   Alcohol ______________________________

9. ______ Correct errors in documentation by scratching out the wrong information and filling in the correct information. True (T) or false (F)?

10. Refusal is the right of any ____________________ adult, meaning any adult who can make rational decisions about his or her care.

11. List at least three reasons to use a special situation report.

    a. ______________________________

    b. ______________________________

    c. ______________________________

12. You have been asked to assist a neighboring EMS agency in developing a minimum data set of information to be collected by their employees during emergency and nonemergency responses.

    a. What are the two categories of information contained in a minimum data set?

    ______________________________

    ______________________________

    b. What components should be included when gathering patient care information?

    ______________________________

    ______________________________

    c. What components should be included when gathering information for administrative purposes?

    ______________________________

    ______________________________

13. You have been dispatched to a local diner for a "possible allergic reaction." On arrival, you find a man in his middle 30s. He is alert and aggravated with the manager for calling EMS. The patient tells you he was feeling a little weak and nauseated and had some trouble catching his breath. He is sure that it is just "a touch of the flu." He refuses to be examined or transported to the hospital.

    a. Does this patient have a legal right to refuse treatment?

    ______________________________

    ______________________________

    b. What might you do to persuade the patient to receive treatment and transportation to the hospital?

    ______________________________

    ______________________________

    c. The patient still refuses care. How should you complete this call?

    ______________________________

    ______________________________

# DIVISION THREE

## Patient Assessment



## DIVISION TEST

**Directions:** *Place the letter of the correct answer in the space provided.*

1. ______ Which of the following statements is *true* regarding BSI precautions?
   a. BSI precautions protect the EMT–Basic from blood-borne pathogens only.
   b. BSI precautions protect the EMT–Basic from air- and blood-borne pathogens.
   c. The need for BSI precautions is determined during the initial assessment.
   d. BSI precautions are necessary only when blood is present.

2. ______ Which of the following is the EMT–Basic's primary concern?
   a. Patient safety
   b. Personal safety
   c. Bystander safety
   d. Crew member safety

3. ______ Which of the following information is obtained during the scene size-up?
   a. Mechanism of injury or nature of illness
   b. The patient's mental status
   c. Determining which hospital the patient should be transported to
   d. The patient's airway, breathing, and circulatory status

4. ______ During the scene size-up, the EMT–Basic should:
   a. Determine the number of patients at the scene.
   b. Wait for additional help to arrive if too many patients need treatment.
   c. Begin to treat patients based on their mechanism of injury.
   d. Determine scene safety after beginning patient care.

5. ______ The best source of information about the responsive medical patient is usually the:
   a. Family
   b. Patient
   c. Medical records
   d. Family physician

6. ______ The first phase of the initial assessment is the:
   a. General impression
   b. Scene size-up
   c. Focused assessment
   d. Determination of severity

7. ______ Which of the following is identified in the general impression?
   a. Assess mental status.
   b. Assess respiratory effort.
   c. Determine if any life threats are present.
   d. Determine if pulse is present.

8. ______ What does the "P" in the acronym AVPU represent?
   a. Provocation
   b. Responds to painful stimuli
   c. Partially responsive
   d. Priority patient

9. ______ While assessing an unresponsive patient, the EMT–Basic determines the patient's respiratory rate is six breaths per minute. What should be done at this time?
   a. Continue assessment from head to toe, and then apply oxygen.
   b. Continue the assessment to the abdomen, then give oxygen via a non-rebreather mask.
   c. Have your partner ventilate the patient.
   d. Immediately place the patient on oxygen at 12 to 15 L/minute via a nonrebreather mask.

10. ______ Where would you initially assess the pulse for an alert adult patient?
   a. Carotid pulse
   b. Radial pulse
   c. Femoral pulse
   d. Brachial pulse

11. ______ Where should the EMT–Basic evaluate the color of the patient's skin to assess perfusion?
   a. Nail beds
   b. Abdomen
   c. Scalp
   d. Extremities

12. ______ Which of the following areas would provide an accurate assessment of the patient's perfusion?
   a. The color of the skin of the extremities
   b. The capillary refill of a 14-year-old boy
   c. The skin temperature of the patient's hand
   d. The comparison of the strength of the carotid and radial pulses in an adult

13. ______ Which of the following is a priority patient requiring immediate care and transport?
   a. An unresponsive patient with no gag reflex
   b. A patient with chest pain and blood pressure of 138/84 mm Hg
   c. A responsive patient who can follow commands
   d. A patient who feels moderate pain in his obviously deformed ankle

14. ______ Which of the following is considered a significant mechanism of injury?
   a. Death of another passenger in the same compartment
   b. Falls greater than 5 feet
   c. A vehicle crash at 15 miles per hour
   d. Penetrating injuries to the upper extremities

15. ______ How long should it take to complete a rapid trauma assessment on most patients?
   a. 10 seconds
   b. 10 to 30 seconds
   c. 60 to 90 seconds
   d. 2 to 3 minutes

16. ______ Which of the following is part of the acronym DCAP-BTLS?
   a. D = deformity
   b. A = amputation
   c. T = time
   d. S = severity of injury

17. ______ During the rapid trauma assessment, assess the abdomen for DCAP-BTLS and:
   a. Paradoxical motion
   b. Crepitation
   c. Distention
   d. Instability

18. ______ For a patient with a twisted ankle and no other injuries or mechanism to suggest injury, how would you assess the patient during the focused history and physical examination?
   a. Perform the rapid trauma assessment.
   b. Assess the pelvis and both extremities.
   c. Assess only the specific injury.
   d. Perform the rapid trauma assessment after inspecting the injury.

19. ______ The acronym OPQRST helps EMT–Basics remember what questions to ask concerning the patient's:
   a. Mechanism of injury
   b. Mental status
   c. Chief complaint
   d. History

20. ______ The "R" in the OPQRST history stands for:
   a. Radiation
   b. Reasons
   c. Risks of complications
   d. Reasonable care

21. ______ Which of the following statements is *true* concerning the focused history and physical examination for the medical patient?
   a. Emergency care is based on signs and symptoms found, in consultation with medical direction.
   b. Unresponsive medical patients are evaluated much the same as responsive medical patients.
   c. Unresponsive medical patients with no signs of trauma should be placed in the prone position.
   d. EMT–Basics do not need to perform an initial assessment on medical patients; include an assessment of the airway, breathing, and circulation in the focused history and physical examination.

22. ______ In the SAMPLE acronym, "S" stands for:
   a. Signs and symptoms
   b. Sensation
   c. Side effects
   d. Severity of the illness

23. ______ The rapid assessment for a responsive medical patient:
   a. Must include a head-to-toe assessment
   b. Requires removal of all patient clothing
   c. Is directed toward the patient's chief complaint
   d. Rules out the possibility of trauma

24. ______ Which of the following is correct care for an unresponsive medical patient?
   a. Perform a trauma assessment only when trauma is known to exist.
   b. Do not immobilize unless you are sure the patient's spine is injured.
   c. Place the patient in the recovery position if you know the spine is injured.
   d. Perform a rapid trauma assessment to determine illness or injury.

25. ______ Which of the following statements is *true* concerning the detailed physical examination?
   a. The detailed physical examination is performed more rapidly than the focused history and physical examination.
   b. The detailed physical examination is designed for trauma patients who may have hidden injuries.
   c. Ideally, the detailed physical examination should be performed on scene.
   d. The detailed physical examination is most often performed on medical patients.

26. ______ Which patient would most likely receive a detailed physical examination?
   a. A responsive medical patient with no injuries
   b. A patient with an isolated injury and no serious mechanism of injury
   c. An unresponsive medical patient
   d. A medical patient with shortness of breath

27. ______ When inspecting the patient's head during the detailed physical examination, you will evaluate for the first time the:
   a. Ears for drainage
   b. Pupil size and reactivity
   c. Airway
   d. Face for instability

28. ______ Which of the following actions is *correct?*
   a. Listen for breath sounds in two places, once at the apices on each side.
   b. Assess the abdomen in two quadrants.
   c. Assess the pelvis if a sign of injury exists.
   d. Assess the neck for jugular vein distention.

29. ______ When evaluating the extremities during the detailed physical examination, assess for DCAP-BTLS and distal:
a. Pain
b. Sensation
c. Distention
d. Crepitation

30. ______ Which of the following is *true* concerning the ongoing assessment?
a. Vital signs are reassessed every 30 minutes during the ongoing assessment.
b. The ongoing assessment repeats the initial assessment except for the mental status check.
c. The ongoing assessment should be performed once during transport.
d. The ongoing assessment allows for evaluation of trends in the patient's condition.

31. ______ Ongoing assessments should be performed on stable patients every:
a. 5 minutes
b. 10 minutes
c. 15 minutes
d. 20 minutes

32. ______ Which of the following statements is *true?*
a. Any intervention that is inadequate should be removed.
b. The ongoing assessment should be repeated one last time approximately 5 minutes away from the receiving facility.
c. EMT–Basics should check factors such as pupil size and mental status to evaluate interventions.
d. The focused assessment does not have to be repeated as part of the ongoing assessment if the patient is unresponsive.

33. ______ Which organization regulates radio frequencies?
a. FAA
b. FCA
c. FCC
d. FDA

34. ______ How far should you hold the radio microphone from your mouth to ensure clear communications?
a. 2 to 3 inches
b. 3 to 5 inches
c. 5 to 7 inches
d. 7 to 9 inches

35. ______ Which of the following statements concerning communications with medical direction is *true?*
a. Medical direction may be at the receiving facility or at a remote site.
b. After receiving an order for a medication or procedure, the communication is complete.
c. Orders that are unclear should not be carried out until arrival at the receiving facility.
d. Reports to medical direction before arrival should be lengthy so personnel at the receiving facility are aware of all details.

36. ______ Which of the following statements is *true* concerning talking on a radio?
a. Speak as soon as you push the "push-to-talk" button to avoid delays.
b. Speak rapidly to minimize airtime.
c. Use clear everyday language instead of codes.
d. Use simple words like "yes" and "no" instead of "affirmative" and "negative" in your discussion.

37. ______ A repeater is:
a. A stationary radio with superior transmission and receiving capabilities
b. A remote receiver that receives a transmission and transmits it at a higher power
c. A digital radio that blocks out radio transmissions
d. The console that a dispatcher uses for communication

38. ______ EMT–Basics should notify dispatch:
    a. With information regarding the assessment findings
    b. Of arrival at the receiving facility after giving a bedside report to the staff
    c. When leaving the scene
    d. To relay patient information to medical direction

39. ______ Which of the following is administrative information obtained for documentation?
    a. Any medications administered to the patient
    b. Time of arrival at the patient's location
    c. Patient's chief complaint
    d. Equipment used at the scene

40. ______ Which of the following are components of the minimum data set for patient information?
    a. Type of location
    b. Time en route to scene
    c. Chief complaint
    d. Response to scene

41. ______ The prehospital care report:
    a. Should contain objective and subjective information
    b. Should not be released for billing purposes
    c. Can be used for case review if patient confidentiality is protected
    d. Should include the EMT–Basic's diagnosis of the patient

42. ______ Which of the following medical abbreviations is *correct?*
    a. Penicillin = Penn
    b. Chief complaint = ChCo
    c. Nothing by mouth = NPO
    d. Every = EV

43. ______ Which of the following procedures regarding documentation is *true?*
    a. Completely scratch out errors in documentation, and write the correct information beside the scratched out information.
    b. Document a patient's refusal of care, and have your partner sign as a witness.
    c. Always document the care that you wished to give, whether it was given or not.
    d. Document situations such as infectious disease exposure on a special report form, submitted in a timely manner.

44. ______ Patient refusal of care documentation should include:
    a. Diagnosis of the patient's condition
    b. Subjective information about the patient's condition
    c. Your explanation to the patient that you are willing to return if more help is needed
    d. The patient's family physician's signature

## CHAPTER 17

# General Pharmacology

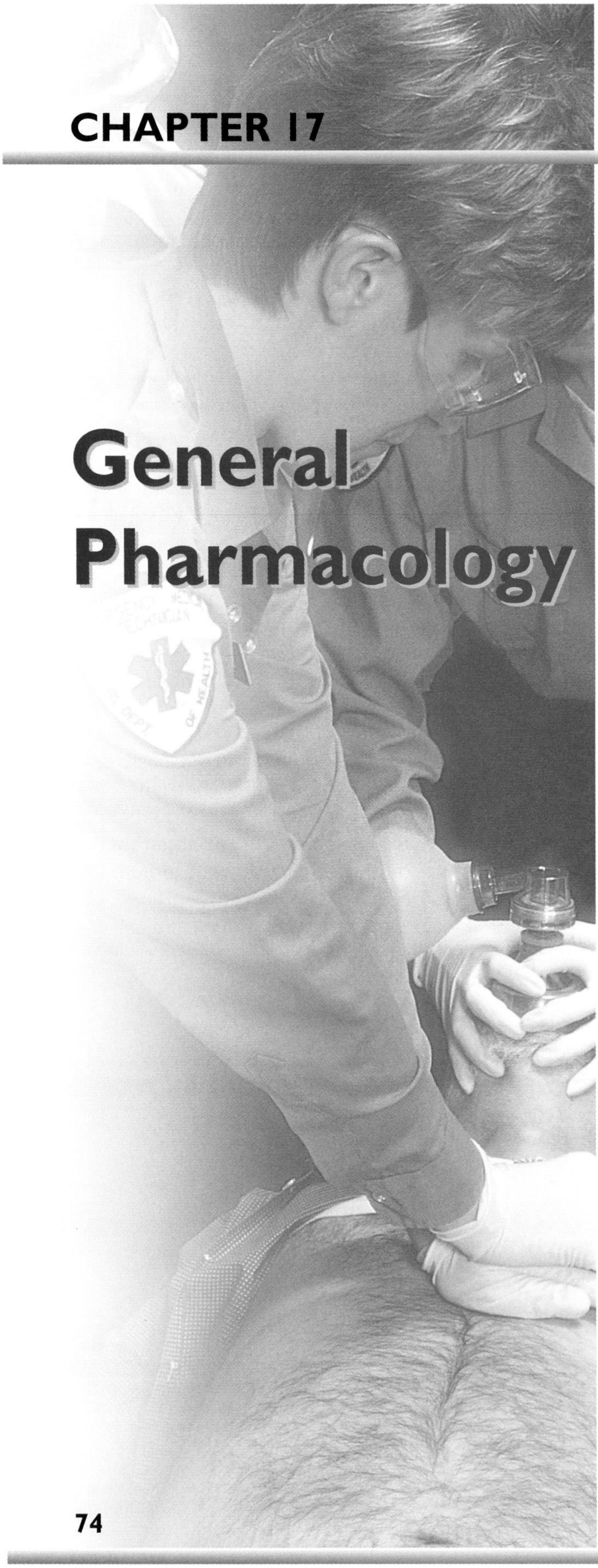

## CHAPTER OUTLINE

## MATCHING 1

*Match the terms in Column 1 with the correct definition in Column 2.*

**Column 1**

1. ______ Contraindication
2. ______ Dose
3. ______ Drug
4. ______ Generic name
5. ______ Indication
6. ______ Trade name

**Column 2**

a. Condition for which a medication may be used
b. Amount of medication that should be administered
c. Any substance that alters the body's functioning when taken into the body
d. Situation in which a medication should not be used
e. Name assigned by the company that sells a medication
f. Name of a medication listed in the *U.S. Pharmacopeia,* the official name assigned to the medication

## MATCHING 2

*Match the terms in Column 1 with the correct definition in Column 2.*

**Column 1**

7. ______ Inhalation
8. ______ Mechanism of action
9. ______ Pharmacology
10. ______ Route of administration
11. ______ Sublingual route

**Column 2**

a. Route of administration for medications in the form of a fine mist or a gas
b. Science of drugs and study of their origin, ingredients, uses, and actions of the body
c. Putting a medication under the patient's tongue
d. How a medication affects the body
e. Method used to administer the medication to the patient

## MATCHING 3

*Match the generic name in Column 1 with the trade name in Column 2.*

**Column 1**

12. ______ Oral glucose
13. ______ Activated charcoal
14. ______ Nitroglycerin
15. ______ Albuterol

**Column 2**

a. Proventil
b. Actidose
c. Glutose
d. Nitrostat

## REVIEW QUESTIONS

1. ______ Medication and pharmacology are interchangeable terms. True (T) or false (F)?

2. EMT–Basic units carry the medications

   ____________________,

   ____________________,

   and ____________________

   on the EMS unit for administration when advised by medical direction.

3. EMT–Basics can assist a patient with what three physician-prescribed medications?

   a. ____________________

   b. ____________________

   c. ____________________

4. ______ When a medication is manufactured and ready for marketing, the manufacturer gives it a ______ name.
   a. Trade
   b. Generic
   c. Common
   d. Drug

5. ______ Medications can have more than one trade name but only one generic name. True (T) or false (F)?

6. List three forms of medications.

   a. ____________________

   b. ____________________

   c. ____________________

7. ______ A contraindication is a factor that prohibits the use of a medication or a procedure. True (T) or false (F)?

8. ______ The dose of a medication may depend on:
   a. Age
   b. Gender
   c. Race
   d. Height

9. ______ Oral medications can be administered to both responsive and unresponsive patients. True (T) or false (F)?

10. ______ The oral route of drug administration has a fast onset of action. True (T) or false (F)?

11. State two drugs the EMT may assist with administration by the oral route.

    a. ____________________

    b. ____________________

12. ______ When drugs are administered sublingually, the medication is rapidly absorbed by:
    a. The vessels in the cheek
    b. Capillaries under the tongue
    c. The digestive tract
    d. Capillaries in the lung

13. ______ Sublingual drugs are delivered under the tongue and then swallowed by the patient. True (T) or false (F)?

14. State one drug the EMT may assist with administration by the sublingual route.

    ____________________

    ____________________

15. List two medications the EMT may assist with administration by the inhalation route.

    a. ____________________

    b. ____________________

16. ______ Inhaled medications typically have a slow onset of action. True (T) or false (F)?

17. ______ The epinephrine autoinjector delivers medication via the __________ route.
    a. Oral
    c. Inhalation
    b. Sublingual
    d. Intramuscular

18. The undesirable actions of a medication are called ____________________________________.

19. ______ Many medications have predictable side effects. True (T) or false (F)?

20. After administering a medication, carefully monitor the patient for __________________________ and _________________________________ of the drug, as well as completing ongoing assessments.

21. Your work shift has just begun, and you are checking out the supplies and equipment in the ambulance.

    a. What medications would you find in the ambulance?

    ________________________________________

    ________________________________________

    b. What physician-prescribed medications can you help a patient administer?

    ________________________________________

    ________________________________________

    c. Define the terms *indication, contraindication,* and *dose.*

    ________________________________________

    ________________________________________

## CHAPTER 18

# Respiratory Emergencies

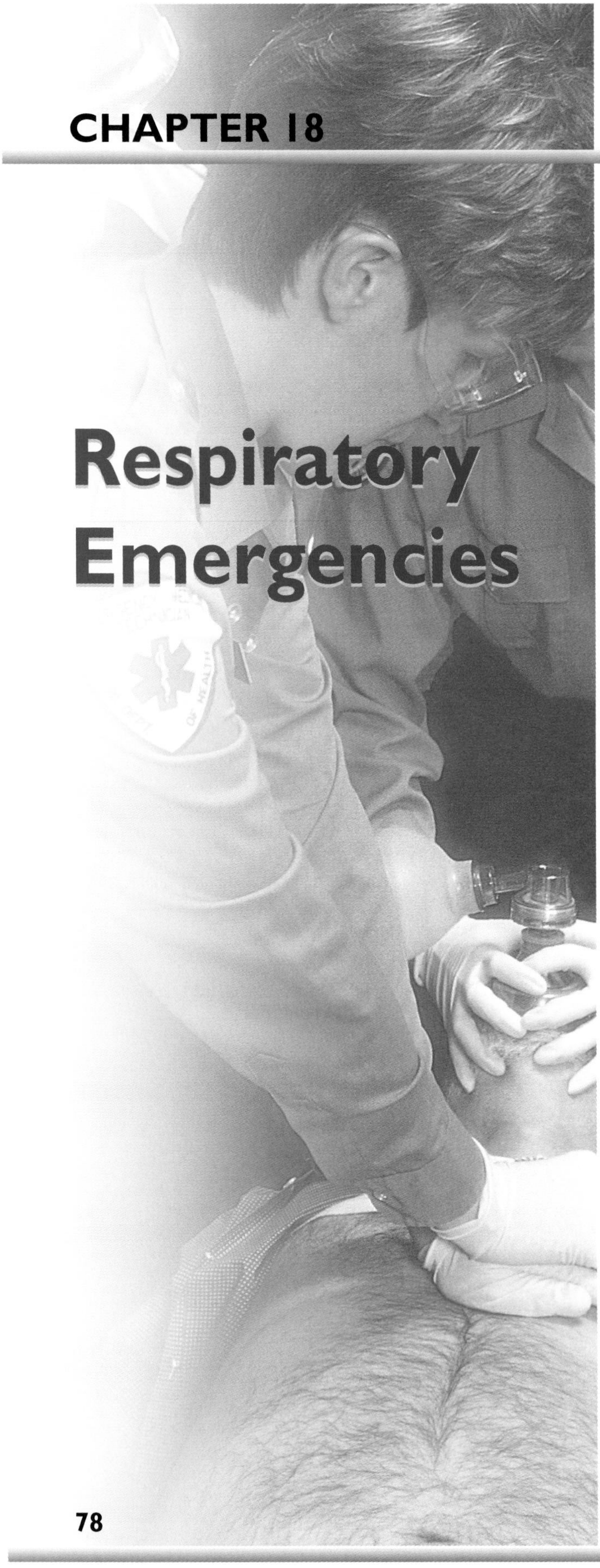

## CHAPTER OUTLINE

I. Respiratory System Review
  A. Anatomy
  B. Physiology
II. Breathing Assessment
  A. Adequate Breathing
  B. Breathing Difficulty
  C. Chronic Obstructive Lung Disease
  D. Focused History and Physical Examination
III. Emergency Medical Care
  A. Oxygen
  B. Position and Transport
  C. Artificial Ventilation
  D. Inhalers

## REVIEW QUESTIONS

1. Label the figure below with the following respiratory structures:

| | | |
|---|---|---|
| Diaphragm | Left bronchus | Right bronchus |
| Epiglottis | Nasopharynx | Trachea |
| Larynx | Oropharynx | Pharynx |

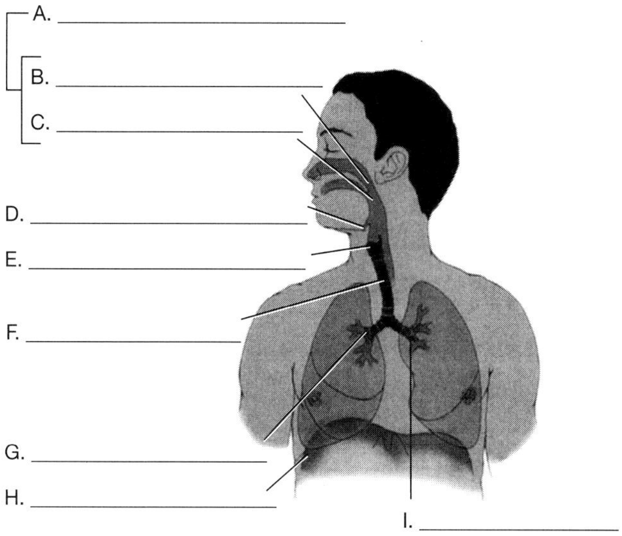


2. When air enters the body, the nose and mouth

______,

______,

and ______ the air.

3. ______ The firm cartilage ring forming the lower portion of the larynx is the:
   a. Thyroid cartilage
   b. Cricoid cartilage
   c. Cricothyroid cartilage
   d. Glottic cartilage

4. ______ During inhalation, the function of the intercostal muscles is to move the ribs:
   a. Down and in
   b. Down and out
   c. Up and in
   d. Up and out

5. ______ The exchange of oxygen and carbon dioxide occurs in the alveoli. True (T) or false (F)?

6. ______ Inhaled air contains high concentrations of ______, whereas exhaled air contains high concentrations of:
   a. Oxygen, carbon dioxide
   b. Air, oxygen
   c. Carbon dioxide, oxygen
   d. Carbon dioxide, air

7. ______ What is the normal respiratory rate for a child?
   a. 25 to 50 breaths per minute
   b. 12 to 20 breaths per minute
   c. 15 to 30 breaths per minute
   d. 20 to 40 breaths per minute

8. List four components of adequate breathing.
   a. ______
   b. ______
   c. ______
   d. ______

9. ______ Inadequate breathing can occur when a patient's rate is too slow, but breathing too fast is not a problem. True (T) or false (F)?

10. ______ Indicate which of the following is a sign or symptom of respiratory distress.
    a. Bilateral chest expansion
    b. Respiratory rate between 12 and 20
    c. Shallow respirations
    d. Speaking in full sentences

11. ______ Noisy respirations are normal and do not require intervention. True (T) or false (F)?

12. List at least three signs and symptoms of difficulty breathing in each of the following categories:

    General

    a. ______________________________

    b. ______________________________

    c. ______________________________

    Visual

    a. ______________________________

    b. ______________________________

    c. ______________________________

    Auditory

    a. ______________________________

    b. ______________________________

    c. ______________________________

13. ______ A barrel chest indicates a new onset of respiratory problems. True (T) or false (F)?

14. ______ Patients in respiratory distress tend to position themselves:
    a. Lying on their back
    b. Lying on their side
    c. In a semi-reclining position
    d. Sitting straight up

15. List three diseases associated with chronic obstructive pulmonary disease.

    a. ______________________________

    b. ______________________________

    c. ______________________________

16. ______ The leading cause of emphysema in the United States is exposure to:
    a. Pesticides
    b. Industrial chemicals
    c. Cigarette smoke
    d. Environmental pollution

17. Define each of the following letters from the OPQRST acronym.

    O ______________________________

    P ______________________________

    Q ______________________________

    R ______________________________

    S ______________________________

    T ______________________________

18. ______ If you encounter a child who is having respiratory distress, you should separate the parent from the child to proceed with the respiratory assessment and treatment. True (T) or false (F)?

19. What is the first medication to administer to a patient in respiratory distress?

    ______________________________

    ______________________________

20. ______ An inhaler is a medication that is carried by EMTs on the EMS unit. True (T) or false (F)?

21. ______ A beta-agonist inhaler is used to ______ bronchioles and ___________ resistance inside airways.
    a. Dilate, increase
    b. Dilate, decrease
    c. Restrict, increase
    d. Restrict, decrease

22. Albuterol and isoetharine are

    ______________________________ names

    for the medication in an inhaler.

23. List three criteria for the use of an inhaler.

    a. ______________________________

    b. ______________________________

    c. ______________________________

24. List at least three contraindications to the use of a prescribed inhaler.

    a. ______________________________

    b. ______________________________

    c. ______________________________

25. ______ The spacer should be removed from an inhaler before administration. True (T) or false (F)?

26. ______ Patients of any age can use an inhaler. True (T) or false (F)?

27. ______ Which of the following is a possible side effect from an inhaler?
    a. Increased heart rate
    b. Altered mental status
    c. Decreased blood pressure
    d. Cyanosis

28. Number the following steps for assisting with a prescribed inhaler in the proper order, with 1 as the first step and 6 as the last.

    ______ Hold breath as long as comfortable

    ______ Check expiration date

    ______ Remove oxygen mask; patient exhales deeply

    ______ Shake vigorously

    ______ Begin inhalation; depress inhaler

    ______ Place mouth over inhaler mouthpiece

29. You have been dispatched to a funeral home where a grieving widow is having difficulty breathing. On arrival, you find a 46-year-old woman sitting in the lobby surrounded by family. Her daughter tells you that the breathing problem came on suddenly and that her mother "can't seem to catch her breath."

    a. What are the general signs and symptoms of difficulty breathing?

    ______________________________

    ______________________________

    b. As your partner applies high-concentration oxygen, what information should you obtain from the patient or family?

    ______________________________

    ______________________________

    c. The patient has no significant medical history, does not take any medications, and has vital signs within normal limits. She agrees to be transported to the hospital for physician evaluation. How will you position this patient for transport?

    ______________________________

    ______________________________

30. You have responded to an elementary school where a 10-year-old student is having a possible asthma attack. On arrival, you find the child and his teacher sitting inside the entryway of the school. The boy is in moderate distress and has audible wheezing. He is holding a metered-dose inhaler in his hand.

    a. What are common trade names for bronchodilators?

    ______________________________

    ______________________________

b. How do bronchodilators decrease resistance inside the airways?

______________________________________________

______________________________________________

c. What information should you obtain from this patient before contacting medical direction?

______________________________________________

______________________________________________

d. What are the three criteria that must be met before assisting this patient with his medication?

______________________________________________

______________________________________________

______________________________________________

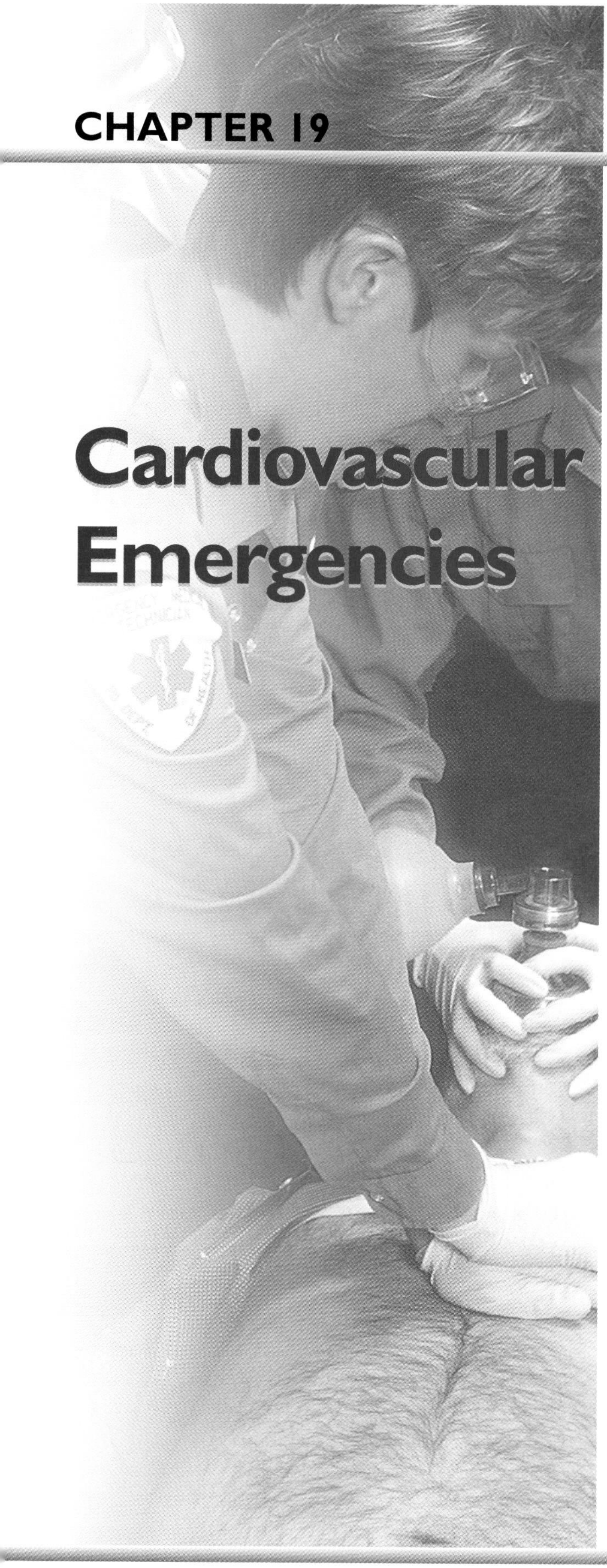

## CHAPTER 19

# Cardiovascular Emergencies

### CHAPTER OUTLINE

I. Review of the Circulatory System
  A. Anatomy
    1. Blood vessels
    2. Blood composition
  B. Physiology
II. Cardiac Compromise
  A. Assessment
  B. Emergency Medical Care
    1. Oxygen and positioning
    2. Nitroglycerin
    3. Basic life support
III. The Automated External Defibrillator
  A. Overview of the Automated External Defibrillator
  B. Advantages of the Automated External Defibrillator
  C. Operation of the Automated External Defibrillator
  D. Postresuscitation Care
  E. Automated External Defibrillator Maintenance
  F. Automated External Defibrillator Skills

## MATCHING 1

*Match the terms in Column 1 with the correct definition in Column 2.*

**Column 1**

1. ______ Angina
2. ______ Diastolic blood pressure
3. ______ Electrodes
4. ______ Ischemia
5. ______ Peripheral
6. ______ Pulse
7. ______ Systolic blood pressure
8. ______ Ventricular fibrillation
9. ______ Ventricular tachycardia

**Column 2**

a. Remote pads attached to the defibrillator and the patient to monitor the electrical activity of the heart
b. Decreased oxygen supply to an area of tissue
c. Chaotic electrical rhythm in the ventricles, with no contraction of the ventricles and no pulse
d. Measurement of the pressure in an artery when the ventricles are contracting
e. Three or more heartbeats in a row at 100 beats or more per minute originating in the ventricles
f. Measurement of the pressure in an artery when the ventricles are at rest
g. Term referring to the extremities
h. Pressure wave felt in an artery when the left ventricle contracts
i. Discomfort felt when the heart does not receive enough oxygen

## MATCHING 2

*Match the arteries in Column 1 with the correct location in Column 2.*

**Column 1**

10. ______ Iliac
11. ______ Coronary
12. ______ Pulmonary
13. ______ Carotid
14. ______ Brachial
15. ______ Femoral
16. ______ Radial
17. ______ Dorsalis pedis

**Column 2**

a. Foot
b. Groin
c. Heart
d. Lungs
e. Pelvis
f. Arm
g. Wrist
h. Neck

## LABELING

*Using arrows, indicate the blood flow through the heart on the figure below.*

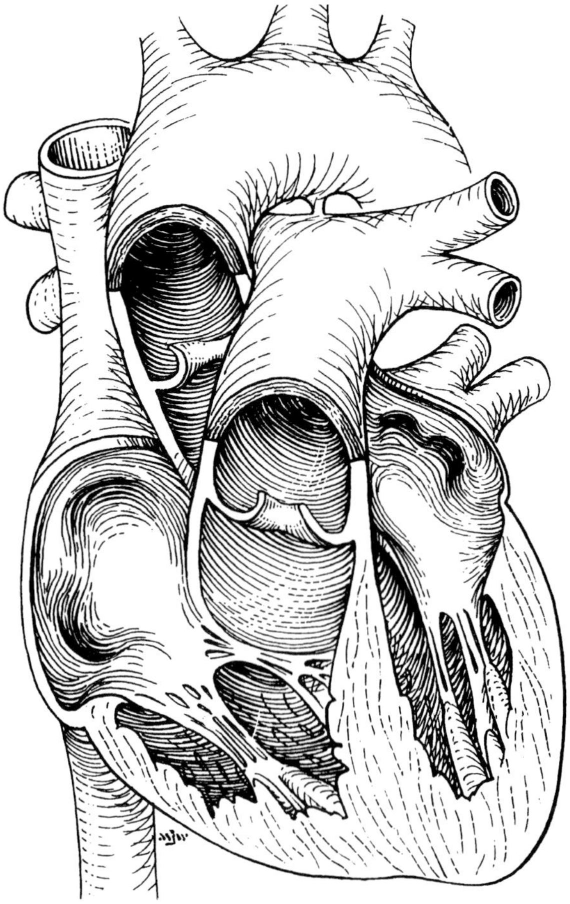

## REVIEW QUESTIONS

1. ______ The heart consists of four chambers with valves between them that work together to circulate blood to the lungs and body. True (T) or false (F)?

2. ______ Blood from the vena cava enters the:
   a. Right atrium
   b. Left atrium
   c. Left ventricle
   d. Right ventricle

3. The tiny blood vessels that connect arterioles to venules are called ______________________.

4. ______ Which of the following blood components are essential in the formation of clots?
   a. White blood cells
   b. Platelets
   c. Red blood cells
   d. Plasma

5. ______ A pulse should be generated every time the left ventricle contracts. True (T) or false (F)?

6. List two sites for locating central pulses and two sites for locating peripheral pulses.

   Central

   a. ______________________

   b. ______________________

   Peripheral

   a. ______________________

   b. ______________________

7. The first number in a blood pressure is the ______________________ value and the second number is the ______________________ value.

8. Another term used to describe shock is ______________________.

9. ______ Which of the following is a sign or symptom of shock?
   a. Full, bounding pulse
   b. High blood pressure
   c. Hot, flushed skin
   d. Anxiety

10. Chest pressure or discomfort that usually goes away with rest is called ______________________.

11. ______ In a heart attack, a blood vessel is blocked and the heart muscle can no longer get _______. This condition is called _______.
    a. Blood, angina
    b. Oxygen, ischemia
    c. White cells, ischemia
    d. Oxygen, tissue damage

12. Respiratory pain is often ______________________ and ______________________ with breathing. Cardiac pain is usually ______________________ and ______________________ with movement.

13. List at least three locations where cardiac pain may radiate.

    a. ______________________

    b. ______________________

    c. ______________________

14. On a scale of 1 to 10, how would a patient rate the worst pain they have ever felt?

    ______________________

    ______________________

15. Define each of the following components of the OPQRST acronym.

O. ______________________________

P. ______________________________

Q. ______________________________

R. ______________________________

S. ______________________________

T. ______________________________

16. The first medication delivered to the cardiac

patient is ______________________________.

17. ______ How would you transport a responsive patient with no trauma, complaining of chest pain?
    a. Sitting up
    b. Lying down
    c. Recovery position
    d. Position of comfort

18. ______ If the patient has nitroglycerin, you should administer it before beginning your assessment. True (T) or false (F)?

19. ______ Nitroglycerin acts by ________ blood vessels, which may ________ blood pressure.
    a. Constricting, decrease
    b. Dilating, decrease
    c. Dilating, increase
    d. Constricting, increase

20. List at least three contraindications to nitroglycerin.

    a. ______________________________

    b. ______________________________

    c. ______________________________

21. ______ All of the following are common side effects of nitroglycerin *except:*
    a. Muscle tremors
    b. Headache
    c. Lowered blood pressure
    d. Burning sensation under the tongue

22. The primary intervention that makes the most

difference in survival from cardiac arrest is

______________________________.

23. ______ The term used to describe a quivering heart muscle is:
    a. Cardiac arrest
    b. Defibrillation
    c. Ventricular fibrillation
    d. Asystole

24. ______ Before placement of an automated external defibrillator (AED), the EMT must confirm that the patient is:
    a. Pulseless, breathing, and unresponsive
    b. Pulseless, breathing, and responsive
    c. Pulseless, not breathing, and unresponsive
    d. Breathing, with a pulse, and with chest pain

25. ______ Coming in contact with the patient or stretcher during defibrillation can result in a shock or burn. True (T) or false (F)?

26. ______ An AED should never be used on a patient younger than 8 years of age. True (T) or false (F)?

27. ______ Each shock should be followed by two ventilations and a pulse check. True (T) or false (F)?

28. You are caring for a 76-year-old man who is complaining of chest pain. The pain began about 30 minutes ago when he was taking his morning walk. He took one nitroglycerin tablet before your arrival. Using a severity scale of 1 to 10, the patient rated his pain as an 8 when it started. After resting and taking a nitroglycerin tablet, he says it is now a 6. You administer high-concentration oxygen by mask and obtain a set of vitals. His blood pressure is 166/84 mm Hg, pulse is 122 beats per minute and regular, and respirations are 16 breaths per minute. The patient looks anxious and is slightly diaphoretic.

a. How would you describe this patient's pain?

_______________________________________________

_______________________________________________

b. What are the three indications for nitroglycerin administration?

_______________________________________________

_______________________________________________

_______________________________________________

c. What are the five contraindications to nitroglycerin administration?

_______________________________________________

_______________________________________________

_______________________________________________

_______________________________________________

_______________________________________________

29. The time is 0300, and your crew has been dispatched for a "possible heart attack." On arrival, you find a 52-year-old woman sitting on a sofa in her living room. She tells you that her chest pain woke her from sleep about an hour ago and has not "let up." Your partner applies high-concentration oxygen and obtains a set of vital signs while you gather a SAMPLE history. Her vitals are within normal range, and she has no significant medical history.

a. What are common signs and symptoms of cardiac compromise?

_______________________________________________

_______________________________________________

b. As you prepare the patient for transport, she tells you that she has some nitroglycerin tablets that belong to a friend. Can you assist her in taking this medication?

_______________________________________________

_______________________________________________

30. Your crew has been dispatched to a possible drug overdose at a local high school. On arrival, you are directed to the gymnasium where you find a 17-year-old student lying on the floor. The coach tells you that the student was acting "a little strange" just before he collapsed. You position the patient supine, open his airway, and assess breathing and circulation. The student is breathless and pulseless. You initiate cardiopulmonary resuscitation, attach the AED, and request advanced life support (ALS) back-up.

a. What two rhythms will the AED recognize as "shockable" rhythms?

_______________________________________________

_______________________________________________

b. Describe proper placement of the AED electrodes.

_______________________________________________

_______________________________________________

## CHAPTER 20

# Diabetes and Altered Mental Status

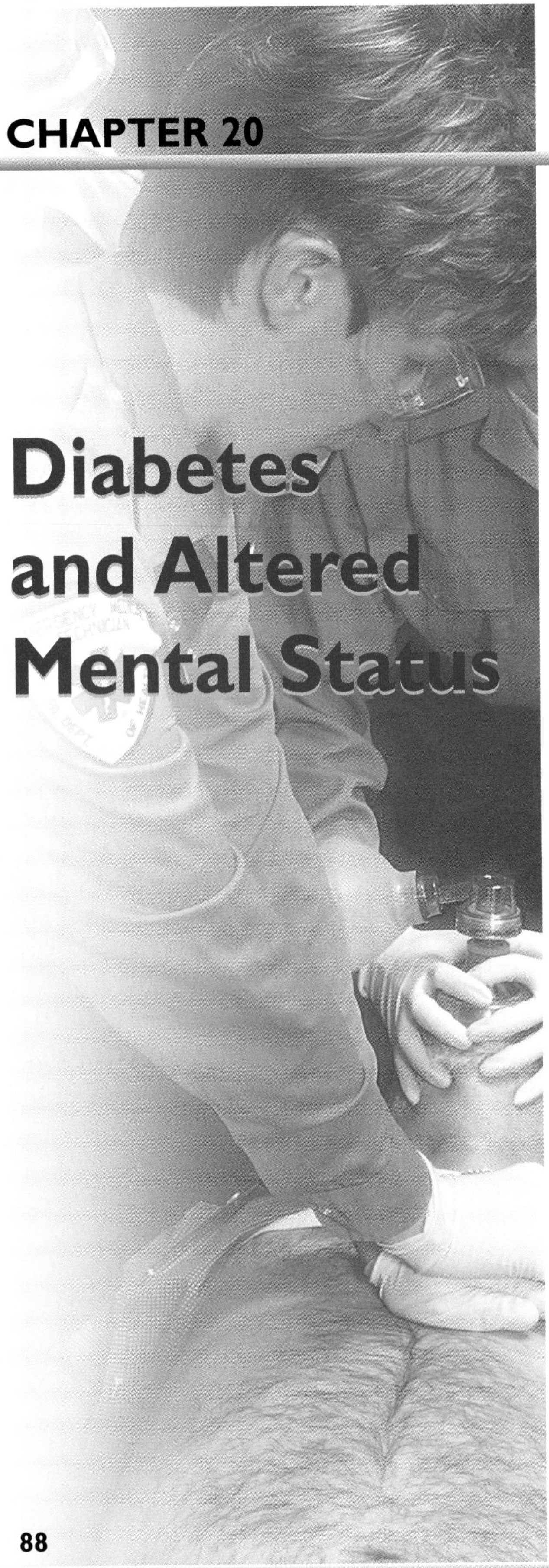

### CHAPTER OUTLINE

I. Causes of Altered Mental Status
   A. Diabetic Emergency
   B. Seizures
   C. Stroke
   D. Other Possible Causes
II. Emergency Care of Patients with Altered Mental Status
   A. Assessment
   B. Airway Management
   C. Treatment for Diabetic Emergency

## MATCHING

*Match the terms in Column 1 with the correct definition in Column 2.*

**Column 1**

1. ______ Altered mental status
2. ______ Diabetes mellitus
3. ______ Glucose
4. ______ Hypoglycemia
5. ______ Insulin-dependent
6. ______ Seizure

**Column 2**

a. Low level of sugar in the blood
b. Diabetic patient who requires hormone injections for the body to use sugar
c. Rapid discharge of nerve cells in the brain causing muscular contractions
d. Disease that prevents insulin from being produced
e. Form of sugar that is converted into usable energy
f. State of mind in which the patient is not oriented to person, place, or time

## REVIEW QUESTIONS

1. ______ Before treating a patient with altered mental status, you must determine the cause. True (T) or false (F)?

2. ______ Altered mental status is related only to medical conditions. True (T) or false (F)?

3. List two common signs and symptoms of hypoglycemia.

   a. ______________________________

   b. ______________________________

4. ______ Seizures can cause full-body jerking or just blank staring into space. True (T) or false (F)?

5. List at least three common causes of seizures.

   a. ______________________________

   b. ______________________________

   c. ______________________________

6. ______ All seizures are life threatening. True (T) or false (F)?

7. One of the most common causes of seizures in children is ______________________________.

8. The time following a seizure when a patient may be disoriented is called the ______________________ period.

9. ______ Most strokes occur from:
   a. Clots in the arteries leading to the brain
   b. Broken blood vessels in the brain
   c. Failure of blood clotting mechanisms
   d. Trauma to the head

10. List three common signs or symptoms of stroke.

    a. ______________________________

    b. ______________________________

    c. ______________________________

11. ______ Which of the following is a positive finding on the Cincinnati stroke scale?
    a. Arms held straight out in front without drifting
    b. Inability to remember the day of the week or month of the year
    c. Slurred speech
    d. Confused responses to questions about the event

12. List at least three common causes of altered mental status.

    a. ______________________________

    b. ______________________________

    c. ______________________________

13. The primary goal of emergency treatment for patients with altered mental status is maintaining a(n) ______________________________.

14. List at least three major points for the focused history and physical examination of a patient with altered mental status.

    a. ______________________________

    b. ______________________________

    c. ______________________________

15. ______ An evaluation of the scene can be an important part of assessing a patient with altered mental status. True (T) or false (F)?

16. ______ Patients with altered mental status are considered ____________ and vital signs are monitored every __________.
    a. Stable, 5 minutes
    b. Unstable, 15 minutes
    c. Unstable, 5 minutes
    d. Stable, 15 minutes

17. List two questions to ask a patient with altered mental status and a history of diabetes.

    a. ______________________________

    b. ______________________________

18. ______ Oral glucose should be used for all patients with altered mental status. True (T) or false (F)?

19. ______ Oral glucose should be used only if the patient can swallow. True (T) or false (F)?

20. ______ Oral glucose is the product's _____ name.
    a. Generic
    b. Trade
    c. Chemical
    d. Brand

21. ______ To administer oral glucose, squirt the tube into the mouth and let the patient swallow. True (T) or false (F)?

22. Absence of a ______________________ is a contraindication to administration of oral glucose.

23. Oral glucose improves the patient's condition by increasing ______________________________.

24. ______ Medical direction must be involved in the decision to administer oral glucose. True (T) or false (F)?

25. You and your partner have had an unusually busy shift. You know that she has insulin-controlled diabetes, and you are concerned because you have missed both breakfast and lunch. Just as you are about to grab a bite to eat, you are dispatched to a car crash.

    a. What type of diabetic reaction might your partner experience and why?

    ______________________________

    ______________________________

    b. What are common signs and symptoms of a diabetic emergency?

    ______________________________

    ______________________________

    c. En route to the scene, your partner eats a candy bar from her purse. If her condition had progressed to an altered mental status, how would you manage this situation?

    ______________________________

    ______________________________

26. Your crew has been dispatched to a possible cardiac arrest. On arrival, you find a man in his middle 20s lying face down on the ground. A passerby found the man in this condition and dialed 911 on his cellular telephone. No patient information is available.

    a. What are your first priorities of care for this patient?

    ______________________________________

    ______________________________________

    b. The patient is breathing but is unresponsive to verbal or painful stimuli. You control his airway and administer high-concentration oxygen. What common causes of altered mental status should you consider?

    ______________________________________

    ______________________________________

    c. How will you manage this patient?

    ______________________________________

    ______________________________________

## CHAPTER 21

# Allergic Reactions

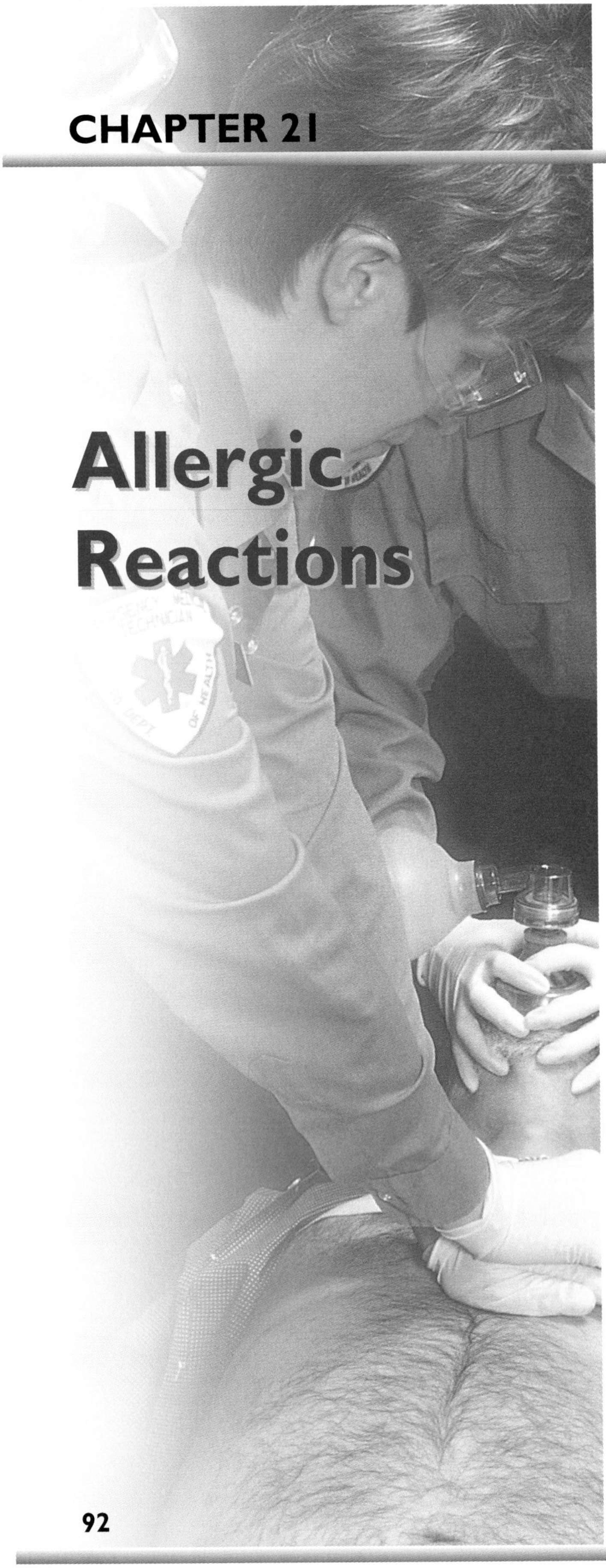

## CHAPTER OUTLINE

## REVIEW QUESTIONS

1. ______ An allergic reaction can best be described as:
   a. A life-threatening emergency
   b. A normal response to an allergen
   c. High blood pressure following a reaction
   d. An exaggerated response to an allergen

2. ______ Allergic reactions are always life threatening and must be treated immediately. True (T) or false (F)?

3. List three common allergens.

   a. ______________________________

   b. ______________________________

   c. ______________________________

4. List five common signs and symptoms of an allergic reaction.

   a. ______________________________

   b. ______________________________

   c. ______________________________

   d. ______________________________

   e. ______________________________

5. Itchy, watery eyes; runny nose; and a headache are all signs and symptoms of a ______________________ allergic reaction.

6. The first sign of hypoperfusion may be a change in ______________________.

7. The term used to describe a significant allergic reaction is ______________________.

8. ______ A true medical emergency exists when the patient shows signs or symptoms of ______ or ______.
   a. Hypoperfusion, high blood pressure
   b. Hypoperfusion, respiratory compromise
   c. Respiratory compromise, nausea
   d. Headache, feeling of doom

9. ______ Epinephrine autoinjectors are used only on patients with signs and symptoms of ______ and ______.
   a. Hypoperfusion, high blood pressure
   b. Hypoperfusion, respiratory compromise
   c. Respiratory compromise, nausea
   d. Headache, feeling of doom

10. A patient with an allergic reaction and signs of respiratory compromise should be assessed at least every ______________________ minutes.

11. ______ Epinephrine works by ______bronchioles and ______ blood vessels.
    a. Dilating, constricting
    b. Dilating, dilating
    c. Constricting, constricting
    d. Constricting, dilating

12. List the three criteria for use of the epinephrine autoinjector.

    a. ______________________________

    b. ______________________________

    c. ______________________________

13. ______ Several contraindications exist to the EMT–Basic administering an epinephrine autoinjector for a patient with life-threatening airway compromise. True (T) or false (F)?

14. ______ An autoinjector consists of a needle and syringe of medication, which is injected when pressed against the skin. True (T) or false (F)?

15. ______ Which of the following is *not* a side effect of epinephrine?
    a. Dizziness
    b. Pale skin
    c. Sleepiness
    d. Nausea and vomiting

16. ______ Airway control is secondary to using the autoinjector in a patient having an allergic reaction. True (T) or false (F)?

17. You have been dispatched to a public swimming pool at the city park. On arrival, you find a 36-year-old man who says he has been stung by a bee. He is near hysterics and tells you that he is highly allergic to stings. He has an epinephrine autoinjector in his bag but is afraid to inject himself.

    a. What are common signs and symptoms of an allergic reaction?

    ______________________________

    ______________________________

    b. The patient has several of the signs and symptoms of an allergic reaction and is complaining of difficulty breathing. What are the criteria for use of an epinephrine autoinjector?

    ______________________________

    ______________________________

    c. Medical direction authorizes you to administer the epinephrine. Describe the steps in drug administration.

    ______________________________

    ______________________________

18. You are working during part of your vacation as a counselor at a youth camp. The administrator knows that you are an EMT–Basic and asks you to look at a child who is feeling sick. The 9-year-old girl is complaining of itchy, watery eyes and has a runny nose and a headache. As you examine her, you notice a rash on her neck and abdomen. Her vital signs are within normal limits, and her lung sounds are clear. The child tells you that she is allergic to "a lot of things" but has no medications.

    a. What are common causes of mild allergic reactions?

    ______________________________

    ______________________________

    b. What assessment findings would reveal a severe allergic reaction in this patient?

    ______________________________

    ______________________________

    c. Would this patient be a candidate for epinephrine administration? Why or why not?

    ______________________________

    ______________________________

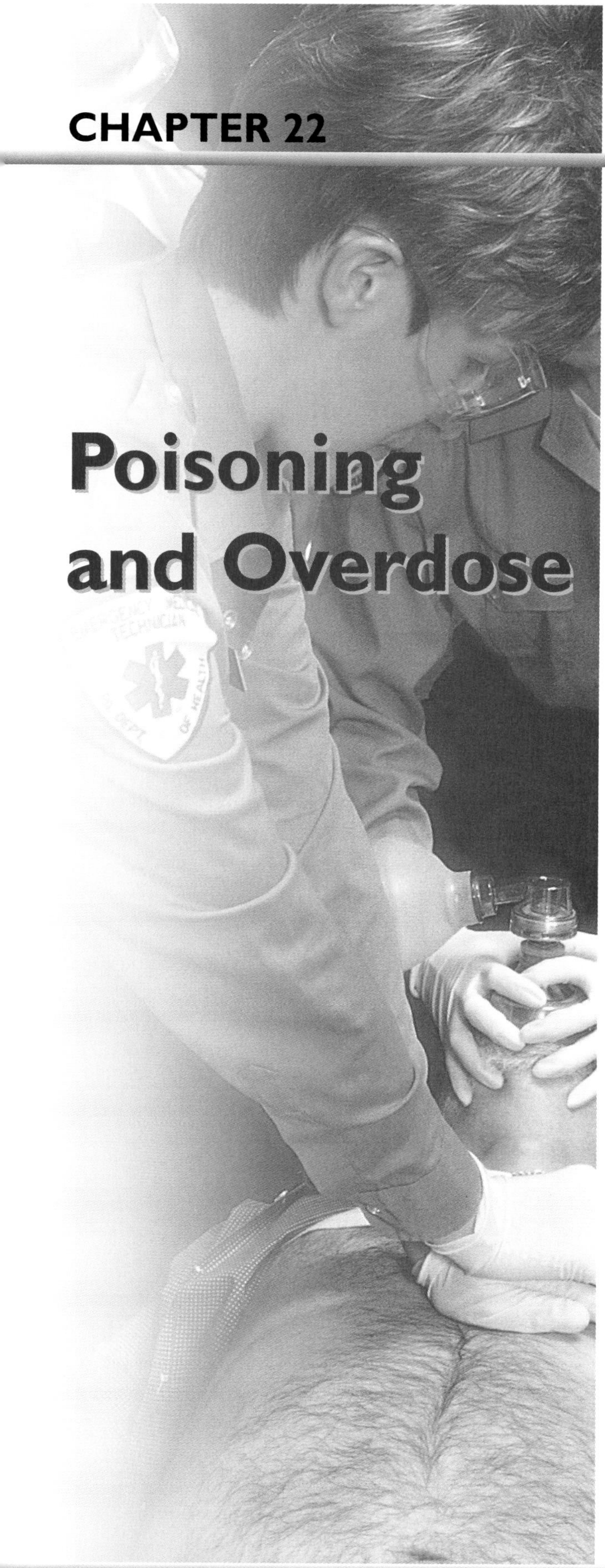

# CHAPTER 22

# Poisoning and Overdose

## CHAPTER OUTLINE

I. History of Poisoning
II. Types of Toxins
  A. Ingested Toxins
  B. Inhaled Toxins
  C. Injected Toxins
  D. Absorbed Toxins
III. Airway Management
IV. Use of Activated Charcoal

## MATCHING

*Match the terms in Column 1 with the correct definition in Column 2.*

**Column I**

1. ______ Absorbed toxin
2. ______ Activated charcoal
3. ______ Ingested toxin
4. ______ Inhaled toxin
5. ______ Injected toxin
6. ______ Toxin

**Column 2**

a. Substance that produces adverse effects when it enters the body
b. Toxin that enters the body through a break in the skin
c. Toxin that enters the body through the skin
d. Toxin that is consumed orally
e. Toxin that is breathed into the lungs where it is absorbed into the bloodstream
f. Medication that medical direction may authorize for management of poisoning caused by an ingested toxin

## REVIEW QUESTIONS

1. ______ A larger than recommended dose of any medication can be considered a poisoning. True (T) or false (F)?

2. Ongoing assessments are performed every __________ minutes for unstable patients and every __________ minutes for stable patients.

3. List four questions to assist you in gathering information about the poisoning or overdose patient.

   a. ____________________
   b. ____________________
   c. ____________________
   d. ____________________

4. ______ Poisoning from medications that are chronic (occurring over weeks or months) is treated the same as poisoning from a single ingestion. True (T) or false (F)?

5. ______ Over-the-counter treatments for poisoning and overdoses are beneficial and should be encouraged. True (T) or false (F)?

6. ______ Diarrhea and peculiar breath odors are common side effects of ______ toxins.
   a. Inhaled
   b. Ingested
   c. Absorbed
   d. Injected

7. If pills or tablets are still in the mouth of an unresponsive patient, how should the EMT–Basic handle the pills?

   ____________________

   ____________________

8. Inhaled toxins usually affect what body systems?

   ____________________

   ____________________

9. List three common signs and symptoms of inhaled toxins.

   a. ____________________
   b. ____________________
   c. ____________________

10. The primary treatment for inhaled poisoning is

______________________________________.

11. Injected toxins reach the body through

______________________________________.

12. ______ Always bring the possible toxin to the receiving facility. True (T) or false (F)?

13. List three factors that affect the rate of absorption of injected poisonings.

a. ______________________________________

b. ______________________________________

c. ______________________________________

14. ______ Powder or liquid on the skin may result in an ______ toxin.
a. Inhaled
b. Ingested
c. Absorbed
d. Injected

15. ______ Dry substances should be ______ away and liquid substances ______ away.
a. Brushed, irrigated
b. Irrigated, irrigated
c. Blown, wiped
d. Irrigated, blotted

16. ______ Activated charcoal is the treatment for ______ toxins.
a. Inhaled
b. Ingested
c. Absorbed
d. Injected

17. Activated charcoal works by ________________

to the toxin in the ________________________.

18. ______ Activated charcoal is the ______ name. LiquiChar and InstaChar are ______ names.
a. Generic, trade
b. Trade, generic
c. Chemical, trade
d. Brand, generic

19. List three contraindications to the use of activated charcoal.

a. ______________________________________

b. ______________________________________

c. ______________________________________

20. ______ Vomiting is a desired effect of administration of activated charcoal. True (T) or false (F)?

21. You have been dispatched to care for a 4-year-old child who has ingested an unknown amount of baby aspirin. On arrival, you find the mother holding the child in her lap. The child appears anxious but is not in obvious distress. The mother tells you that she found the child playing with two empty aspirin bottles about 20 minutes ago. She does not know how many pills were in the bottles. You contact medical direction and give your patient report. The physician advises you to administer activated charcoal.

a. What is the normal dose of activated charcoal for infants and children?

______________________________________

______________________________________

b. What are the indications and contraindications for administering activated charcoal?

______________________________________

______________________________________

c. You administer the activated charcoal as directed. En route to the hospital, the patient vomits. What should you do?

______________________________________

______________________________________

22. You are caring for a patient who has attempted suicide. He was found in his car by a neighbor who noticed the car's engine was running while the garage door was closed. You and your partner move the patient outside and perform an initial assessment of his airway, breathing, and circulation. He is unresponsive and has a pulse and shallow respirations at six per minute.

    a. What treatment is indicated first for this patient?

    ______________________________

    ______________________________

    b. Describe the characteristics of carbon monoxide and the general symptoms of exposure.

    ______________________________

    ______________________________

    c. In what other scenario is carbon monoxide commonly present?

    ______________________________

    ______________________________

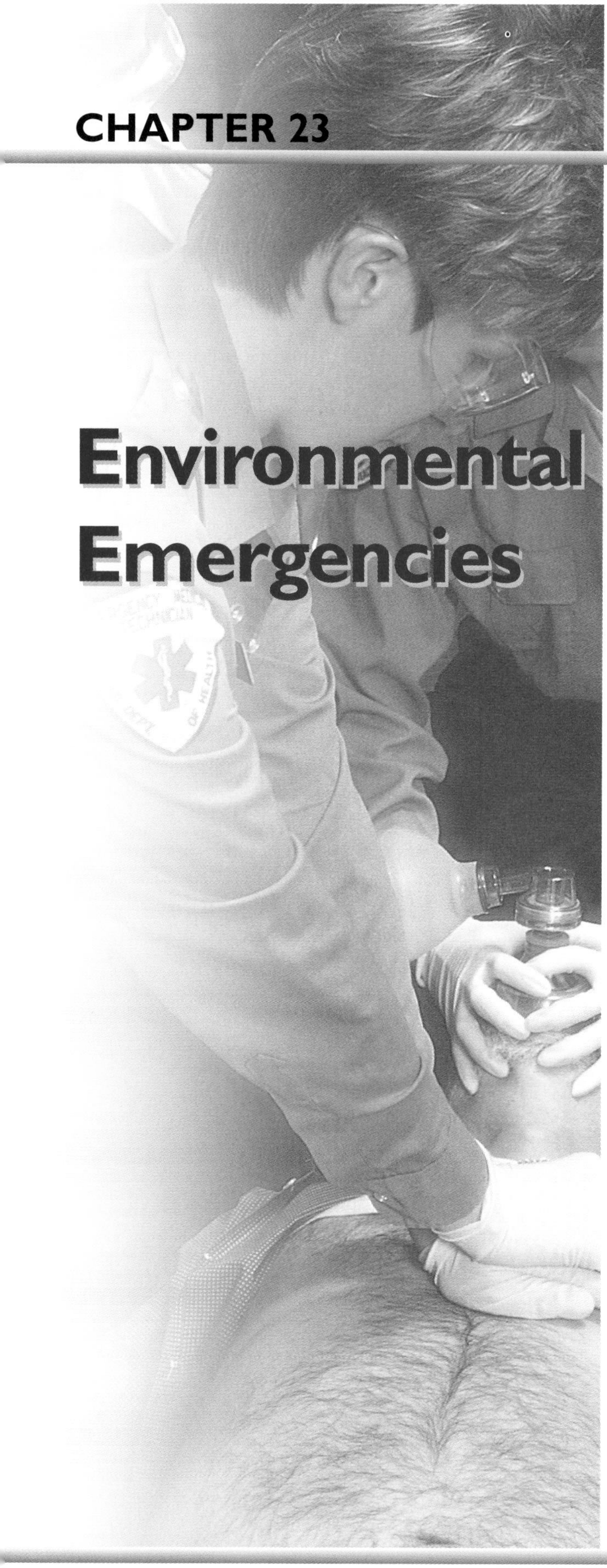

## CHAPTER 23

# Environmental Emergencies

## CHAPTER OUTLINE

I. Thermoregulatory Emergencies
   A. Temperature Regulation in the Body
   B. Exposure to the Cold
      1. Generalized hypothermia
         a. Predisposing factors
         b. Signs and symptoms of generalized hypothermia
         c. Emergency care for patients with generalized hypothermia
      2. Local cold injuries
         a. Predisposing factors
         b. Signs and symptoms of local cold injuries
         c. Emergency care for patients with local cold injuries
   C. Exposure to Heat
      1. Predisposing factors
      2. Signs and symptoms of generalized hyperthermia
      3. Emergency care for patients with generalized hyperthermia
      4. Rescuing the rescuer

II. Drowning and Near Drowning
   A. Emergency Medical Care of the Near-Drowning Patient

III. Bites and Stings
   A. Signs and Symptoms
   B. Emergency Medical Care for Bites and Stings

## MATCHING

*Match the terms in Column 1 with the correct definition in Column 2.*

**Column 1**

1. ______ Conduction
2. ______ Convection
3. ______ Evaporation
4. ______ Hyperthermia
5. ______ Hypothermia
6. ______ Radiation
7. ______ Thermoregulatory emergency

**Column 2**

a. Any condition involving a significant change in temperature of the body
b. Condition in which the body temperature is above normal (98.6° F or 37° C)
c. Loss of heat, in the form of infrared energy, to cooler surroundings
d. Transfer of heat directly from one object to another
e. Transfer of heat to moving air or liquid
f. Transfer of heat that occurs when a liquid changes into a gas
g. Condition in which the body temperature is below normal (98.6° F or 37° C)

## REVIEW QUESTIONS

1. ______ The temperature of the body needs to remain fairly constant to maintain vital chemical functions. True (T) or false (F)?

2. The human body loses heat by evaporation, conduction, radiation, ______________________, and ________________________________.

3. When body temperature begins to decrease, the body produces heat by ______________________.

4. ______ When the body temperature begins to rise, the blood vessels react by:
   a. Constricting
   b. Dilating
   c. Reducing blood flow through the vessels
   d. Diverting blood to the body's core

5. When body temperature begins to increase, the body produces ______________________, which cools the body by evaporation.

6. ______ Any time the body temperature drops below normal, the patient is hypothermic. True (T) or false (F)?

7. ______ The most common cause of generalized hypothermia is submersion in water. True (T) or false (F)?

8. List at least five predisposing factors for generalized hypothermia.
   a. ______________________
   b. ______________________
   c. ______________________
   d. ______________________
   e. ______________________

9. List two reasons why elderly patients are at increased risk of developing hypothermia.
   a. ______________________
   b. ______________________

10. An unreliable sign of hypothermia is cool ______________________.

11. Where should you assess skin temperature to determine if the patient is hypothermic?

_______________________________________

_______________________________________

12. ______ Which of the following is a sign or symptom of early hypothermia?
    a. Normal blood pressure
    b. Slow pulse
    c. Slow respirations
    d. Pale skin

13. ______ A rapid pulse and respirations are common early in the body's attempt to increase heat production. True (T) or false (F)?

14. Define active rewarming and passive rewarming.

Active rewarming:

_______________________________________

_______________________________________

Passive rewarming:

_______________________________________

_______________________________________

15. Heat packs at the axillae and groin are a form of

_______________________________ rewarming.

16. ______ Active rewarming is a vital part of treatment for the patient in late hypothermia with decreased level of responsiveness. True (T) or false (F)?

17. A pulse check for a severely hypothermic patient should be between __________ and __________ seconds.

18. List five body areas most susceptible to localized cold injuries.

a. _______________________________________

b. _______________________________________

c. _______________________________________

d. _______________________________________

e. _______________________________________

19. ______ Which of the following is a sign or symptom of early, localized cold damage?
    a. Waxy or white skin
    b. Swelling, blisters
    c. Tingling sensation
    d. Firm feeling when touched

20. ______ Rubbing and massaging a cold injury is beneficial because it causes blood flow to return to the area. True (T) or false (F)?

21. List four predisposing factors for heat emergencies.

a. _______________________________________

b. _______________________________________

c. _______________________________________

d. _______________________________________

22. List four signs or symptoms of generalized heat emergency.

a. _______________________________________

b. _______________________________________

c. _______________________________________

d. _______________________________________

23. ______ Hot skin is a late sign of an extreme heat emergency. True (T) or false (F)?

24. The steps for the care of the patient with generalized hyperthermia and hot skin include:

    a. ______________________________

    b. ______________________________

    c. ______________________________

25. Define drowning and near drowning.

    Drowning

    ______________________________

    ______________________________

    Near drowning

    ______________________________

    ______________________________

26. ______ Patients found unresponsive in the water should be treated and evaluated for possible spinal injury. True (T) or false (F)?

27. ______ The first priority in a bite or sting emergency is to remove the stinger from the patient. True (T) or false (F)?

28. ______ For an extremity bite or sting, position the injured area:
    a. At heart level
    b. Below heart level
    c. Above heart level
    d. Positioning of the extremity is not important

29. ______ Credit cards or rigid cardboard can be used to scrape out a stinger. True (T) or false (F)?

30. You have been dispatched to a nearby ski resort to care for an accident victim. On arrival, you find a 30-year-old woman who was injured on one of the ski slopes. Her friends had reported her missing for several hours. She was rescued and brought to the lodge by members of the ski patrol. She has an injury to her right lower extremity and appears to be suffering from hypothermia.

    a. What are the predisposing factors for generalized hypothermia?

    ______________________________

    ______________________________

    b. What mental status and motor function changes may be caused by hypothermia?

    ______________________________

    ______________________________

    c. What are general principles for treating all hypothermic patients?

    ______________________________

    ______________________________

31. Your crew has been dispatched to standby at a rescue operation where a car has been submerged in a lake. Shortly after your arrival, one of the divers becomes trapped beneath the water. While trying to free himself, his air hose is cut by the car's wreckage. He is brought to the surface by other members of the rescue team. He is unresponsive and in respiratory arrest.

    a. What are your first priorities in managing this patient?

    ______________________________________

    ______________________________________

    b. During resuscitation, the patient's abdomen swells and begins to interfere with ventilation. What should you do?

    ______________________________________

    ______________________________________

    c. Should attempts always be made to relieve gastric distention in victims of near drowning? Why or why not?

    ______________________________________

    ______________________________________

# CHAPTER 24

# Behavioral Emergencies

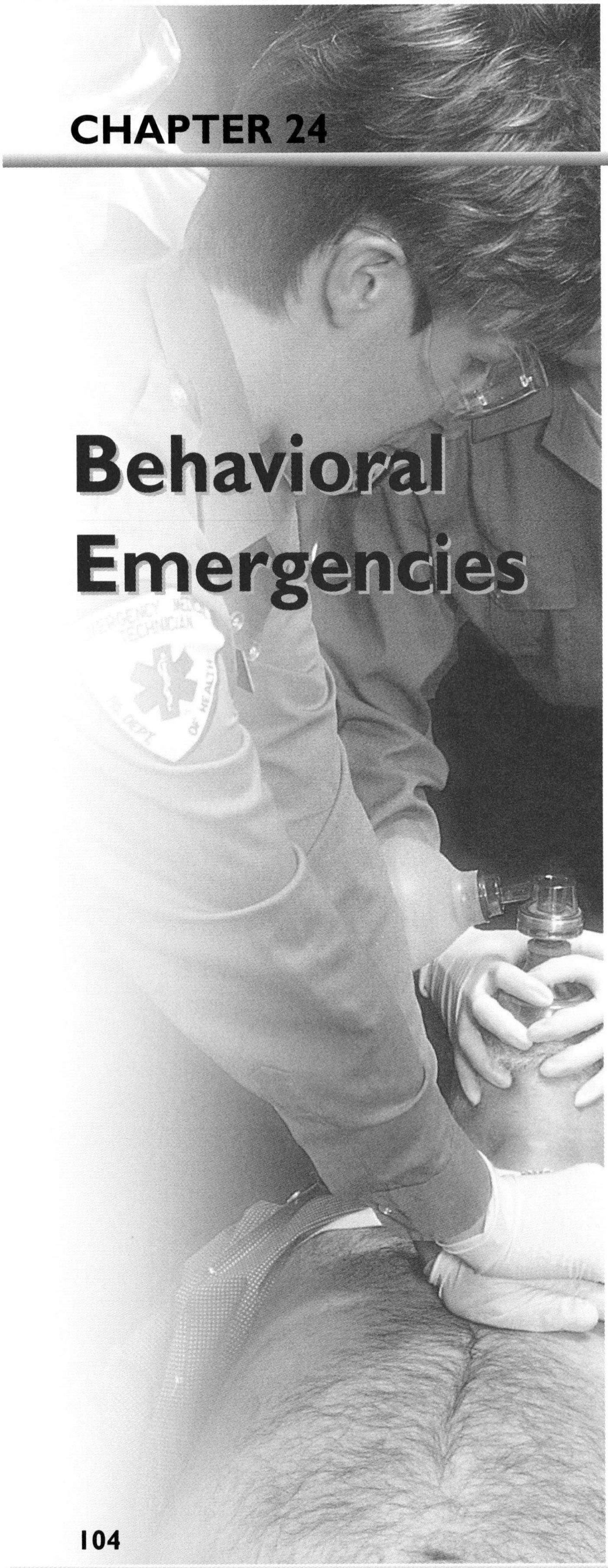

## CHAPTER OUTLINE

## MATCHING

*Match the terms in Column 1 with the correct definition in Column 2.*

**Column 1**

1. ______ Abnormal behavior
2. ______ Behavioral emergency
3. ______ Domestic dispute
4. ______ Psychotic
5. ______ Reasonable force

**Column 2**

a. Form of violence that results from a family argument and may result in abuse of spouse or children
b. Refers to behavior by a person who has lost touch with reality
c. Power necessary to keep a person from injuring him or herself or others
d. Actions exhibited by a person that is outside of the norm for the situation and is socially unacceptable
e. Situation in which a person acts in a manner that is unacceptable or intolerable to the person, family members, or the community

## REVIEW QUESTIONS

1. The way people act on a day-to-day basis is called their ______________________________.

2. List three factors that can alter a person's behavior.

   a. ______________________________

   b. ______________________________

   c. ______________________________

3. ______ Patients experiencing psychotic thinking should be treated:
   a. As any other patient
   b. Carefully and calmly
   c. Loudly so as to get their attention
   d. With rapid actions and speaking

4. List three risk factors associated with suicide.

   a. ______________________________

   b. ______________________________

   c. ______________________________

5. ______ Suicidal patients will demonstrate at least one risk factor. True (T) or false (F)?

6. ______ The scene size-up is the most important part of entering a scene with a potential behavioral emergency. True (T) or false (F)?

7. List three signs of potential violence.

   a. ______________________________

   b. ______________________________

   c. ______________________________

8. ______ If the patient has a history of behavioral problems, he or she will not require evaluation for medical or trauma-related problems. True (T) or false (F)?

9. ______ Avoid agreeing with patients who appear to have disturbed thinking patterns. True (T) or false (F)?

10. Patients who do not calm down or are showing signs of destructive behavior may need to be ______________________________.

11. Restraints may help you provide adequate care to the patient; however, if used incorrectly, they can cause ____________________________.

12. ______ Restraints should be removed as soon as the patient begins to calm down to avoid injury. True (T) or false (F)?

13. ______ If a combative patient is spitting, restraining the patient in a prone position on the stretcher is acceptable. True (T) or false (F)?

14. ______ No patient can be transported against his or her will. True (T) or false (F)?

15. List three points that must be documented for behavioral emergencies.

    a. ____________________________

    b. ____________________________

    c. ____________________________

16. Assistance in determining the need for transport of a patient refusing care should be obtained through ____________________________.

17. The amount of force required to keep patients from injuring themselves or others is called ____________________________ force.

18. Local law enforcement personnel have requested EMS to transport a patient to the hospital for psychological evaluation. You arrive at the scene and find a 30-year-old man who claims that the FBI is trying to kill him. The police have placed him in protective custody, and the scene is safe.

    a. What type of communication should you attempt with this patient? Provide examples of questions you should ask.

    ____________________________

    ____________________________

    b. What methods can you use to calm this patient?

    ____________________________

    ____________________________

    c. What type of documentation is considered important when caring for a patient with a behavioral emergency?

    ____________________________

    ____________________________

## CHAPTER 25

# Obstetrics and Gynecology

## CHAPTER OUTLINE

I. Reproductive Anatomy and Physiology
  A. Labor
II. Contents of the Childbirth Kit
III. Predelivery Emergencies
  A. Miscarriage
    1. Emergency care for miscarriage
  B. Seizure During Pregnancy
    1. Emergency care for seizure during pregnancy
  C. Vaginal Bleeding Late in Pregnancy
    1. Emergency care for bleeding late in pregnancy
  D. Trauma
    1. Emergency care for trauma in pregnancy
IV. Normal Delivery
  A. Predelivery Considerations
  B. Precautions
  C. Delivery Procedure
  D. Initial Care of the Newborn
V. Abnormal Deliveries and Complications
  A. Prolapsed Cord
    1. Emergency care for prolapsed cord
  B. Breech Presentation
    1. Emergency care for breech presentation
  C. Limb Presentation
    1. Emergency care for limb presentation
  D. Multiple Births
    1. Emergency care for multiple births
  E. Meconium
    1. Emergency care when meconium is present
  F. Premature Birth
    1. Emergency care for premature birth
VI. Gynecological Emergencies
  A. Vaginal Bleeding
  B. Trauma to External Genitalia
  C. Sexual Assault

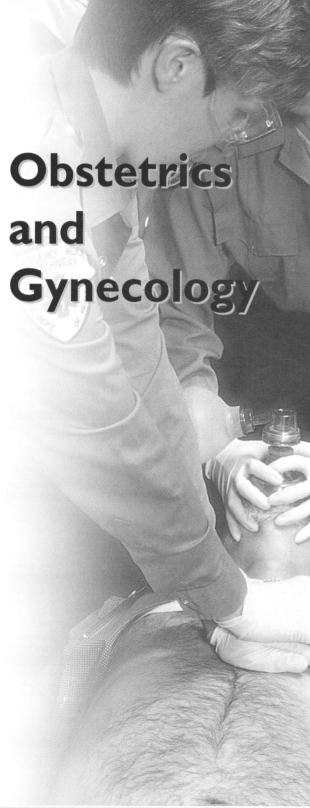

## MATCHING 1

*Match the terms in Column 1 with the correct definition in Column 2.*

**Column 1**

1. ______ Abortion
2. ______ Bloody show
3. ______ Cesarean section
4. ______ Fetus
5. ______ Meconium
6. ______ Miscarriage

**Column 2**

a. Expulsion of the mucous plug as the cervix dilates
b. An unborn, developing baby
c. Spontaneous delivery of a human fetus before it is able to live on its own
d. Medical term for any delivery or removal of a human fetus before it can live on its own
e. Fetal stool that may be present in the amniotic fluid
f. Surgical delivery in which the muscles of the abdomen are cut and the baby is delivered through the abdomen

## MATCHING 2

*Match the terms in Column 1 with the correct definition in Column 2.*

**Column 1**

7. ______ Amniotic sac
8. ______ Birth canal
9. ______ Cervix
10. ______ Perineum
11. ______ Uterus
12. ______ Vagina

**Column 2**

a. The canal that leads from the uterus to the external opening in women
b. The lower part of the uterus and the vagina
c. Membrane forming a closed, fluid-filled pouch around a developing fetus
d. Area of skin between the vagina and anus
e. Neck of the uterus
f. Female reproductive organ in which a baby grows and develops

## MATCHING 3

*Match the terms in Column 1 with the correct definition in Column 2.*

**Column 1**

13. ______ Breech presentation
14. ______ Cephalic
15. ______ Crowning
16. ______ Placenta
17. ______ Presenting part
18. ______ Prolapsed cord
19. ______ Umbilical cord

**Column 2**

a. Connects the placenta to the fetus
b. Presentation of the baby's feet or buttocks first in delivery
c. Fetal and maternal organ through which the fetus absorbs oxygen and nutrients and excretes wastes
d. Stage in which the head of the baby is seen at the vaginal opening
e. Situation in which the umbilical cord delivers through the vagina before any presenting part
f. Presentation of baby's head first in delivery
g. Area of the fetus that appears at the vaginal opening first

## REVIEW QUESTIONS

1. The fetus grows and develops in the

    ______________________________.

2. During pregnancy, the fetus receives nutrition

    from the mother through the ______________.

3. ______ The placenta is always present in a woman's uterus but is used only during pregnancy. True (T) or false (F)?

4. ______ The fetus rests in a sac filled with 1 to 2 L of:
    a. Blood
    b. Water
    c. Amniotic fluid
    d. Plasma

5. ______ The usual length of a pregnancy is ______ or ______.
    a. 6 months, 40 weeks
    b. 9 months, 40 weeks
    c. 9 months, 36 weeks
    d. 8 months, 36 weeks

6. During pregnancy, a woman's blood volume

    ____________________ to accommodate for

    the needs of the baby.

7. ______ The delivery of the baby ends the second stage of labor. True (T) or false (F)?

8. ______ Crowning is a sign that delivery is approximately 30 to 45 minutes away. True (T) or false (F)?

9. List three pieces of equipment in the obstetrics kit and how they are used.

    a. ______________________________

    b. ______________________________

    c. ______________________________

10. ______ The care for a woman who is experiencing a predelivery emergency is the same as for any patient exhibiting similar signs and symptoms. True (T) or false (F)?

11. Labor pains are associated with the contraction of

    the ______________________________.

12. ______ Personal protective equipment needed during a delivery is usually limited to gloves. True (T) or false (F)?

13. A miscarriage usually occurs in the first

    ____________________ months of a pregnancy.

14. List three of the questions that will be important to ask to determine if time is sufficient to transport the patient before delivery of the baby.

    a. ______________________________

    b. ______________________________

    c. ______________________________

15. How would you prepare the mother for delivery?

    ______________________________

    ______________________________

16. ______ Apply gentle pressure to the ______ to prevent a rapid or explosive delivery.
    a. Head of the fetus
    b. Perineum
    c. Vagina
    d. Abdomen

17. ______ As the infant's head is delivered, check the neck for the presence of the:
    a. Umbilical cord
    b. Placenta
    c. Tissue
    d. Amniotic fluid

18. Suction the baby's mouth and nose with a

    ____________________ before delivery of the torso.

19. ______ The umbilical cord should be cut:
    a. After pulsations stop in the cord
    b. Immediately after the baby delivers
    c. Before the placenta delivers
    d. At the receiving facility

20. ______ After the baby delivers, gently pull on the umbilical cord until the placenta delivers. True (T) or false (F)?

21. ______ The placenta should be wrapped and discarded before transport of the mother and infant. True (T) or false (F)?

22. If the mother loses more than 500 ml of blood during the delivery, to help the uterus contract, the EMT–Basic should provide ________________.

23. ______ Which of the following is part of the initial and ongoing assessment of the newborn?
    a. Amniotic fluid
    b. Smile
    c. Reflex assessment
    d. Pulse

24. The heart rate of a newborn should be greater than ________________ beats per minute.

25. ______ A newborn baby has slow and shallow respirations, and the EMT–Basic provides ventilations with a bag-valve-mask (BVM). The heart rate is 68 beats per minute. The EMT–Basic should:
    a. Provide free-flow oxygen
    b. Flick the soles of the baby's feet
    c. Provide chest compressions along with ventilation
    d. Continue with BVM ventilations only

26. ______ To transport a patient with prolapsed cord:
    a. Turn her on her side and transport.
    b. Elevate her hips or place her in a head-down position.
    c. Lay her on her stomach.
    d. Lay her flat on her back with legs flat.

27. ______ To prevent suffocation during a breech presentation:
    a. With a gloved hand, form a "V" around the baby's face.
    b. Rotate the baby to be face up.
    c. Pull gently on the baby until it delivers.
    d. Nothing can be done.

28. ______ Which of the following statements is true concerning multiple births?
    a. Babies from multiple births are often smaller and premature.
    b. Mothers will always know they are having twins.
    c. Complications are not common with multiple births.
    d. Cut the umbilical cords only after both babies have been born.

29. ______ A limb presentation is a true emergency and the mother should be transported immediately. True (T) or false (F)?

30. ______ Meconium in the amniotic fluid may present a respiratory problem for a newborn. True (T) or false (F)?

31. Infants born at less than 37 weeks or weighing less than 5.5 pounds are considered to be ________________________.

32. ______ Resuscitation, including cardiopulmonary resuscitation, is more likely to be required for a premature infant rather than a full-term infant. True (T) or false (F)?

33. ______ Discourage a sexual assault patient from bathing or cleaning until after evaluation at the receiving facility. True (T) or false (F)?

34. Your crew is dispatched to an "OB case." En route, you are advised that the patient is full term and that her water has broken. On arrival at the scene, you find a 36-year-old woman in labor. She tells you this is her third pregnancy and that the baby is "on the way."

   a. What questions should you ask the mother when deciding whether to transport or assist in delivery on the scene?

   ______________________________________

   ______________________________________

   b. You prepare for delivery on the scene and advise medical direction. Within a few minutes, the infant's head is being delivered. You find the umbilical cord is wrapped around the infant's neck. What should you do?

   ______________________________________

   ______________________________________

   c. What are the last steps in the delivery process?

   ______________________________________

   ______________________________________

35. You are assisting in the delivery of a multiple birth. The first infant has been delivered, and the baby and mother are doing fine. As the second infant delivers, you note that the color of the infant's neck and trunk is blue and dusky. The baby is not crying, and the mother senses that something is wrong. You suction the mouth and nose, dry the infant, and stimulate breathing. Spontaneous respirations remain inadequate.

   a. What is your next step in resuscitation?

   ______________________________________

   ______________________________________

   b. After a few ventilations the infant begins to cry. What is your next assessment?

   ______________________________________

   ______________________________________

   c. The baby's color improves, and the baby is beginning to respond appropriately. What is your next step in managing this infant?

   ______________________________________

   ______________________________________

# CHAPTER 26

# Geriatrics

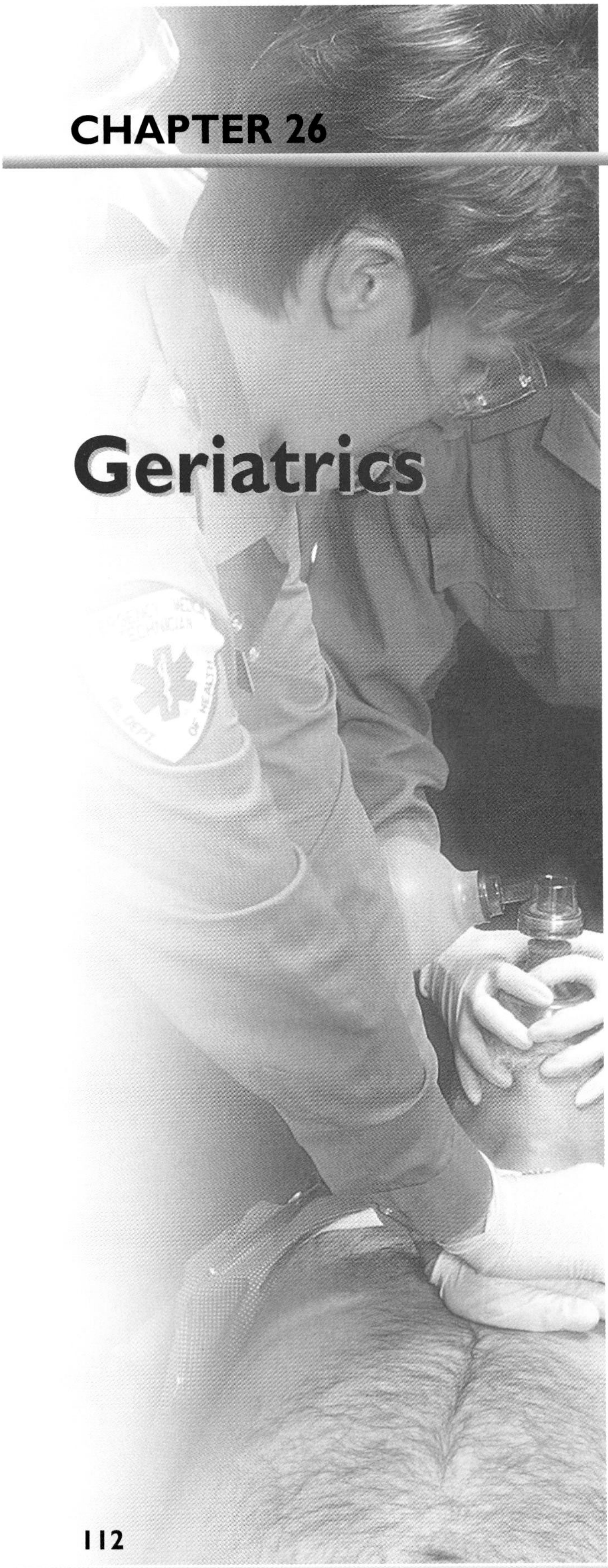

## CHAPTER OUTLINE

I. Anatomy and Physiology Related to Common Medical Emergencies
   A. Respiratory System
   B. Cardiovascular System
   C. Renal System
   D. Nervous System
   E. Musculoskeletal System
   F. Gastrointestinal (GI) System
II. Environmental Emergencies
III. Psychiatric Disorders
IV. Special Trauma Considerations in the Elderly
V. Assessment of the Geriatric Patient
VI. Other Considerations
   A. Medication Considerations
   B. Abuse and Neglect
   C. Expanding the Role of EMS

## MATCHING I

*Match the terms in Column 1 with the correct definition in Column 2.*

**Column 1**

1. ______ Delirium
2. ______ Dementia
3. ______ Pathologic
4. ______ Syncope
5. ______ Vital capacity

**Column 2**

a. An acute change in mental status, usually involving a serious medical condition
b. The maximum volume of air the lungs will hold when a patient forcefully breathes in
c. A steady decline in mental performance, usually occurring over several months or years
d. Refers to an abnormal process resulting from disease or injury
e. A condition usually referred to as a simple faint

## REVIEW QUESTIONS

1. List three reasons why older adults are the fastest-growing population in the United States.

   a. ______________________________

   b. ______________________________

   c. ______________________________

2. A generalized decline in body function begins as early as age ______________________.

3. ______ From 30 to 80 years of age, the respiratory system shows a 10% decrease in vital capacity. True (T) or false (F)?

4. An elderly patient having a myocardial infarction (MI) may have atypical symptoms such as:

   a. ______________________________

   b. ______________________________

   c. ______________________________

5. Almost one half of elderly patients with acute MI present with ____________________ instead of chest pain.

6. Decreasing renal function in older adults can lead to problems with ______________________.

7. The two major cardiovascular diseases are:

   a. ______________________________

   b. ______________________________

8. ______ Another term for ministroke is:
   a. TIA
   b. PEA
   c. RST
   d. DAL

9. ______ Patients experiencing vertigo report feeling:
   a. A spinning or whirling sensation
   b. Lightheadedness
   c. Darkening vision
   d. Weakness in the muscles of the upper body

10. ______ Dementia is a normal process of aging. True (T) or false (F)?

11. ______ Delirium is:
    a. The same as dementia
    b. A minor problem with no significant consequences
    c. A final diagnosis
    d. A syndrome

12. ______ Older patients have a decrease in height averaging:
    a. 2 to 3 inches
    b. 4 to 5 inches
    c. 6 to 7 inches
    d. 8 to 9 inches

13. List one social and one physiologic reason why older adults have less tolerance for extremes of temperature.

    Social: ______________________________

    Physiologic: ______________________________

14. ______ Which of the following psychiatric disorders is most common in aging?
    a. Organic brain syndrome
    b. Schizophrenia
    c. Multiple personality disorder
    d. Bipolar disorder

15. ______ Older adults have a much higher risk of death and disability from trauma, especially multisystem trauma, than do younger individuals. True (T) or false (F)?

16. ______ Elderly patients commonly make suicidal gestures but are unlikely to successfully commit suicide. True (T) or false (F)?

17. List three changes in spinal immobilization techniques you should consider for elderly patients.

    a. ______________________________

    b. ______________________________

    c. ______________________________

18. ______ If an elderly patient with difficulty hearing cannot understand your speech, you should:
    a. Shout to be heard.
    b. Write notes.
    c. Speak to the patient's spouse instead of the patient.
    d. Not worry about assessing the patient's medical history.

19. ______ Which of the following statements on elder abuse is *true?*
    a. Most victims of elder abuse are of low socioeconomic status.
    b. Elder abuse becomes a problem when an older person loses his or her independence.
    c. Elder abuse usually manifests as violent abuse.
    d. Unlike child abuse, elder abuse carries no mandatory reporting.

20. List two ways an EMS provider can have an expanded role in caring for older adults.

    a. ______________________________

    b. ______________________________

# DIVISION FOUR

## Medical/Behavioral Emergencies, Obstetrics, and Gynecology



## DIVISION TEST

**Directions:** *Place the letter of the correct answer in the space provided.*

1. ______ Which of the following medications is carried on the EMS unit?
   a. Nitroglycerin
   b. Activated charcoal
   c. Epinephrine autoinjectors
   d. Inhalers

2. ______ What name of a medication is listed in the U.S. Pharmacopeia?
   a. Chemical name
   b. Generic name
   c. Trade name
   d. Brand name

3. ______ A(n) ________ is a situation in which a medication should not be used because it may cause harm to the patient or offer no effect in improving the patient's condition or illness.
   a. Indication
   b. Contraindication
   c. Complication
   d. Association

4. ______ What form of medication is activated charcoal?
   a. Tablet
   b. Gel
   c. Suspension
   d. Sublingual spray

5. ______ Oral medications:
   a. Are sprayed under the tongue
   b. Are useful for unresponsive patients
   c. Have a slow onset of action
   d. Should not be given to alert children

6. ______ Which of the following statements is *true?*
   a. Knowing the side effects of a drug will help the EMT–Basic anticipate the onset of these side effects.
   b. Side effects are the helpful effects of a drug.
   c. The mechanism of action of a drug describes how the drug is eliminated from the body.
   d. EMT–Basics can help a patient take any medication if the patient is in acute distress.

7. ______ The larynx is also known as the:
   a. Oropharynx
   b. Diaphragm
   c. Windpipe
   d. Voice box

8. ______ Which of the following statements is *true?*
   a. Stridor is the noise heard when liquid is in the back of the throat.
   b. Agonal respirations are normal in pediatric patients.
   c. A barrel chest may indicate long-term respiratory problems.
   d. Do not apply high-flow oxygen to a patient who normally receives low-concentration oxygen.

9. ______ Which of the following is a sign or symptom associated with adequate breathing?
   a. Shortness of breath for a 44-year-old patient
   b. Increased pulse rate for a 65-year-old patient
   c. Retractions in a 10-year-old patient
   d. Rate of 15 breaths per minute for an 18-year-old patient

10. ______ Medication names such as Proventil and Ventolin are examples of ______ names.
   a. Generic
   b. Trade
   c. Official
   d. Chemical

11. ______ Which of the following is an indication for assisting a patient with a prescribed inhaler?
   a. The patient is unresponsive and cannot use the device without assistance.
   b. Medical direction orders the EMT–Basics to administer an inhaler carried on the EMS unit.
   c. The patient has signs and symptoms of a respiratory emergency.
   d. The patient has not yet been diagnosed with a respiratory problem requiring an inhaler.

12. ______ Common side effects of prescribed inhalers include:
   a. Hypotension
   b. Cyanosis
   c. Increased pulse rate
   d. Memory disturbances

13. ______ The right ventricle pumps blood to the:
   a. Body  c. Right atrium
   b. Lungs  d. Aorta

14. ______ Signs and symptoms of shock (hypoperfusion) include:
   a. Slow, full pulse
   b. Bright red skin
   c. High temperature
   d. Rapid, shallow breathing

15. ______ How should a patient with a cardiac history and no suspicion of trauma be positioned for transport?
   a. Sitting
   b. Lying down
   c. 30 degrees upright
   d. In a position of comfort

16. ______ Which of the following is an indication or a condition that must be met before assisting a patient with administration of nitroglycerin?
   a. The patient has no chest pain now but had chest pain earlier today.
   b. The patient has his or her own physician-prescribed sublingual tablets.
   c. The patient has taken the maximum dose with no relief.
   d. The patient's blood pressure is 94/60 mm Hg.

17. ______ An AED can be used for which of the following patients?
   a. An 80-year-old, 100-pound woman with no pulse
   b. A 50-year-old, 220-pound man who complains of chest pain
   c. A 1-month-old child who is found unresponsive and pulseless
   d. A 90-year-old, 75-kg unresponsive man with a pulse

18. ______ How long should the EMT–Basic perform CPR after the AED delivers a shock?
   a. 30 seconds  c. 90 seconds
   b. 60 seconds  d. 120 seconds

19. ______ Signs and symptoms of a diabetic emergency include:
   a. Lack of appetite
   b. Intoxicated appearance
   c. Normal heart rate
   d. Hot, dry skin

20. ______ Which of the following medications in a patient's home would alert you that the patient has a history of diabetes?
    a. Ventolin
    b. Humulin
    c. Dilantin
    d. Procardia

21. ______ Which of the following is a common cause of seizures?
    a. Hypothermia
    b. Infections
    c. Near drowning
    d. Decreased levels of carbon dioxide

22. ______ Which of the following is an indication for the administration of oral glucose?
    a. Patient with a history of diabetes who is unresponsive
    b. Patient with signs and symptoms of hypoglycemia who is unable to swallow
    c. Patient with an altered mental status and a history of diabetes
    d. Patient with an altered mental status with no medical history

23. ______ What dose of glucose should be given to a patient who is unresponsive?
    a. One tube, placed between the patient's cheek and gum
    b. Two tubes, under the tongue
    c. One tube, under the tongue
    d. Oral glucose is not indicated

24. ______ Which of the following best defines an allergic reaction?
    a. Coughing with dry mucous membranes
    b. A rash on the extremities
    c. Swelling of the face and throat
    d. Exaggerated immune response to any substance

25. ______ When do you assess the SAMPLE history for a patient with an allergic reaction?
    a. During the initial assessment
    b. During the focused history and physical examination
    c. During the detailed physical examination
    d. During the ongoing assessment

26. ______ What dose of epinephrine is found in an adult epinephrine autoinjector?
    a. 0.15 mg
    b. 0.3 mg
    c. 5.0 mg
    d. 10.0 mg

27. ______ Where is the tip of the autoinjector placed on the patient?
    a. Lateral arm
    b. Lower leg
    c. Lateral thigh
    d. Forearm

28. ______ What should be done with the auto-injector after use?
    a. Retract the needle into the injector.
    b. Keep with the patient until you reach the hospital.
    c. Place in sharps container.
    d. Dispose of the needle separate from the injector.

29. ______ Which of the following is a side effect of epinephrine?
    a. Increased heart rate
    b. Red, itchy skin
    c. Warm, dry skin
    d. Difficulty breathing

30. ______ Which of the following should be determined while caring for a poisoning or overdose patient?
    a. If the poisoning was intentional or accidental
    b. If the parents were negligent, if the patient is a child
    c. How much substance was ingested
    d. Whose medication was taken

31. ______ If the patient exhibits signs and symptoms that include diarrhea, abdominal pain, chemical burns around the mouth, and unusual breath odors, which route of poisoning would you suspect?
    a. Inhaled
    b. Ingested
    c. Injected
    d. Absorbed

32. ______ Which of the following routes for poisoning is an indication for activated charcoal?
a. Inhaled
b. Injected
c. Absorbed
d. Ingested

33. ______ What is the dose of activated charcoal for children?
a. 0.5 g/kg
b. 1 g/kg
c. 2 g/kg
d. 5 g/kg

34. ______ Which of the following is a common side effect of activated charcoal?
a. Elevated heart rate
b. Vomiting
c. Cyanosis around the mouth
d. Unresponsiveness

35. ______ Which of the following is a method of heat loss?
a. Shivering
b. Condensation
c. Conduction
d. Conversion

36. ______ Where should the EMT–Basic feel the patient's skin to determine signs and symptoms of generalized hypothermia?
a. Forehead
b. Upper arm
c. Abdomen
d. Lower leg

37. ______ What are the early signs and symptoms associated with generalized hypothermia?
a. Rapid pulse, rapid breathing, and red skin
b. Slow pulse, rapid breathing, and pale skin
c. Rapid pulse, slow breathing, and cyanotic skin
d. Slow pulse, slow breathing, and red skin

38. ______ Which of the following is the most serious sign or symptom of generalized hyperthermia?
a. Muscular cramps
b. Rapid heart rate
c. Hot, dry skin
d. Abdominal cramps

39. ______ Which of the following statements is *true?*
a. The term "drowning" indicates that a patient has lived after an immersion incident.
b. The incidence of spinal injuries is high in water-related emergencies.
c. Gastric distention should be relieved as soon as possible for near-drowning patients.
d. Immersion in warm water will make resuscitation more likely.

40. ______ How should you care for an extremity that has a stinger in place from an insect?
a. Leave it in.
b. Use tweezers to remove it.
c. Use the edge of a card to remove it.
d. Rub it off with your finger.

41. ______ Patients considered to be at risk for suicide include:
a. Patients who are 30 years of age and single
b. Adolescents
c. Patients who have had a serious illness for many years
d. Patients who have lost their job

42. ______ Which of the following is a method for calming a patient with a behavioral emergency?
a. Tell the patient what you are doing.
b. Move close to the patient quickly to gain the patient's trust.
c. Do not answer questions that may upset the patient.
d. Separate the patient from family members or friends.

43. ______ Which of the following statements is *true?*
a. Do not assess behavioral emergency patients for injury or illness.
b. Do not question the patient about medical history because this may upset the patient.
c. Do not use metal handcuffs as restraints.
d. Do not use same-gender attendants for behavioral emergency patients.

44. ______ How much force should be used to restrain a patient?
   a. Minimal force
   b. Maximal force
   c. Reasonable force
   d. Force should not be used

45. ______ What is the name of the organ in which the fetus grows and matures?
   a. Amniotic sac
   b. Uterus
   c. Birth canal
   d. Perineum

46. ______ Which of the following statements is *true?*
   a. The first stage of labor begins with regular contractions of the uterus.
   b. The second stage of labor ends when the baby enters the birth canal.
   c. The third stage of labor begins with the delivery of the placenta.
   d. The second stage of labor ends when the cervix is fully dilated.

47. ______ Which of the following is usually found in an obstetrical kit?
   a. Infant BVM
   b. Bulb syringe
   c. Magill forceps
   d. Broselow tape

48. ______ Which of the following is a consideration for normal delivery?
   a. Prepare the patient for transport if the contractions are less than 2 minutes apart.
   b. Do not let the mother go to the bathroom.
   c. Do not let the mother push until you arrive at the hospital.
   d. If crowning is present, prepare for transport immediately.

49. ______ How far from the infant should the cord be cut after delivery?
   a. Two finger widths
   b. Four finger widths
   c. Equal distances between mother and infant
   d. Very close to the mother

50. ______ If the mother loses 750 ml of blood during the delivery and she is still bleeding, how should the EMT–Basic manage this patient?
   a. No special management is required; losing up to 1000 ml of blood during childbirth is normal.
   b. Place gauze into the vaginal opening, and replace the gauze when it becomes soaked with blood.
   c. Massage the uterus in a kneading motion.
   d. Massage the perineum until the bleeding stops.

51. ______ What is the name of the condition when the cord presents through the birth canal before delivery of the head?
   a. Breech cord
   b. Prolapsed cord
   c. Presenting cord
   d. Meconium birth

52. ______ The leading cause of death in the geriatric population is:
   a. Cardiovascular disease
   b. Diabetes
   c. Cancer
   d. Chronic obstructive pulmonary disease

53. ______ Nitroglycerin is effective in relieving pain from:
   a. COPD
   b. Respiratory infections
   c. Angina
   d. Cancer

54. ______ An ischemic stroke means that brain damage results from:
   a. Narrowing blood vessels in the brain
   b. Burst blood vessels in the brain
   c. Decreased pumping action of the heart
   d. Decreased blood pressure

55. ______ Dementia is diagnosed by:
   a. A blood test
   b. CT scan
   c. PET scan
   d. Excluding other diseases

## CHAPTER 27

# Bleeding and Shock

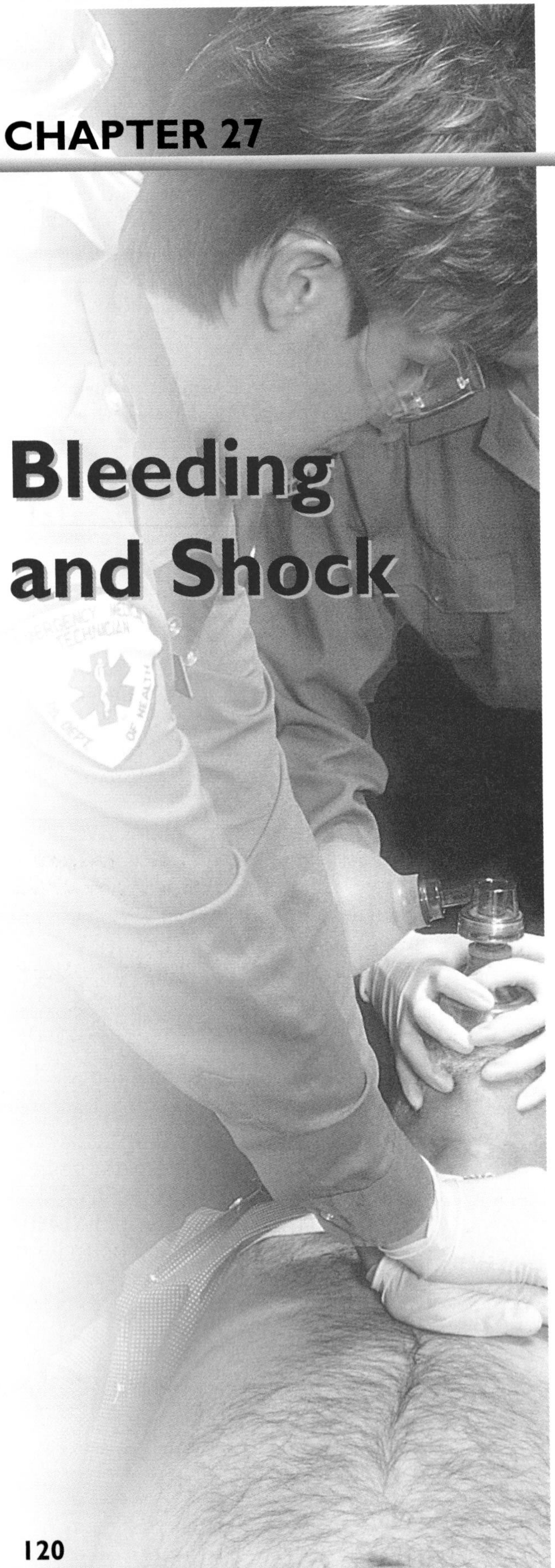

### CHAPTER OUTLINE

I. Review of the Cardiovascular System
II. Shock
  A. Assessing Shock
  B. Emergency Care for Shock
III. External Bleeding
  A. Body Substance Isolation Precautions
  B. Assessing Blood Loss
  C. Types of Bleeding
    1. Arterial bleeding
    2. Venous bleeding
    3. Capillary bleeding
  D. Emergency Care for External Bleeding
    1. Concentrated direct pressure
    2. Diffuse direct pressure
    3. Extremity elevation
    4. Pressure points
    5. Splints
    6. Tourniquets
  E. Bleeding from the Ears, Nose, and Mouth
IV. Internal Bleeding
  A. Assessing Blood Loss
  B. Signs and Symptoms of Internal Bleeding
  C. Emergency Care for Internal Bleeding

## MATCHING

*Match the terms in Column 1 with the correct definition in Column 2.*

**Column 1**

1. ______ Capillary refill
2. ______ Circumferential pressure
3. ______ Epistaxis
4. ______ Hemorrhagic shock
5. ______ Hypoperfusion
6. ______ Hypovolemic shock
7. ______ Perfusion
8. ______ Pressure point
9. ______ Shock

**Column 2**

a. Measure of the perfusion of the skin in a child under 6 years of age
b. Hypoperfusion
c. State that results when cells are not receiving adequate blood flow
d. Hypoperfusion that results from an inadequate volume of blood
e. Bleeding from the nose
f. Place in an extremity where a major artery lies close to a bone
g. Pressure around an extremity
h. Hypoperfusion that results from bleeding
i. Process of delivering oxygen and nutrients to, and removing metabolic waste products from, the body's cells

## REVIEW QUESTIONS

1. The cardiovascular system delivers ____________ through a system of ___________________________, ___________________________, and capillaries.

2. ______ The average adult has approximately _____ L of blood in the body.
   a. 2
   b. 3
   c. 6
   d. 10

3. ______ The body delivers an equal amount of blood to all parts of the body. True (T) or false (F)?

4. ______ The ______ pressure is measured during contraction of the heart; the ____ pressure is measured during the heart's resting phase.
   a. Systolic, diastolic
   b. Diastolic, systolic
   c. Systolic, resting
   d. Beating, diastolic

5. Good perfusion of the body requires an adequate ___________________________________.

6. A decrease in perfusion to the cells in the body results in hypoperfusion or ________________.

7. When tissues are not adequately perfused, they are damaged by lack of __________________ and a buildup of _________________________.

8. The four major organs easily damaged by hypoperfusion are:
   a. ______________________________
   b. ______________________________
   c. ______________________________
   d. ______________________________

9. List three causes of hypovolemic shock.

   a. ______________________________

   b. ______________________________

   c. ______________________________

10. ______ Early, subtle signs of shock are anxiety and:
    a. Anger
    b. Restlessness
    c. Sleepiness
    d. Responsiveness only to pain

11. ______ Vasoconstriction causes blood vessels in the extremities to dilate, producing warm skin. True (T) or false (F)?

12. ______ Reduced blood flow to arms and legs results in weaker peripheral pulses compared with central pulses. True (T) or false (F)?

13. ______ When assessing the capillary refill of a child, the color will return in less than ________ for a patient with adequate perfusion.
    a. 2 seconds
    b. 3 seconds
    c. 4 seconds
    d. 5 seconds

14. ______ Another early sign of shock is an increased:
    a. Blood pressure
    b. Temperature
    c. Heart rate
    d. Mental status

15. A late sign of shock is a ____________________ blood pressure.

16. The first priority with any patient is to ensure an ______________________________.

17. The legs can be elevated only if the patient has no serious injuries to the: *(Mark all that apply with a checkmark.)*

    a. ______ Spine

    b. ______ Upper extremities

    c. ______ Pelvis

    d. ______ Lower extremities

    e. ______ Head

    f. ______ Chest

    g. ______ Abdomen

18. ______ Body substance isolation precautions are important when caring for a patient with external injuries. True (T) or false (F)?

19. For an adult, a sudden loss of ____________ L of blood is serious.

20. ______ When bleeding is from an artery the blood will:
    a. Drip
    b. Ooze
    c. Spurt
    d. Flow

21. ______ Venous bleeding will usually:
    a. Drip
    b. Ooze
    c. Spurt
    d. Flow

22. Bleeding that involves the capillaries will usually ______________________________.

23. ______ The most effective method of controlling bleeding from one main artery or major vein is with:
    a. Diffuse direct pressure
    b. Concentrated direct pressure
    c. Pressure points
    d. Extremity elevation

24. List three ways bleeding from multiple sites on an extremity can be controlled.

    a. ______________________________

    b. ______________________________

    c. ______________________________

25. If pain, swelling, or deformity is absent, ____________________ can decrease blood flow to an injury.

26. ______ Which type of bleeding control will slow bleeding but rarely stop it completely?
    a. Diffuse direct pressure
    b. Concentrated direct pressure
    c. Pressure points
    d. Extremity elevation

27. ______ Splinting an extremity injury stabilizes bone ends and reduces potential for further damage to blood vessels and nerves. True (T) or false (F)?

28. ______ An injury to the chest is a contraindication for use of the pneumatic antishock garment (PASG). True (T) or false (F)?

29. The last resort for bleeding control is a ______________________________.

30. ______ Which of the following is a principle of tourniquet use?
    a. It must apply enough continuous circumferential pressure to stop the bleeding.
    b. It should be removed once the bleeding has been stopped for 10 minutes.
    c. It should be used as a primary measure for control of serious bleeding.
    d. Use a thin wire or string.

31. If a tourniquet is used, always avoid placing it over a ______________________________.

32. Bleeding from the ears and nose can be a sign of a ____________________ in a trauma patient.

33. ______ Direct pressure should be applied to bleeding from the nose and ears. True (T) or false (F)?

34. If a patient has signs and symptoms of shock (hypoperfusion) and a serious mechanism of injury, with no obvious bleeding, you should suspect ______________________________.

35. List six signs and symptoms of internal bleeding.

    a. ______________________________

    b. ______________________________

    c. ______________________________

    d. ______________________________

    e. ______________________________

    f. ______________________________

36. If you suspect a patient is bleeding internally from an injured femur, how would you treat this patient?

    ______________________________

    ______________________________

37. When should the PASG be applied?

    ______________________________

    ______________________________

38. You and your crew have been dispatched to an automobile-pedestrian collision. On arrival, you find an elderly man lying in the roadway at a busy intersection. Police are directing traffic, and the scene is safe. According to witnesses, a vehicle traveling 10 to 20 miles per hour struck the patient head-on. Profuse bleeding occurs from the patient's lower extremities and an obvious open injury to his left thigh with visible bone ends protruding. Because of the patient's age, his apparent blood loss, and the mechanism of injury, you suspect the patient may soon have hypoperfusion.

    a. Airway control and spinal immobilization are your first priorities in caring for this patient. What role does providing oxygen play in managing shock?

    ______________________________________

    ______________________________________

    b. You attempt to control bleeding by applying diffuse direct pressure to the patient's wounds. The bleeding, however, continues. What will be your next step in providing hemorrhage control?

    ______________________________________

    ______________________________________

    c. The patient obviously needs rapid transport for definitive care. Medical direction advises you to apply and inflate the PASG. How will the PASG benefit this patient?

    ______________________________________

    ______________________________________

39. You are caring for an elderly patient who has had bloody stools for the last 12 hours. She is pale, diaphoretic, and extremely weak. She describes the bloody stools as "bright-red diarrhea." She has no significant medical history and denies any pain. Her vital signs are blood pressure 106/70 mm Hg, pulse 120 beats per minute, and respirations 22 breaths per minute and shallow.

    a. Based on the patient's description of her bleeding, where do you suspect to be the source of her bleeding?

    ______________________________________

    ______________________________________

    b. What is the significance of the patient's vital signs?

    ______________________________________

    ______________________________________

    c. How would you manage this patient?

    ______________________________________

    ______________________________________

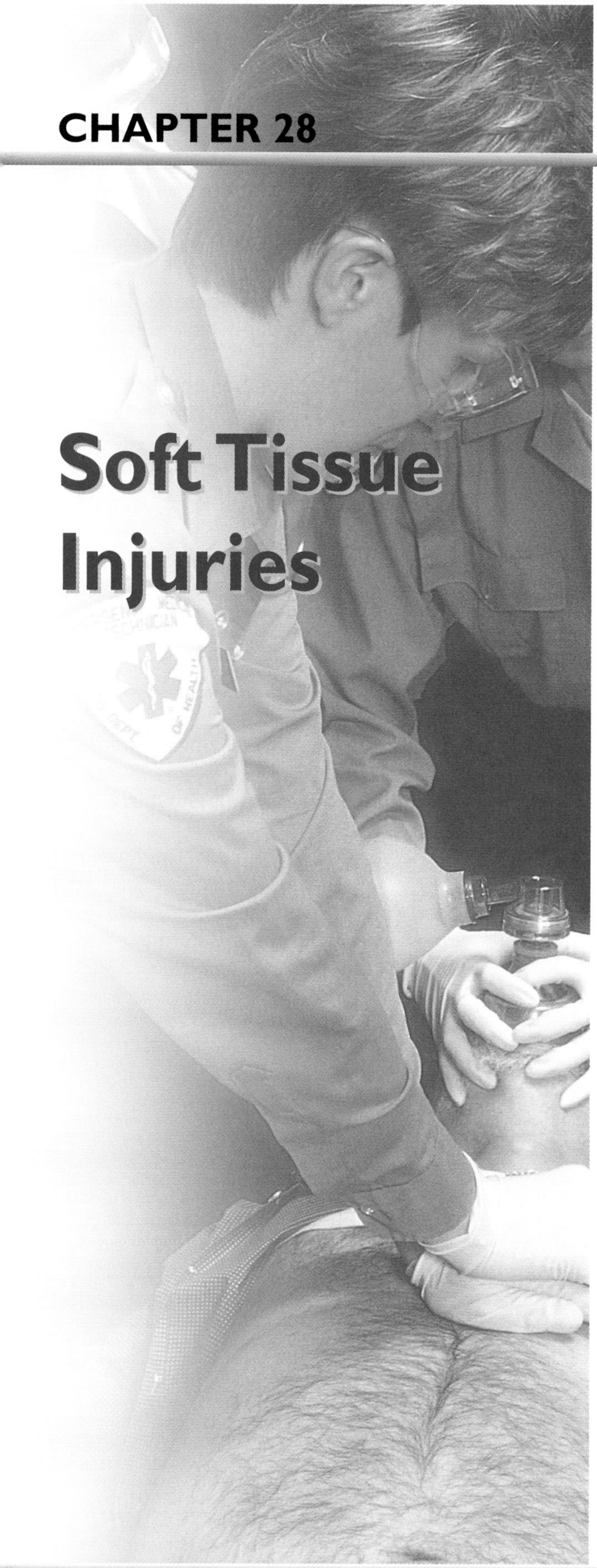

## CHAPTER 28

# Soft Tissue Injuries

### CHAPTER OUTLINE

I. The Skin
  A. Function
  B. Layers
II. Injuries
  A. Closed Injuries
    1. Contusion
    2. Hematoma
    3. Closed crush injury
  B. Open Injuries
    1. Abrasion
    2. Laceration
    3. Avulsion
    4. Penetration or puncture
    5. Amputation
    6. Open crush injury
  C. Emergency Medical Care for Patients With Soft Tissue Injuries
    1. Dressings and bandages
    2. Injuries requiring special consideration
III. Burns
  A. Classification of Burns
  B. Severity of Burns
    1. Critical burns
    2. Moderate burns
    3. Minor burns
  C. Emergency Medical Care for Burn Victims
  D. Special Considerations in Burn Care
    1. Chemical burns
    2. Electrical burns
    3. Burns involving the airway

## MATCHING 1

*Match the terms in Column 1 with the correct definition in Column 2.*

**Column 1**

1. ______ Abrasion
2. ______ Amputation
3. ______ Avulsion
4. ______ Contusion
5. ______ Crush injury
6. ______ Hematoma
7. ______ Laceration
8. ______ Penetration or puncture

**Column 2**

a. Open soft tissue injury resulting from a scraping force
b. Open or closed soft tissue injury resulting from blunt force trauma
c. Flap of skin that is torn or pulled loose
d. Break in the skin of varying depth caused by a sharp object; a cut
e. Removal of an appendage from the body
f. Open soft tissue injury caused by an object being pushed into skin
g. Type of closed soft tissue injury; a bruise
h. Closed soft tissue injury with a collection of blood under the skin

## MATCHING 2

*Match the terms in Column 1 with the correct definition in Column 2.*

**Column 1**

9. ______ Bandage
10. ______ Dressing
11. ______ Evisceration
12. ______ Full-thickness burn
13. ______ Occlusive
14. ______ Partial-thickness burn
15. ______ Superficial burn

**Column 2**

a. Sterile material used to control bleeding and protect soft tissue injury
b. Open wound in the abdomen through which organs are protruding
c. Material used to secure a wound covering in place
d. Burn that affects only the epidermis
e. Burn that affects all layers of the skin
f. Burn that affects the epidermis and dermis
g. Referring to protection from the air

## REVIEW QUESTIONS

1. List three functions of the skin.

   a. ____________________

   b. ____________________

   c. ____________________

2. ______ Nerve endings can be found in which layer of the skin?
   a. Epidermis
   b. Dermis
   c. Subcutaneous
   d. Muscular

3. Define a closed injury.

   ____________________

   ____________________

4. ______ A discoloration to the skin with minimal pain and swelling is called a(n):
   a. Contusion
   b. Hematoma
   c. Crush injury
   d. Abrasion

5. ______ A large collection of blood under the skin is called a(n):
   a. Contusion
   b. Hematoma
   c. Crush injury
   d. Abrasion

6. Define an open injury.

______________________________________

______________________________________

7. ______ The scraping wound caused by falling on asphalt is a(n):
   a. Penetration or puncture
   b. Abrasion
   c. Crush injury
   d. Amputation

8. ______ The type of wound commonly called a "cut" is a(n):
   a. Avulsion
   b. Abrasion
   c. Laceration
   d. Amputation

9. ______ A gunshot wound is an example of a(n):
   a. Penetration or puncture
   b. Abrasion
   c. Crush injury
   d. Amputation

10. ______ The loss of a finger is called a(n):
   a. Penetration or puncture
   b. Abrasion
   c. Laceration
   d. Amputation

11. ______ Body substance isolation precautions are a necessary part of preparing to care for a soft tissue injury. True (T) or false (F)?

12. ______ An appropriately sized dressing should just barely cover the wound. True (T) or false (F)?

13. List three ways to apply a pressure dressing.

   a. ______________________________________

   b. ______________________________________

   c. ______________________________________

14. An occlusive dressing, taped on ____________ sides, allows air to ____________________ but not ____________________ the wound.

15. ______ Protect eviscerated organs with a dry, sterile dressing. True (T) or false (F)?

16. List two of the conditions under which an impaled object should be removed.

   a. ______________________________________

   b. ______________________________________

17. ______ For an impaled object in the eye, the uninjured eye is also covered to:
   a. Keep the patient quiet
   b. Reduce movement of both eyes
   c. Keep the patient from seeing the injury
   d. Reduce sensory stimulus

18. ______ Amputated parts should be placed in cold water for transport. True (T) or false (F)?

19. When caring for a patient with an evisceration, chest injury, or burn, the priority for care is always to maintain the patient's ____________________.

20. ______ Partial amputations should be ______ and ______.
   a. Splinted, completed
   b. Immobilized, bandaged
   c. Completed, bandaged
   d. Cooled, splinted

21. Direct pressure can be used on the head only if no evidence of a ______________________ exists.

22. ______ Injuries to the mouth should be evaluated for ______ and ______.
    a. Bleeding, foreign objects
    b. Loose teeth, bleeding
    c. Dentures, impaled objects
    d. Foreign objects, airway obstruction

23. List five criteria used to determine the severity of a burn.
    a. ______________________________
    b. ______________________________
    c. ______________________________
    d. ______________________________
    e. ______________________________

24. A sunburn is a type of ________________ burn.

25. Dry, leathery, charred skin with little or no pain describes a __________________________ burn.

26. If blisters form, the burn is considered to be a ______________________________________ burn.

27. In the "rule of nines," the head of an adult is __________% of the body surface area and the head of an infant is ______________________%.

28. ______ A circumferential burn of the torso wraps all the way around and can cause respiratory difficulty. True (T) or false (F)?

29. List five areas of the body that are considered critical if burned.
    a. ______________________________
    b. ______________________________
    c. ______________________________
    d. ______________________________
    e. ______________________________

30. Determine the severity of each burn described below *(c = critical; mod = moderate; min = minor).*

    ______ A partial-thickness burn of the face

    ______ A child with a partial-thickness burn of less than 10%

    ______ A full-thickness burn of less than 2%

    ______ A partial-thickness burn covering 27% of the body

31. Because of skin loss with a burn, patients must be protected from ____________________________.

32. ______ Jewelry and clothing should be removed when treating a burn patient. True (T) or false (F)?

33. If a patient has suffered a chemical burn from dry powder, first ____________________ the powder, then ___________________________ with water.

34. When treating a patient with _________________ burns, be prepared with the automated external defibrillator (AED) because cardiac arrest is a possibility.

35. You are caring for a worker who has fallen from a mowing tractor. As he fell, his right foot was caught in the machine, producing a large open wound to his foot and ankle. The bones of his ankle and lower extremity are exposed, and the wound is full of grass and debris. He is in extreme pain and says that he cannot feel or move his toes. You begin to remove his shoe when you realize that his foot is nearly amputated.

   a. Describe general principles of emergency care for patients with soft-tissue injury.

   ______________________________________

   ______________________________________

   b. You attempt to control his bleeding with direct pressure, but the dressing continues to become saturated with blood. What should you do?

   ______________________________________

   ______________________________________

   c. The patient is starting to look a little "shocky." What should you do?

   ______________________________________

   ______________________________________

36. You are caring for a firefighter who was trapped in a burning building. She has partial- and full-thickness burns over her anterior chest and abdomen, right arm, and leg.

   a. Define partial-thickness and full-thickness burns.

   ______________________________________

   ______________________________________

   b. Using the "rule of nines," what percentage of body area is burned?

   ______________________________________

   ______________________________________

   c. Describe emergency care for burn patients.

   ______________________________________

   ______________________________________

CHAPTER 29

# Musculoskeletal Care

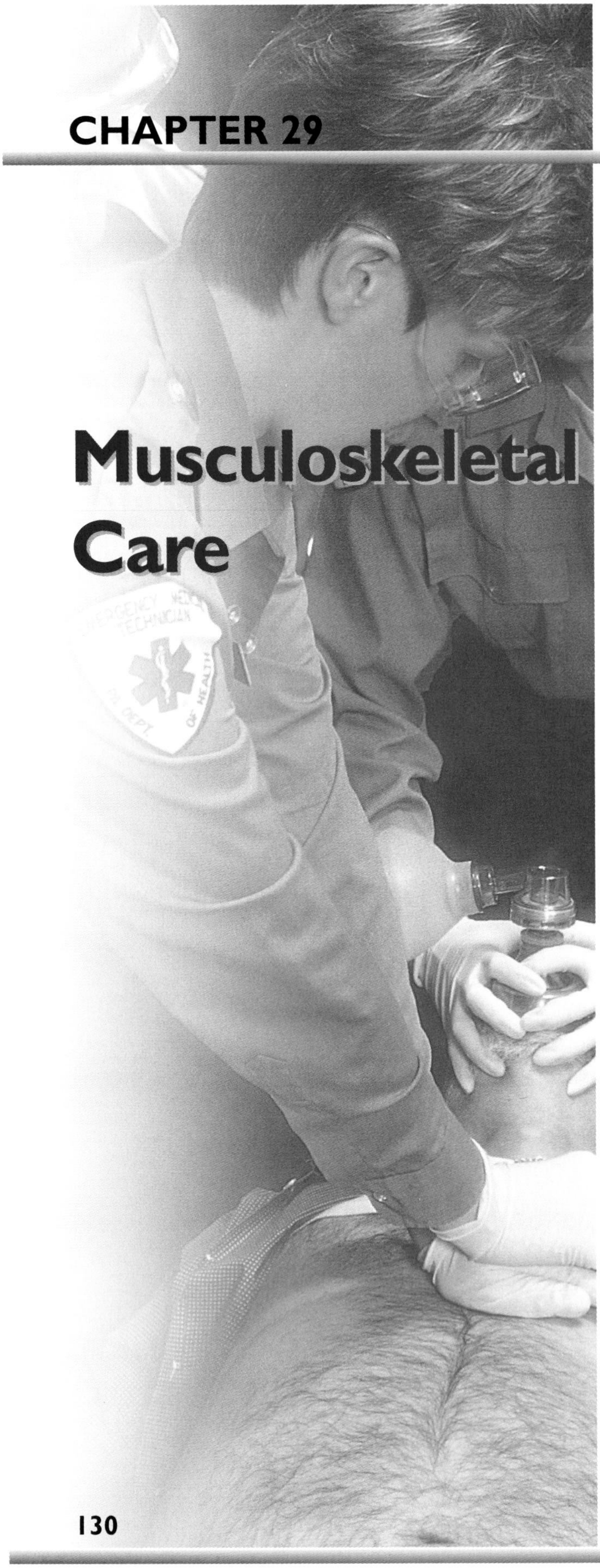

## CHAPTER OUTLINE

## MATCHING 1

*Match the terms in Column 1 with the correct definition in Column 2.*

**Column 1**

1. ______ Angulation
2. ______ Crepitation
3. ______ Pneumatic splints
4. ______ Position of function
5. ______ Rigid splints
6. ______ Sling and swathe
7. ______ Traction splints

**Column 2**

a. Type of splint that does not conform to the body
b. Sound made when bone ends rub together or when air is inside the tissue
c. Bandaging used to immobilize an injured shoulder or arm
d. Special device used to immobilize a closed midfemur injury
e. Injury that is deformed (bent) at the site
f. Devices such as air or vacuum splints that conform to the injury
g. Relaxed position of the hand or foot in which minimal movement or stretching of muscle occurs

## MATCHING 2

*Match the terms in Column 1 with the correct definition in Column 2.*

**Column 1**

8. ______ Closed injury
9. ______ Direct injury
10. ______ Indirect injury
11. ______ Mechanism of injury
12. ______ Open injury
13. ______ Twisting injury

**Column 2**

a. Injury that results from a force that comes in contact with an area of the body
b. Injury in one body area that results from a force that comes in contact with a different part of the body
c. Injury that breaks the continuity of the skin
d. Force that acts on the body to produce an injury
e. Injury that does not break the continuity of the skin
f. Injury that results from a turning motion of the body in opposite directions

## MATCHING 3

*Match the mechanism of injury in Column 1 with the correct example in Column 2.*

**Column 1**

14. ______ Direct injury
15. ______ Twisting injury
16. ______ Indirect injury

**Column 2**

a. Fist to the jaw
b. Internal organs against the chest in an automobile crash
c. Running back tackled after turning from a catch

## LABELING

1. Label the figure below with the following terms:

| | | |
|---|---|---|
| Clavicle | Ribs | Femur |
| Tibia | Humerus | Ulna |
| Thorax | Vertebral column | Patella |
| Fibula | Radius | |

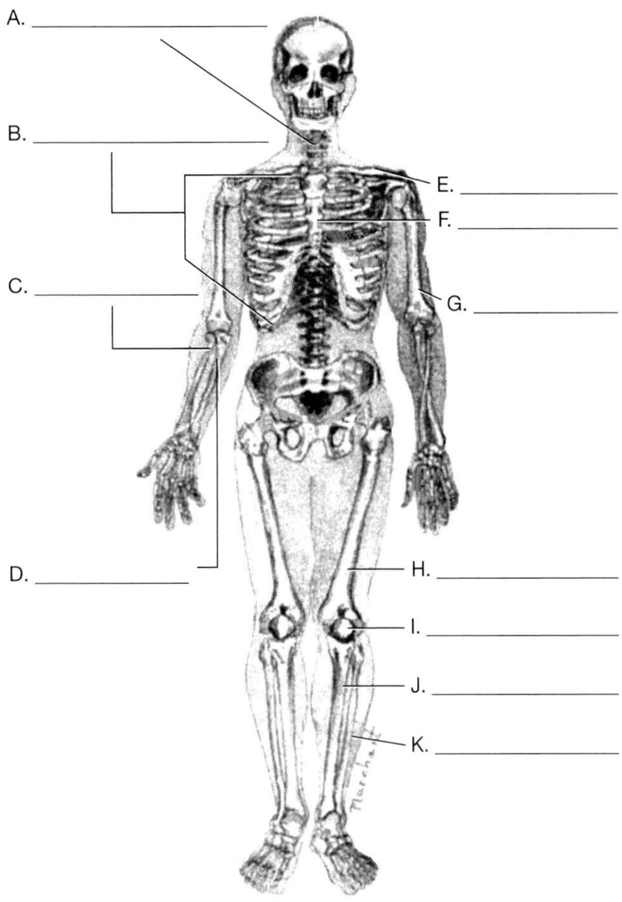


2. Label the figure below with the following terms:

| | |
|---|---|
| Cervical vertebrae | Fused coccyx |
| Sacral vertebrae | Lumbar vertebrae |
| Thoracic vertebrae | |

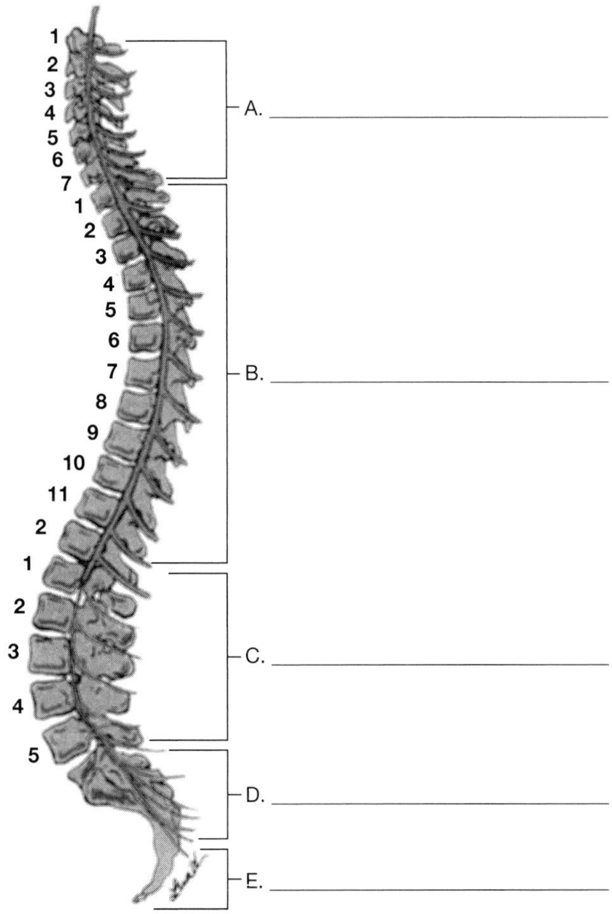

## REVIEW QUESTIONS

1. List three functions of muscles.

   a. ______________________

   b. ______________________

   c. ______________________

2. Skeletal muscles are attached to ______________ and are responsible for ______________________.

3. Muscles that we have no direct control over are called ______________________, or ______________________ muscles.

4. Automaticity is a characteristic only found in ______________________ muscle.

5. List three functions of the skeletal system.

   a. ______________________

   b. ______________________

   c. ______________________

6. The knee is an example of a ______________ joint, and the hip is a ______________ joint.

7. Why do we determine the mechanism of injury?

   ______________________

   ______________________

8. List four signs and symptoms of a musculoskeletal injury.

   a. ______________________

   b. ______________________

   c. ______________________

   d. ______________________

9. _____ Splinting painful, swollen extremities should always begin after an evaluation of airway and breathing. True (T) or false (F)?

10. Splinting ______________________ movement of bone fragments and ______________________ damage to muscles and nerves.

11. Pulse, motor function, and sensation must be evaluated ______________________ and ______________________ splinting.

12. If the distal pulse changes after splinting, ______________________ the splint and reassess.

13. _____ The position of function for the hand is with the fingers extended. True (T) or false (F)?

14. To be effective, a splint must immobilize the joint ______________ and ______________ a long bone injury.

15. Full-body immobilization should be used if ______________________ trauma is suspected.

16. _____ A traction splint can be used if the injury:
    a. Is at or near a joint
    b. Is closed and near midfemur
    c. Involves the lower leg
    d. Is open with exposed bone ends

17. Pneumatic splints are flexible and good for immobilization of ______________ injuries.

18. List at least two advantages of a pneumatic splint.

    a. ______________________

    b. ______________________

19. ______ The pneumatic antishock garment (PASG) can be used as an immobilization device. True (T) or false (F)?

20. Shoulder injuries usually require a

    ______________________________ for stabilization.

21. List three risks of splints that are too tight, too loose, or improperly applied.

    a. ______________________________

    b. ______________________________

    c. ______________________________

22. You have been dispatched to the local skating rink where a 12-year-old boy has fallen and injured his arm. He tells you that he lost his balance and tried to "catch himself" as he fell backward. His right arm is angulated and swollen and deformed at the wrist. No other injuries are apparent. He denies hitting his head or losing responsiveness.

    a. What are signs and symptoms of a bone or joint injury?

    ______________________________

    ______________________________

    b. What type of assessment is required for this injury?

    ______________________________

    ______________________________

    c. Describe how you would splint this injury.

    ______________________________

    ______________________________

## CHAPTER 30

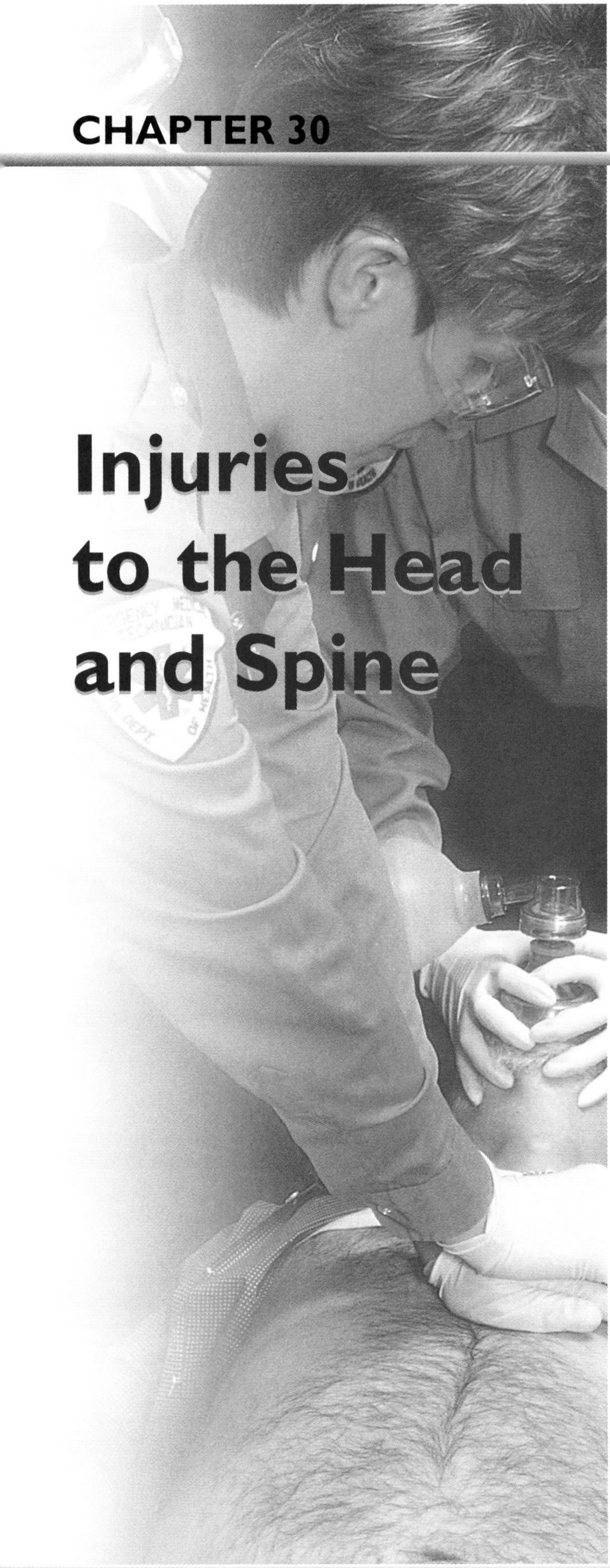

# Injuries to the Head and Spine

### CHAPTER OUTLINE

- I. Review of the Nervous and Skeletal Systems
  - A. The Nervous System
  - B. The Skeletal System
- II. Devices for Immobilization
  - A. Cervical Spine
  - B. Short Backboards
  - C. Long Backboards (Full-Body Spinal Immobilization Devices)
- III. Injuries to the Spine
  - A. Mechanism of Injury
  - B. Assessment
    - 1. Signs and symptoms
    - 2. Responsive patients
    - 3. Unresponsive patients
  - C. Complications
  - D. Emergency Medical Care of the Spine-Injured Patient
- IV. Injuries to the Brain and Skull
  - A. Head and Skull Injuries
  - B. Emergency Medical Care of the Head-Injured Patient
- V. Special Considerations
  - A. Rapid Extrication
  - B. Helmet Removal
  - C. Infants and Children
  - D. Geriatric Patients

## MATCHING 1

*Match the following terms in Column 1 with the correct definition in Column 2.*

**Column 1**

1. ______ Cervical spine immobilization device
2. ______ Kendrick extrication device (KED)
3. ______ Long backboard
4. ______ Log roll
5. ______ Rapid extrication
6. ______ Short backboard

**Column 2**

a. A full-body spinal immobilization device
b. Method used to move a lying patient onto a long board
c. Technique used to rapidly move a patient from a scene
d. Device used to maintain immobilization of the head, neck, and torso
e. Device used to maintain immobilization of the head and neck
f. Type of short board used to immobilize a seated patient

## MATCHING 2

*Match the type of incident in Column 1 with the mechanism of injury in Column 2.*

**Column 1**

7. ______ Hanging
8. ______ Shallow water diving
9. ______ Rear-end automobile crash

**Column 2**

a. Compression
b. Distraction
c. Excessive flexion, extension

## REVIEW QUESTIONS

1. The components of the central nervous system are the ______________________________ and the ______________________________.
2. Cerebrospinal fluid surrounds the ____________ and spinal cord and acts as a ________________.
3. Sensory nerves carry information ______________________ (to/from) the body ______________________ (to/from) the brain.
4. The spinal column contains ________________ bones.
5. Indicate the number of bones in each section of the vertebral column.

   ______ Cervical
   ______ Coccygeal
   ______ Sacral
   ______ Lumbar
   ______ Thoracic

6. ______ Cervical spine immobilization devices provide adequate immobilization for the head, and the patient requires no manual stabilization. True (T) or false (F)?
7. A short backboard is used to immobilize the head, neck, and torso when the patient is in a ______________________ position.

8. Long backboards provide ____________________ body immobilization.

9. ______ Adequate immobilization of the spine requires only a cervical spine immobilization device and long backboard. True (T) or false (F)?

10. Define mechanism of injury.

________________________________________

________________________________________

11. ______ The mechanism of injury helps you understand:
    a. If the patient truly could be hurt
    b. If a significant force was applied to the body
    c. If you should be concerned about the patient
    d. If the patient needs to be assessed

12. List four significant mechanisms of injury.
    a. ________________________________________
    b. ________________________________________
    c. ________________________________________
    d. ________________________________________

13. Describe the forces that are involved in a "whiplash" injury.

________________________________________

________________________________________

14. ______ Never ask a patient to move an injured body part to determine if he or she has pain in a particular area. True (T) or false (F)?

15. Injuries to the shoulder and chest may indicate the possibility of an injury to the ________________________________________.

16. Numbness, tingling, or weakness are possible signs and symptoms of a ____________________.

17. List five important questions to ask during an assessment of a responsive trauma patient.
    a. ________________________________________
    b. ________________________________________
    c. ________________________________________
    d. ________________________________________
    e. ________________________________________

18. Define each of the letters in the acronym DCAP-BTLS.

D ________________________________________

C ________________________________________

A ________________________________________

P ________________________________________

B ________________________________________

T ________________________________________

L ________________________________________

S ________________________________________

19. What items should you reassess after every intervention?

________________________________________

________________________________________

20. ______ You must document all findings and any changes in patient status during care and treatment. True (T) or false (F)?

21. Completing the assessment of the cervical region

    ________________ *(before/after)*

    application of the cervical spine immobilization device is helpful.

22. Why is monitoring the respirations of a potentially spine-injured patient especially important?

    ________________

    ________________

23. ______ Which of the following statements about cervical spine immobilization devices is *true?*
    a. They should be used for patients who may have sustained head, neck, or back injuries.
    b. Most do not need to be sized.
    c. The patient's head must be straightened to measure for it, even if this action causes pain.
    d. Manual spinal stabilization can be released once it is in place.

24. ______ Which of the following statements about log rolls and spinal immobilization is *true?*
    a. The EMT–Basic controlling the patient's shoulders is responsible for calling out when to move the patient.
    b. If the patient is not on the center of the long backboard after log-rolling, move the patient by pushing on the shoulder and hip until the patient is centered.
    c. The patient's head should be immobilized to the board after the shoulders and hips.
    d. The patient's legs should be immobilized to the board before immobilizing the shoulders.

25. Number the steps in the immobilization of a patient with a short backboard in order, with 1 as the first step and 7 as the last.

    ______ Secure the torso to the board.

    ______ Place the spine board behind the patient.

    ______ Reassess pulse, motor function, and sensation.

    ______ Secure the arms, legs, and feet.

    ______ Pad the voids behind the patient's head.

    ______ Attach the straps to the board.

    ______ Secure the head to the board.

26. List two types of immobilization devices that can be used for a seated patient.

    a. ________________

    b. ________________

27. After extricating a patient with a short spine board, what is the next step before transport?

    ________________

    ________________

28. Spinal injuries also may involve injuries to the

    ________________ and

    ________________.

29. ______ Scalp wounds bleed little because few blood vessels are located in the scalp. True (T) or false (F)?

30. The best indicator of a traumatic head injury is

    ________________.

31. List five signs and symptoms of a traumatic head injury.

    a. ______________________________

    b. ______________________________

    c. ______________________________

    d. ______________________________

    e. ______________________________

32. List three situations when rapid extrication should be used.

    a. ______________________________

    b. ______________________________

    c. ______________________________

33. ______ In which of the following situations should a helmet be left in place?
    a. When the patient complains of neck pain
    b. Any time the patient is unresponsive
    c. When removal would cause further injury
    d. When the helmet fits loosely and is comfortable for the patient

34. ______ Which of the following statements is true regarding helmets and helmet removal?
    a. Sports helmets are typically open in the front, making the airway easy to access.
    b. Full face shield helmets typically should be left in place.
    c. If the helmet is left in place, a commercial cervical spine immobilization device will provide good immobilization of the helmet to the long backboard.
    d. Shoulder pads should be left in place when a football helmet is removed.

35. ______ How is the head immobilized while the helmet is being removed?
    a. With one hand on the forehead and one under the jaw
    b. With both hands under the neck
    c. With one hand on the mandible and the other on the occipital region
    d. By placing one hand on either side of the helmet, without touching the face or head

36. For an infant or small child, padding may have to be placed under the ______________________ to ______________________ to maintain neutral alignment.

37. ______ Neutral alignment in the elderly may be difficult because of changes in the spine from disease. True (T) or false (F)?

38. You have been dispatched to the scene of an "injured child." En route, you are advised that a 10-year-old girl has fallen from the back of a moving pick-up truck. On arrival, the distraught father is holding the child in his arms. She is unresponsive and has noisy respirations, and an open scalp wound with moderate bleeding is obvious. With spinal precautions, you and your partner move the child to a spine board and place her in the ambulance.

    a. What is your first priority of care in managing this patient?

    ______________________________

    ______________________________

    b. You suction the child's airway and assist her respirations with a bag-valve-mask (BVM) device. How would you control the bleeding from her scalp?

    ______________________________

    ______________________________

c. En route to the emergency department, you continue your assessment and management of this patient. What signs and symptoms of traumatic head injury should you anticipate?

________________________________________

________________________________________

# DIVISION FIVE

## Trauma



## DIVISION TEST

**Directions:** *Place the letter of the correct answer in the space provided.*

1. ______ Which of the following statements is *true?*
   a. All organs need to be equally perfused to function properly.
   b. The average adult has approximately 10 L of blood in the body.
   c. Hypovolemic shock occurs when blood in the body is insufficient.
   d. The brain, heart, lungs, and kidneys tolerate an interruption in blood supply.

2. ______ Changes in mental status:
   a. Are caused by changes in perfusion of the brain
   b. Occur late in shock
   c. Typically occur after a drop in blood pressure
   d. Are a sign of good brain perfusion

3. ______ Signs and symptoms of shock include:
   a. Strong, regular peripheral pulses with weak central pulses
   b. Capillary refill greater than 0.5 second in children
   c. Dry skin
   d. Restlessness

4. ______ When treating a patient with signs and symptoms of shock including a low blood pressure:
   a. Position the patient sitting upright to make breathing easier.
   b. Provide high-flow oxygen.
   c. Keep the patient cool.
   d. Splint all extremity injuries on scene to minimize blood loss.

5. ______ Which of the following statements is *true?*
   a. Blood loss of 1 L is considered serious in adult patients.
   b. Geriatric patients tolerate blood loss better than younger patients.
   c. Children bleed more slowly than adults.
   d. Infants can lose up to 500 ml of blood before the condition is considered serious.

6. ______ Which type of bleeding is bright red in color, may spurt with each heartbeat, and is difficult to control?
   a. Venous bleeding
   b. Arterial bleeding
   c. Capillary bleeding
   d. Pulmonary bleeding

7. ______ What is the most effective method to control bleeding from one main source?
   a. Fingertip pressure directly on the point of bleeding
   b. Elevation of the extremity
   c. Pressure points
   d. Tourniquet

8. ______ Which of the following statements about tourniquets is *true?*
   a. Tourniquets are usually needed in cases of amputation.
   b. A piece of rope or wire is an effective tourniquet.
   c. Tourniquets cause little tissue damage if left in place less than 10 hours.
   d. Areas distal to a tourniquet may need to be amputated.

9. ______ Which of the following is *true?*
   a. Care for epistaxis includes having the patient tilt his or her head back.
   b. Up to 1 L of blood may be lost in a closed injury to the tibia.
   c. Patients should be treated for hemorrhagic shock only if external bleeding is observed.
   d. Vomit that appears as coffee grounds may be a sign of internal bleeding.

10. ______ The outer layer of the skin is the:
   a. Epidermis
   b. Dermis
   c. Endodermis
   d. Subcutaneous

11. ______ A(n) _______ is an injury in which the outermost layers of the skin are scraped away, with little bleeding.
   a. Contusion
   b. Crush injury
   c. Abrasion
   d. Avulsion

12. ______ Which of the following is an example of a closed injury?
   a. Abrasion
   b. Laceration
   c. Contusion
   d. Avulsion

13. ______ In this type of injury, the skin or tissue is torn loose or pulled completely off.
   a. Laceration
   b. Amputation
   c. Contusion
   d. Avulsion

14. ______ Which of the following statements is *true?*
   a. Dressings are used to secure bandages in place.
   b. An occlusive dressing is made of porous material to allow air to pass through.
   c. Splint extremity injuries to minimize bleeding.
   d. Straighten a joint that is injured before applying bandaging.

15. ______ A(n) _______ is an abdominal injury in which the organs are protruding through the wound.
   a. Evisceration
   b. Amputation
   c. Avulsion
   d. Penetration

16. ______ How should you treat a patient with an impaled object in the cheek that is obstructing the airway?
   a. Leave the impaled object as found.
   b. Remove the impaled object.
   c. Stabilize the object from inside the mouth.
   d. Stabilize the object from outside the mouth.

17. ______ How should you care for an amputated finger?
   a. Place the finger in a hot pack to keep it warm.
   b. Place the finger in plastic and keep it cool.
   c. Place the finger on ice so that it freezes as soon as possible.
   d. Place the finger in a bag of ice and water so it will be cool without freezing.

18. ______ What type of burn is characterized by intense pain, white to red skin, and blisters?
   a. Superficial burn
   b. Partial-thickness burn
   c. Full-thickness burn
   d. Full-contact burn

19. ______ You are assessing a 2-month-old patient who has circumferential burns on both legs and one arm. Using the rule of nines, what percentage body surface is burned?
    a. 24%
    b. 30%
    c. 37%
    d. 43%

20. ______ Which of the following statements about burns is *true?*
    a. A partial-thickness burn involving the feet is a critical burn.
    b. A burn caused by dry lime should be flushed with large amounts of water.
    c. Electrical burns cause extensive skin damage but little internal damage.
    d. Keep burn patients cool to minimize pain.

21. ______ Involuntary muscles:
    a. Are attached to bones to provide movement
    b. Have automaticity and cause the heart to beat
    c. Carry out automatic muscular functions of the body
    d. Are also known as skeletal muscles

22. ______ Which of the following is an example of a direct injury?
    a. Injury to the knee caused by striking the dashboard
    b. Injury to the pelvis caused by the knees striking the dashboard
    c. Injury to an arm caused by pulling and twisting
    d. Injury to the spine caused when landing on the feet from a fall

23. ______ Crepitation is the:
    a. Sound when water is under an injury
    b. Sound of bone ends rubbing together
    c. Sound of fluid in the lungs
    d. Sound made when swelling occurs in the airway

24. ______ Which of the following statements about splinting is *true?*
    a. Assess proximal pulse, sensation, and motor function before/after splinting.
    b. Splint the bone above and below a joint injury.
    c. Replace protruding bone ends before splinting.
    d. Leave clothing in place to minimize pain when splinting.

25. ______ What should be done for a patient who has multiple extremity injuries and signs and symptoms of shock?
    a. Splint each extremity before transport.
    b. Splint the extremities to the long backboard.
    c. Splint the upper extremities before transport.
    d. Splint the lower extremities before transport.

26. ______ For which of the following injuries would you use a traction splint?
    a. Closed injury of the midthigh
    b. Injury to thigh and knee
    c. Injury to lower leg
    d. Injury to hip

27. ______ The central nervous system is composed of:
    a. Brain and spinal cord
    b. Brain and peripheral nerves
    c. Spinal cord and sensory nerves
    d. Sensory and motor nerves

28. ______ A properly sized cervical spine immobilization device:
    a. Allows the chin to move in and out of the chin rest
    b. Restricts the patient's side-to-side head motion only
    c. Will immobilize the patient's head in a neutral position
    d. Will provide complete immobilization of the head

29. ______ What should be done for the patient if you do not have the proper size cervical spine immobilization device?
    a. Instruct the patient not to move his or her head.
    b. Use a towel roll and tape.
    c. Use a device that is one size too large.
    d. Use a device that is one size too small.

30. ______ Which of the following statements about short and long backboards is *true?*
   a. Secure the patient's head to the short board, then secure the body.
   b. When using a long backboard, a cervical spine immobilization device need not be used.
   c. When using a Kendrick extrication device (KED), buckle the top chest strap before the other chest straps.
   d. Reassess distal pulses after immobilizing a patient with a long backboard.

31. ______ If a patient hit his or her head on the bottom of a pool while diving, the mechanism of injury to the spine would be:
   a. Extension
   b. Compression
   c. Distraction
   d. Flexion

32. ______ Which of the following statements is *true?*
   a. Patients with no neck or back pain most likely do not have spinal cord damage.
   b. Begin manual stabilization of the head after completing the initial assessment.
   c. Reassess pulse, motor function, and sensation after every intervention.
   d. If the patient's injury is to the pelvis, spinal trauma can be ruled out.

33. ______ Use rapid extrication when:
   a. The scene is unsafe for the EMT–Basic to enter.
   b. The patient complains of pain in the neck or back.
   c. You cannot care for the patient in his or her current position.
   d. The patient has a head injury.

34. ______ Which of the following statements about helmet removal is *true?*
   a. Football helmets should always be removed.
   b. Remove the helmet if it restricts head movement.
   c. Only athletic trainers should remove helmets.
   d. Helmets are removed if the head cannot be immobilized.

35. ______ Which of the following statements is *true?*
   a. When immobilizing children, place a pad under the head to achieve a neutral position.
   b. Attempt to straighten the spine of geriatric patients for good immobilization.
   c. Leave the straps loose when immobilizing children so they do not struggle.
   d. Children have larger heads in proportion to their body, requiring special immobilization techniques.

## CHAPTER 31

# Infant and Child Emergency Care

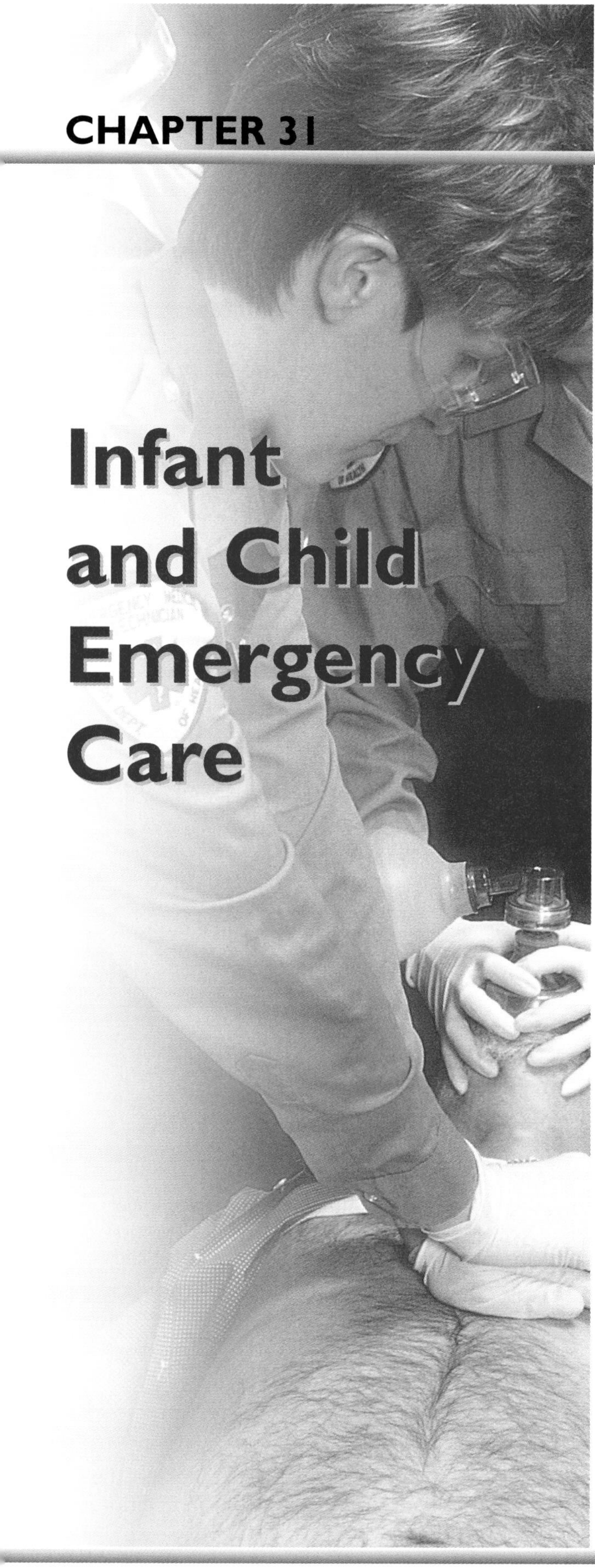

## CHAPTER OUTLINE

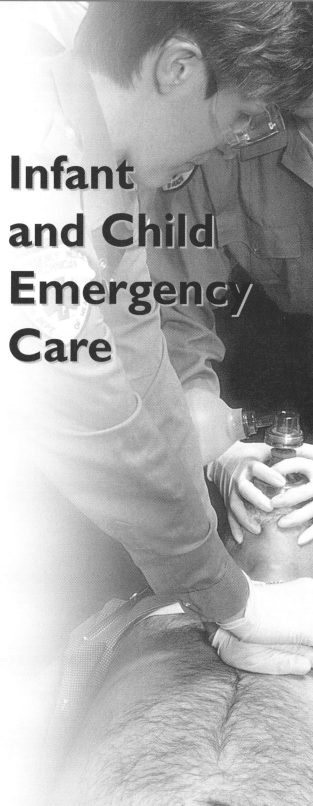

## CHAPTER OUTLINE—cont'd



## MATCHING 1

*Match the terms in Column 1 with the correct definition in Column 2.*

| Column 1 | | Column 2 |
|---|---|---|
| 1. ______ | Adolescent | a. Child from 12 to 18 years of age |
| 2. ______ | Infant | b. Child from 6 to 12 years of age |
| 3. ______ | Newborn | c. Term for an infant from birth to 1 month of age |
| 4. ______ | Preschool child | d. Child from 3 to 6 years of age |
| 5. ______ | School-age child | e. Child younger than 1 year of age |
| 6. ______ | Toddler | f. Child from 1 to 3 years of age |

## MATCHING 2

*Match the terms in Column 1 with the correct definition in Column 2.*

| Column 1 | | Column 2 |
|---|---|---|
| 7. ______ | Blow-by oxygen | a. Clinical condition in which the infant or child begins to increase the work of breathing |
| 8. ______ | Central lines | b. Used for feeding as a way to place food directly into the stomach |
| 9. ______ | Gastric tube | c. Tube running from the brain to the abdomen to drain excess cerebrospinal fluid |
| 10. ______ | Grunting | d. Sound made when patient in respiratory distress attempts to trap air to keep alveoli open |
| 11. ______ | Nasal flaring | e. Use of accessory muscles to increase the work of breathing |
| 12. ______ | Respiratory failure | f. Attempt by the infant to increase the size of the airway by expanding the nostrils |
| 13. ______ | Respiratory distress | g. Method of oxygen delivery for infants and children without a mask on the face |
| 14. ______ | Retractions | h. Intravascular lines placed near the heart for long-term use |
| 15. ______ | Shunt | i. Clinical condition when the patient is continuing to work hard to breathe, the effort of breathing is increased, and the patient's condition begins to deteriorate |

## MATCHING 3

*Match the terms in Column 1 with the correct definition in Column 2.*

**Column 1**

16. ______ Child abuse
17. ______ Drowning
18. ______ Near drowning
19. ______ Neglect
20. ______ Secondary drowning
21. ______ Sudden infant death syndrome

**Column 2**

a. Survival past 24 hours after suffocation resulting from submersion
b. Improper or excessive action by parents, guardians, or caretakers that injures or causes harm to children
c. Not giving attention to a child's essential needs
d. Rapid deterioration of respiratory status from several hours to 96 hours after resuscitation
e. Death within the first 24 hours of submersion in liquid
f. Sudden, unexplained death of an infant with no discernible cause

## MATCHING 4

*Match the developmental age of the child in Column 1 to the child's need for parents in Column 2.*

**Column 1**

22. ______ School-age
23. ______ Adolescent
24. ______ Toddler
25. ______ Infant

**Column 2**

a. Will not be separated from parents
b. Wants to be separated from parents
c. Will be okay without parents but wants them there
d. Better in parent's arms

## REVIEW QUESTIONS

1. ______ Infants must be assessed and treated in a manner to avoid hypothermia. True (T) or false (F)?

2. What part of the infant's body should you assess first?

______________________________

______________________________

3. List three way to evaluate a child's respirations without touching the patient.

a. ______________________________

b. ______________________________

c. ______________________________

4. ______ Most toddlers do not mind being touched by strangers. True (T) or false (F)?

5. ______ The parent can be the most help in the evaluation of a toddler. True (T) or false (F)?

6. ______ Preschool children like to:
   a. Be touched by strangers
   b. Have their clothes removed
   c. Be apart from their parents
   d. Explore

7. ______ Unlike toddlers and preschoolers, school-age children are able to relate a good history about what happened. True (T) or false (F)?

8. The most important anatomic and physiological differences between infants and children and adults involve the ______________________________.

9. ______ Compared with an adult, the airway of a child is ______ and ______ blocked by secretions and swelling.
   a. Larger, more easily
   b. Smaller, more easily
   c. Larger, not easily
   d. Smaller, not easily

10. ______ In infants and children, the ______ is(are) relatively ______ in relation to the mouth as compared with adults.
    a. Teeth, large
    b. Mouth, large
    c. Gums, small
    d. Tongue, large

11. In children, drowsiness and tolerance with examination procedures can be a sign of ______________________________.

12. To prevent occlusion or kinking of the airway, a head-tilt, chin-lift maneuver should put the head into a ______________________________ position in which the nose points straight up.

13. ______ Whenever you suction an infant or child, measure the catheter before insertion and suction only as far as you can see. True (T) or false (F)?

14. Suctioning should be limited to ______ seconds, and you should always apply ______________ before and after.

15. To insert an oropharyngeal airway in an infant or child, first ______________________ (depress/lift) the tongue and insert the airway ______________________ (with/without) rotation.

16. What airway adjunct can you use when the patient has a gag reflex and will not tolerate an oropharyngeal airway?

    ______________________________

    ______________________________

17. ______ Blow-by oxygen allows delivery of oxygen to an infant or child without placing a mask directly on the child's face. True (T) or false (F)?

18. ______ For infants, the rate of flow for blow-by oxygen should be ______ L/min and ______ L/min for children.
    a. 5, 8
    b. 5, 10
    c. 4, 8
    d. 6, 12

19. ______ The recommended rate for artificial ventilation in infants and children is once every ______ seconds or ______ times a minute.
    a. 3, 12
    b. 3, 20
    c. 2, 28
    d. 4, 15

20. Besides the gentle rise of the chest, list other indicators of adequate ventilation in children.

    ______________________________

    ______________________________

21. With children, when should you consider examining painful areas?

_______________________________________________

_______________________________________________

22. Define the following letters associated with the mental status acronym.

A _____________________________________________

V _____________________________________________

P _____________________________________________

U _____________________________________________

23. Indicate if the patients described have a partial (P) upper airway obstruction, complete (C) upper airway obstruction, or lower (L) airway obstruction.

_____ Stridor on inspiration

_____ Expiratory wheeze

_____ Unable to cough or speak

_____ Skin may appear normal or cyanotic

_____ Skin may appear pale or cyanotic

24. _____ Which of the following statements concerning foreign body airway obstruction is *true?*
    a. Unresponsive infants should receive back blows and abdominal thrusts for complete airway obstruction.
    b. Use abdominal thrusts for a responsive child with an obstruction as you would for an adult.
    c. Blind finger sweeps should be performed for infants when a history of foreign body obstruction is known.
    d. When performing abdominal thrusts on the unresponsive child, use the heel of two hands and give 6 to 10 thrusts before inspecting the airway.

25. More than 80% of all cardiac arrests in children begin as _______________________ arrests.

26. List four signs of early respiratory distress in children.

    a. _____________________________________________

    b. _____________________________________________

    c. _____________________________________________

    d _____________________________________________

27. List four signs of respiratory failure in children.

    a. _____________________________________________

    b. _____________________________________________

    c. _____________________________________________

    d _____________________________________________

28. A seizure can be caused by a rapid rise in a

_______________________________________________.

29. _____ Which of the following statements is *true* concerning seizures in pediatric patients?
    a. Always place patients in the recovery position following seizures because associated trauma is rare.
    b. A bite block inserted into the patient's mouth can be helpful in controlling the airway.
    c. A nasopharyngeal airway can be helpful in keeping the tongue off of the back of the throat following a seizure.
    d. Seizures are rarely dangerous, even if they last for 30 minutes or more.

30. List three common signs and symptoms of shock in an infant or child.

    a. ______________________________

    b. ______________________________

    c. ______________________________

31. What are the top priorities in the treatment of near-drowning cases?

    ______________________________

    ______________________________

32. ______ Sudden infant death syndrome usually occurs in patients less than _____ months of age.
    a. 12
    b. 18
    c. 20
    d. 24

33. Because the ____________________ is larger and heavier than the other parts of the body, it is the most frequently injured part of a child's body.

34. ______ When a child has been burned, the biggest concern after airway and breathing is:
    a. Hyperthermia
    b. Hypovolemia
    c. Hypothermia
    d. Vomiting

35. List an indication for using the pneumatic anti-shock garment in a child.

    ______________________________

    ______________________________

36. List three signs of child abuse.

    a. ______________________________

    b. ______________________________

    c. ______________________________

37. ______ Most parents feel a sense of loss of control and helplessness when their child is sick or injured. True (T) or false (F)?

38. You have been dispatched to a "child with seizures." On arrival, a grandparent is holding the listless child. The grandmother tells you that the 4-year-old child had an earache and has been "running a high fever" most of the day. She was seen by the pediatrician yesterday and is taking medication for an infection. The seizure lasted only a few minutes.

    a. What questions should you ask the grandparents regarding the child's medical history?

    ______________________________

    ______________________________

    b. What medications should alert you to the likelihood of previous seizures?

    ______________________________

    ______________________________

    c. What emergency care is required for this patient?

    ______________________________

    ______________________________

39. You are caring for 9-year-old child who lost control of his bicycle while riding down a gravel road. He was thrown over the handlebars and is complaining of severe abdominal pain. He is alert and denies hitting his head or losing responsiveness. Aside from minor scrapes and abrasions, no apparent injuries have occurred. His mother asks you to transport him to the hospital immediately. You perform initial and focused assessments, immobilize the child on a long backboard with spinal precautions, apply oxygen, and obtain a set of vital signs. His blood pressure is 104/70 mm Hg, pulse rate is 126 beats per minute, and respirations are 22 breaths per minute and shallow.

   a. En route to the hospital, you note that the patient's stomach appears distended. The boy tells you that he feels cold and asks for a blanket. He also says that he is a little sick to his stomach. What do you suspect?

   ______________________________________________

   ______________________________________________

   b. You reassess his vital signs, which are blood pressure 92/64 mm Hg, pulse rate 130 beats per minute, and respirations 24 breaths per minute and shallow. What does the second set of vital signs suggest to you?

   ______________________________________________

   ______________________________________________

   c. What should you do?

   ______________________________________________

   ______________________________________________

   d. The child begins to wretch and vomit. How will you manage his airway?

   ______________________________________________

   ______________________________________________

# DIVISION SIX

## Infants and Children

Chapter 31 Infant and Child Emergency Care

## DIVISION TEST

**Directions:** *Place the letter of the correct answer in the space provided.*

1. ______ Which age group, developmentally, does not like to be separated from the parents but otherwise tolerates assessment well?
   a. Newborns and infants
   b. Toddlers
   c. Preschool children
   d. School-age children

2. ______ Which age group, developmentally, fears permanent injury, is modest, fears disfigurement, and should be treated as adults?
   a. Toddlers
   b. Preschool children
   c. School-age children
   d. Adolescents

3. ______ Which of the following statements is *true?*
   a. Infants are obligate nose breathers.
   b. A child's tongue is relatively small in comparison with the mouth.
   c. Children compensate for respiratory compromise by decreasing their respiratory rate.
   d. An infant's airway is less developed and less flexible compared with an adult's.

4. ______ Which of the following statements about oral and nasal airways is *true?*
   a. The preferred method of inserting an oral airway for a child is by rotating the airway 180 degrees into place.
   b. The nasopharyngeal airway in the child is more likely to stimulate vomiting than the oral airway.
   c. Nasal airways are useful in children following seizures.
   d. The nasal airway can be inserted only into the right nostril.

5. ______ Which of the following statements about oxygen delivery for infants and children is *true?*
   a. Blow-by oxygen means the oxygen is blown directly into the patient's mouth and nose by placing a mask on the patient's face.
   b. Parents can be used to assist in delivering oxygen to the patient.
   c. Nonrebreather masks should not be used for infants because the oxygen concentration is too high.
   d. The flow rate for oxygen delivery via a nonrebreather mask is 4 L/minute in children.

6. ______ When ventilating a child patient:
   a. Ventilate the patient until you see a gentle chest rise.
   b. The ventilation rate is 30 breaths per minute or one breath every 2 seconds.
   c. Use a BVM with a 250-ml bag.
   d. Make sure the BVM is equipped with a pop-off valve to reduce gastric distention.

7. ______ Which of the following statements about assessing an infant or child is *true?*
   a. Patients should be considered "V—responsive to voice" in the AVPU categories only if they follow commands.
   b. Infants and children generally have mottled skin before they have cyanosis.
   c. Capillary refill should take less than 4 seconds if the patient is perfusing adequately.
   d. Assess the child patient from the head to trunk then from toes to trunk.

8. ______ Where would you assess the pulse of a responsive 6-month-old patient?
   a. Radial artery
   b. Carotid artery
   c. Posterior tibial artery
   d. Brachial artery

9. ______ EMT–Basics should assess blood pressure for patients older than ______ years of age.
   a. 1
   b. 2
   c. 3
   d. 5

10. ______ How should a complete obstruction of the airway be cleared for a responsive 3-year-old child?
   a. Back blows
   b. Abdominal thrusts
   c. Back blows and abdominal thrusts
   d. Back blows and chest thrusts

11. ______ Which of the following signs indicates a complete upper airway obstruction?
   a. The patient is unable to cough.
   b. The skin is pink.
   c. The patient has expiratory wheezes.
   d. The patient has a history of airway disease.

12. ______ Which of the following is a sign of early respiratory distress?
   a. Wheezing
   b. Limp muscle tone
   c. Cyanosis
   d. Weak or absent distant pulses

13. ______ Which of the following is *true?*
   a. The patient's response to care provided for a seizure should help the EMT–Basic determine what caused the seizure.
   b. Providing good chest compressions is the priority for a near-drowning patient.
   c. Altered mental status may be caused by head trauma or infection.
   d. Activated charcoal should not be administered to children.

14. ______ Which of the following statements is *true* concerning SIDS?
   a. SIDS is most common in the third year of life.
   b. Do not attempt to resuscitate these patients with basic life support measures.
   c. Question the parents about care and neglect.
   d. SIDS deaths do not have an apparent cause or significant history.

15. ______ What type of injury is most common in children?
   a. Penetrating trauma
   b. Blunt trauma
   c. Burns
   d. Drowning

16. ______ What area of the body is most commonly injured in children?
    a. Head
    b. Chest
    c. Abdomen
    d. Extremities

17. ______ What is the most common cause of hypoxia in the unresponsive patient with head injury?
    a. The head injury itself
    b. Failure of EMS personnel to ventilate the patient
    c. The tongue of the patient obstructing the airway
    d. Damage to the trachea

18. ______ Which of the following is true regarding child abuse and neglect?
    a. Neglect is an improper action that injures a child.
    b. Physical abuse is more serious compared with emotional abuse.
    c. One sign of abuse is parents who seem inappropriately unconcerned about their child.
    d. If abuse is suspected, question the parents at the scene.

19. ______ What is the name of the tube placed directly into the stomach for feeding?
    a. Central line
    b. Shunt
    c. Gastric tube
    d. Tracheostomy tube

20. ______ Parents are often anxious because:
    a. They do not trust the EMT–Basic caring for their child.
    b. They are trying to hide abuse or neglect.
    c. They feel helpless.
    d. They do not want their child to be treated.

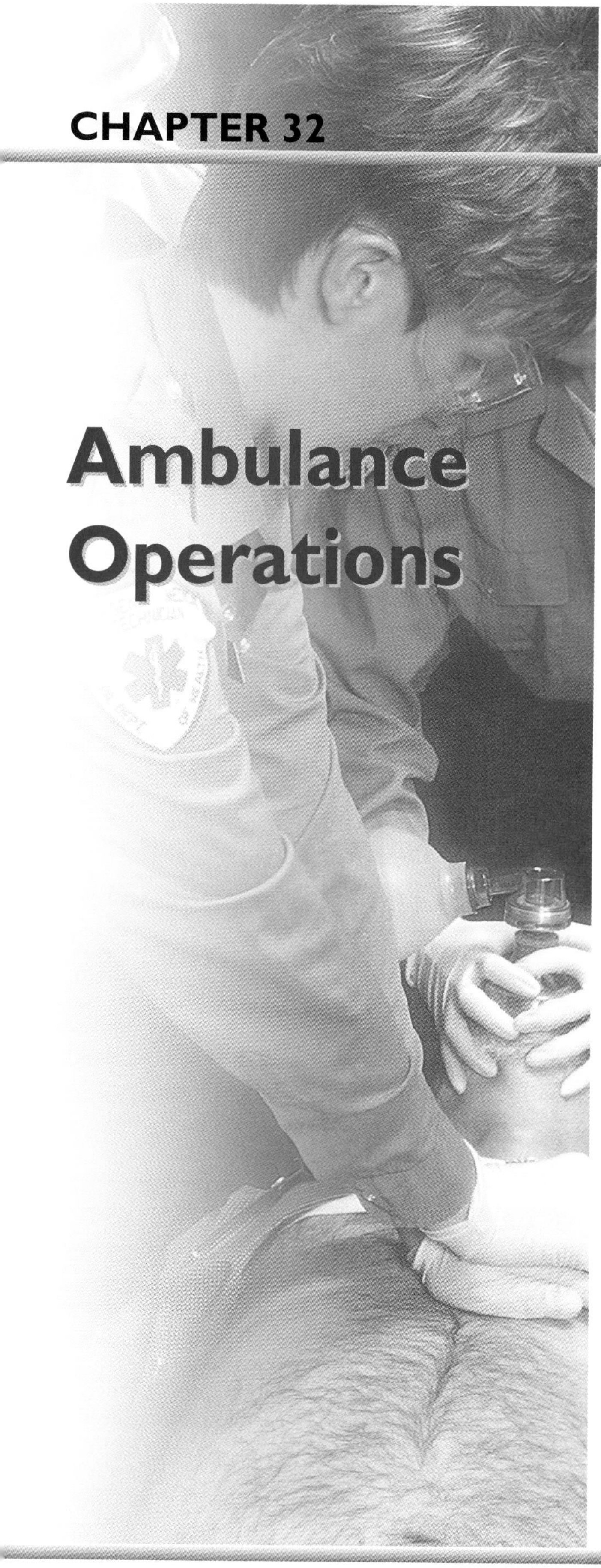

## CHAPTER 32

# Ambulance Operations

### CHAPTER OUTLINE

## MATCHING

*Match the terms in Column 1 with the correct definition in Column 2.*

**Column 1**

1. ______ Decontamination
2. ______ Disinfection
3. ______ Due regard
4. ______ Escort
5. ______ Infection control
6. ______ Sterilization

**Column 2**

a. Measures that EMTs take to help prevent the transmission of infection from patients to EMTs, from one patient to another, and from EMTs to patients
b. Another emergency vehicle that accompanies the ambulance to the scene or from the scene to the receiving facility
c. Process of killing microorganisms on a surface or item
d. Disinfecting process that destroys all microorganisms, including bacterial spores
e. Principle that a reasonable and careful person in similar circumstances would act in a way that is safe for and considerate of others
f. Use of physical or chemical means to remove, inactivate, or destroy blood-borne pathogens on a surface or item so that it can no longer transmit infection

## REVIEW QUESTIONS

1. Preparation for the call includes checking availability and readiness of ____________________, ____________________, and ____________________.

2. ______ Participating in continuing education is also considered part of preparing for a call. True (T) or false (F)?

3. List three items of personal protective equipment.
   a. ____________________
   b. ____________________
   c. ____________________

4. ______ Personal protective gear is part of the nonmedical equipment that should be on every ambulance. True (T) or false (F)?

5. ______ Dispatch information typically includes the number of patients, their chief complaint, and location. True (T) or false (F)?

6. ______ A safe emergency vehicle driver always:
   a. Anticipates actions of others
   b. Plans alternative routes for different times of the day
   c. Uses vehicle warning devices wisely
   d. All of the above

7. ______ Drivers typically respond in a predictable manner when an emergency vehicle approaches. True (T) or false (F)?

8. List three factors that contribute to emergency vehicle crashes.
   a. ____________________
   b. ____________________
   c. ____________________

9. ______ En route to a call is also a time to:
   a. Discuss the previous call.
   b. Get more information from dispatch.
   c. Plan for equipment and personal needs.
   d. A and B
   e. B and C

10. The first priority in parking at the scene is

_______________________________________.

11. ______ Arrival at the scene is a good time to:
    a. Plan for equipment needs.
    b. Reach the patient as soon as possible.
    c. Call for additional resources based on scene size-up.
    d. Remove all patients immediately to your vehicle.

12. ______ Patient transport to a receiving facility is always with lights and siren. True (T) or false (F)?

13. ______ The EMT in the patient compartment should use transport time to perform the:
    a. Focused history and physical examination
    b. Initial assessment
    c. Detailed and ongoing assessment
    d. Care for life-threatening injuries

14. Patient transfer includes putting the patient in

the appropriate room and giving the

________________________________ report.

15. ______ Documentation can be done after returning to the station. True (T) or false (F)?

16. ______ Which type of disinfection is recommended for routine cleaning when no body fluids are present?
    a. High-level disinfection
    b. Sterilization
    c. Low-level disinfection
    d. Intermediate-level disinfection

17. ______ Which type of disinfection is recommended for equipment that is in contact with areas of the body that are normally sterile?
    a. High-level disinfection
    b. Sterilization
    c. Low-level disinfection
    d. Intermediate-level disinfection

18. Restocking and rechecking inventory occur

during the ________________________ phase.

19. List three mechanisms of injury that would be possible candidates for air medical transport.

    a. ________________________________

    b. ________________________________

    c. ________________________________

20. ______ Always approach a helicopter from the front, avoiding the pilot's blind areas. True (T) or false (F)?

21. You are transporting a cardiac patient to the hospital. His condition stabilized after you applied high-concentration oxygen and assisted him in taking his nitroglycerin. Everything on this call just "seemed to click," and you wish they all would run so smoothly.

    a. As part of your preparation for this call, what emergency equipment did you arrange to take to the patient's side while en route to the scene?

    ________________________________

    ________________________________

    b. Your partner carefully drove to the scene with due regard for others. What does due regard require during an emergency response?

    ________________________________

    ________________________________

    c. What are your responsibilities during transfer of this patient at the receiving facility?

    ________________________________

    ________________________________

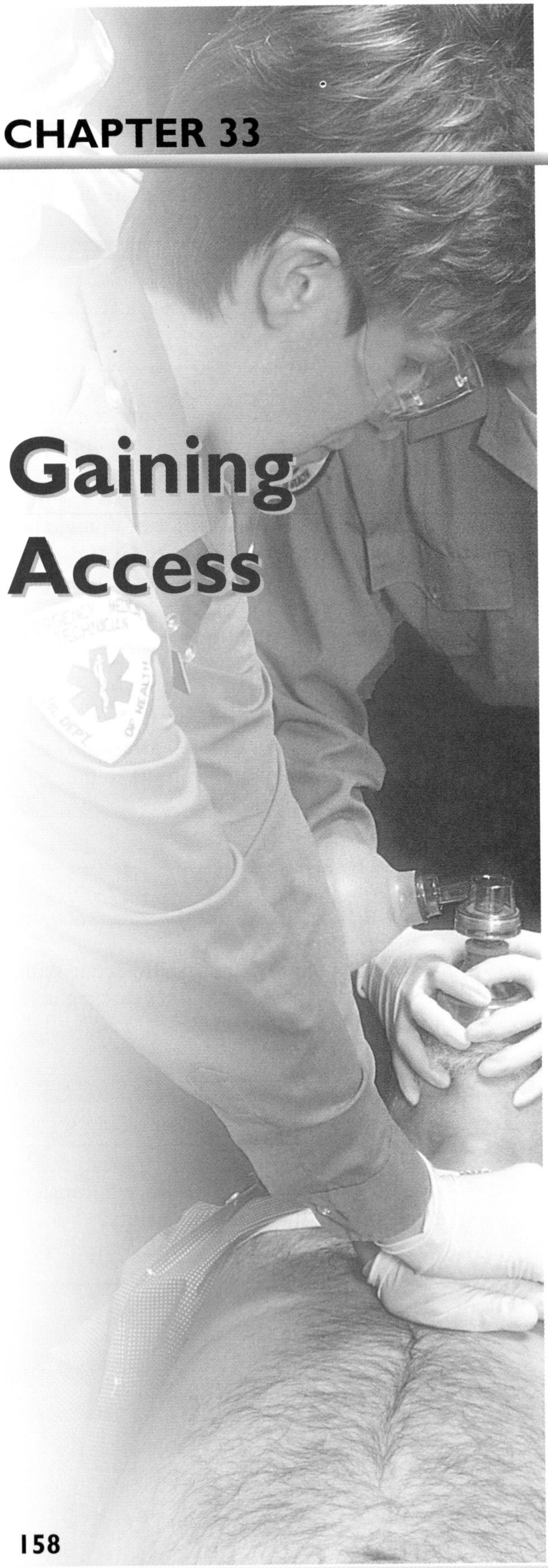

## CHAPTER 33

# Gaining Access

## CHAPTER OUTLINE

I. Fundamentals of Extrication
II. Safety and Equipment
   A. Personal Safety
   B. Patient Safety
   C. Other Safety Issues
III. Accessing the Patient
IV. Removing the Patient

## REVIEW QUESTIONS

1. Define the term *extrication.*

 ______________________________________

 ______________________________________

2. The role of the incident commander is to

 ____________________ efforts of medical

 and rescue personnel.

3. ______ Extrication requires specialized education and equipment. True (T) or false (F)?

4. In all cases of entrapment, what actions precede extrication?

 ______________________________________

 ______________________________________

5. ______ EMS and rescue personnel should work together to:
 a. Remove the patient as quickly as possible.
 b. Provide critical interventions.
 c. Prepare the necessary equipment for immobilization.
 d. None of the above are correct.

6. Place the following statements about safety during extrication in order of priority.

 ______ Bystander safety

 ______ Personal safety

 ______ Crew safety

 ______ Patient safety

7. List five pieces of protective gear necessary for extrication.

 a. ______________________________________

 b. ______________________________________

 c. ______________________________________

 d. ______________________________________

 e. ______________________________________

8. ______ During extrication cover the patient to:
 a. Lessen the noise
 b. Protect from debris
 c. Keep the patient from being scared
 d. Keep the patient from being identified

9. ______ Bystanders and onlookers can be helpful during extrication. True (T) or false (F)?

10. List three issues or potential hazards at the scene of an automobile crash.

 a. ______________________________________

 b. ______________________________________

 c. ______________________________________

11. The safety officer is a(n) ____________________

 observer who helps identify additional

 ______________________________ not readily

 apparent to the EMTs.

12. Define simple and complex access.

 ______________________________________

 ______________________________________

13. List three types of specialized rescue.

    a. ______________________________

    b. ______________________________

    c. ______________________________

14. ______ Which of the following is a reason for extrication before spinal immobilization?
    a. The patient has no pain to the neck.
    b. The patient cannot be treated in his or her current position.
    c. The initial assessment revealed no injuries.
    d. The patient has no feeling in his or her legs.

15. ______ Removing a patient from a vehicle usually requires only two people. True (T) or false (F)?

16. You have been dispatched to a helicopter crash. While en route, police on the scene inform you that two victims are trapped in the wreckage. A second ambulance and fire and rescue personnel have also been dispatched.

    a. What is your first priority at this scene?

    ______________________________

    ______________________________

    b. Because you will arrive before fire and rescue personnel, what minimal personal protective equipment should you have available?

    ______________________________

    ______________________________

    c. During scene size-up, you see downed power lines around the wreckage. What should you do?

    ______________________________

    ______________________________

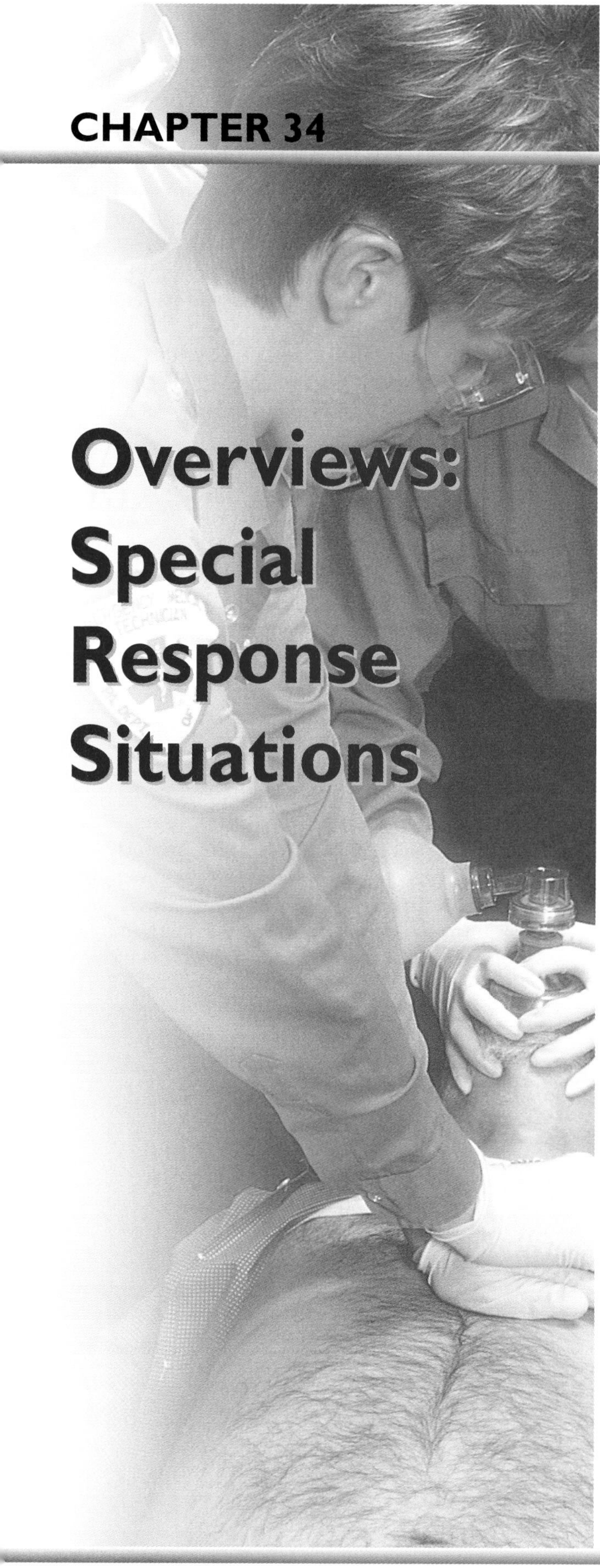

## CHAPTER 34

# Overviews: Special Response Situations

**CHAPTER OUTLINE**

I. Hazardous Materials
   A. Extent of the Problem
   B. Safety Concerns
   C. Approaching the Scene
   D. Information Resources
   E. Procedures
   F. Education for Emergency Medical Services Responders
II. Incident Management Systems
   A. Structure of Responsibilities
   B. Role of the Emergency Medical Technician
III. Multiple Casualty Situations
   A. Triage
   B. Procedures

## MATCHING

*Match the terms in Column 1 with the correct definition in Column 2.*

**Column 1**

1. ______ Extrication sector
2. ______ Hazardous material
3. ______ Incident management system
4. ______ Material safety data sheets
5. ______ Placard
6. ______ Staging sector
7. ______ Support or supply sector
8. ______ Transportation sector
9. ______ Treatment sector
10. ______ Triage
11. ______ Triage sector

**Column 2**

a. Information sign with symbols and numbers to assist in identifying the hazardous material or class of material
b. Sector in the incident management system that is responsible for dealing with removing patients who are trapped at the scene
c. Sector in the incident management system that coordinates with the transportation sector for the movement of vehicles to and from the transportation sector
d. Sector of the incident management system that coordinates resources, including receiving hospitals, air medical resources, and ambulances
e. Coordinating procedures to assist in the control, direction, and coordination of emergency response resources
f. Sector in the incident management system that is responsible for obtaining additional resources—including disposable supplies, personnel, and equipment—for other sectors
g. Optional sector in the incident management system that prioritizes patients for treatment and transport
h. Any substance or material that can pose an unreasonable risk to health, safety, or property
i. Method of categorizing patients into treatment or transport priorities
j. Sector in the incident management system that provides care to patients received from the triage and extrication sector
k. Information required by the U.S. Department of Labor that list properties and hazards associated with chemicals and compounds to assist in management of incidents involving them

## REVIEW QUESTIONS

1. ______ Hazardous materials scenes occur only at industrial sites. True (T) or false (F)?

2. The primary concern at any hazardous material scene is ________________________________.

3. Always approach a hazardous material scene from a(n) ______________________________ and ______________________________ direction.

4. ______ Container ______ and ______ are helpful in identifying the possible chemical.
   a. Size, color
   b. Shape, texture
   c. Size, shape
   d. Color, texture

5. ______ Always maintain a safe distance from and do not enter an unsafe area. True (T) or false (F)?

6. ______ Every EMT should be educated to at least the ______________ level of hazardous materials knowledge.
   a. First Responder awareness
   b. First Responder operations
   c. Hazardous materials technician
   d. Hazardous materials specialist

7. List the steps the EMT–Basic should take when approaching a potential hazardous materials scene.

   a. ______________________________
   b. ______________________________
   c. ______________________________
   d. ______________________________
   e. ______________________________
   f. ______________________________
   g. ______________________________
   h. ______________________________

8. List at least three sources of information and assistance with a hazardous material incident.

   a. ______________________________
   b. ______________________________
   c. ______________________________

9. ______ Incident management systems provide: *(Mark all that apply.)*

   a. ______ A group leader
   b. ______ An orderly method for communications
   c. ______ Unlimited resources
   d. ______ Efficient interaction with other agencies
   e. ______ Orderly decision making

10. List two situations in which a major incident should be declared.

    a. ______________________________
    b. ______________________________

11. The ______________________ sector provides care for patients as they are received from triage and extrication.

12. The ______________________ sector provides resources, supplies, personnel, and equipment.

13. Within each sector, a ______________________ runs the operation of the sector.

14. ______ During a major incident or a mass casualty situation, what should the EMT–Basic who arrives after the incident command system has been established do first?
    a. Report to the triage sector.
    b. Begin transporting the most critically ill patients.
    c. Begin caring for the most critically injured patients.
    d. Report to the staging area for assignment.

15. A method of categorizing patient treatment and transport needs is called ____________________.

16. Explain the purpose of triage tags.

____________________________________________

____________________________________________

17. Indicate the correct priority for each of the following conditions. (A = highest, B = second, and C = lowest.)

______ Severed artery in leg

______ Contusion and laceration to forearm

______ Circumferential burn to chest

______ Absent pulse and respirations

______ Deformity to one wrist with contusions

______ Burns to arms, hands, and feet

______ Cool, clammy skin, low blood pressure, rapid heart rate

______ Pain, swelling, and deformity to thigh

______ Severe back and neck pain, motor, sensory functions intact

18. You and your partner have just witnessed a train derailment where multiple patients have been injured. Your department just completed an education program for mass casualty management, and you believe that you are prepared for "the big one." The first step in managing a major incident is to declare that one exists. You advise dispatch and mentally prepare to manage the scene.

a. Describe situations in which a major incident should be declared.

____________________________________________

____________________________________________

b. As other emergency services arrive on the scene, you establish EMS sectors. What are seven generally recognized EMS sectors?

____________________________________________

____________________________________________

c. A person more qualified to manage the incident arrives and assumes command. She assigns you to the triage sector as the triage officer. What are your new responsibilities?

____________________________________________

____________________________________________

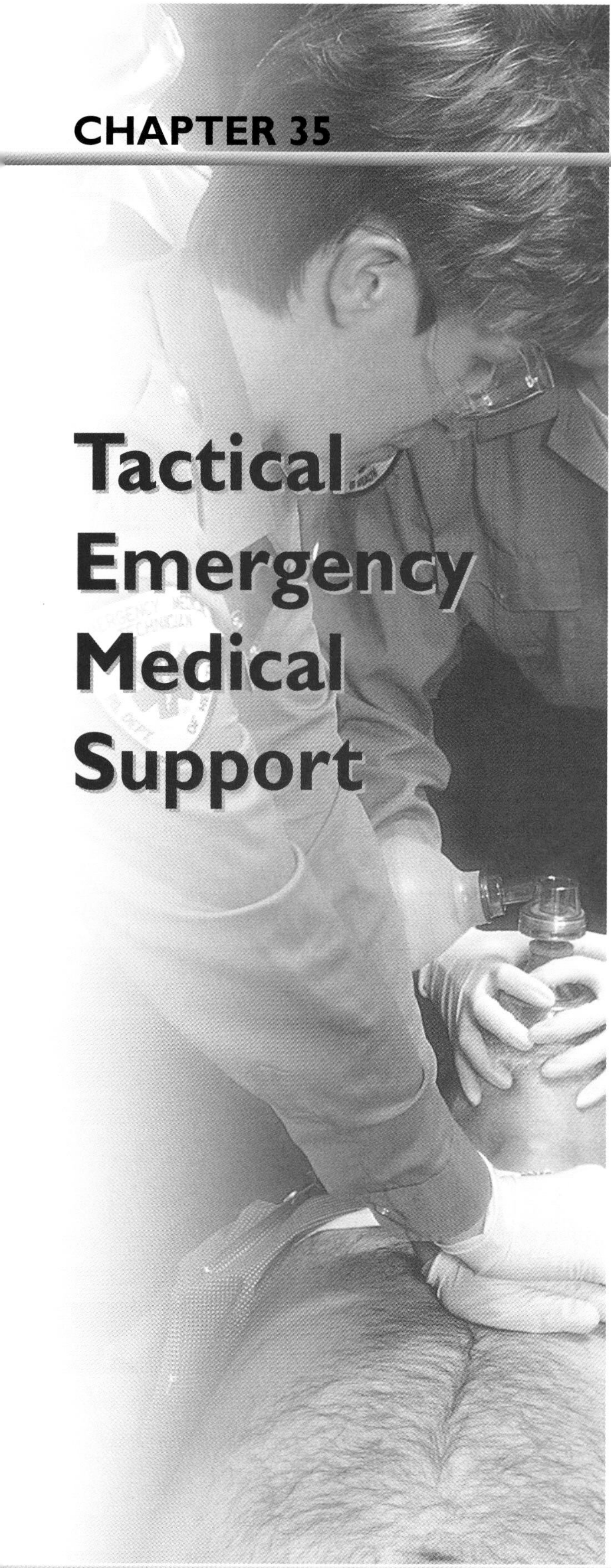

## CHAPTER 35

# Tactical Emergency Medical Support

### CHAPTER OUTLINE

I. Role of Tactical Emergency Medical Support
II. Tactical Field Care and Triage
  A. Scene Awareness
    1. Awareness
    2. Cover and concealment
    3. Evacuation
  B. Tactical Medical Care
    1. Hot zone
    2. Warm zone
    3. Cold zone
  C. Special Considerations

## MATCHING I

*Match the terms in Column 1 with the correct definition in Column 2.*

**Column 1**

1. ______ Cold zone
2. ______ Concealment
3. ______ Cover
4. ______ Hot zone
5. ______ Warm zone

**Column 2**

a. The area in which persistent or unknown threat exists
b. A physical barrier for protection from a perpetrator
c. The area in which direct contact with the suspect is unlikely but tactical operators are still at risk
d. An area considered to be safe from threats
e. Obstruction from view

## REVIEW QUESTIONS

1. Define a medical threat assessment.

_______________________________________

_______________________________________

2. ______ The hot zones, warm zones, and cold zones of a tactical setting do not change once they are designated. True (T) or false (F)?

3. ______ In tactical EMS (TEMS), the "A" in the acronym ACE stands for:
   a. Announcement
   b. Assessment
   c. Awareness
   d. Amplification

4. Define *cover* and *concealment.*

   a. Cover: ______________________________

   _______________________________________

   b. Concealment: _________________________

   _______________________________________

5. Further medical care provided in the warm zone is routinely called _______________________.

6. What should TEMS providers who have multiple patients use when working in the cold zone?

_______________________________________

_______________________________________

7. What does the acronym START stand for?

S ______________________________

T ______________________________

A ______________________________

R ______________________________

T ______________________________

CHAPTER 36

# Weapons of Mass Destruction

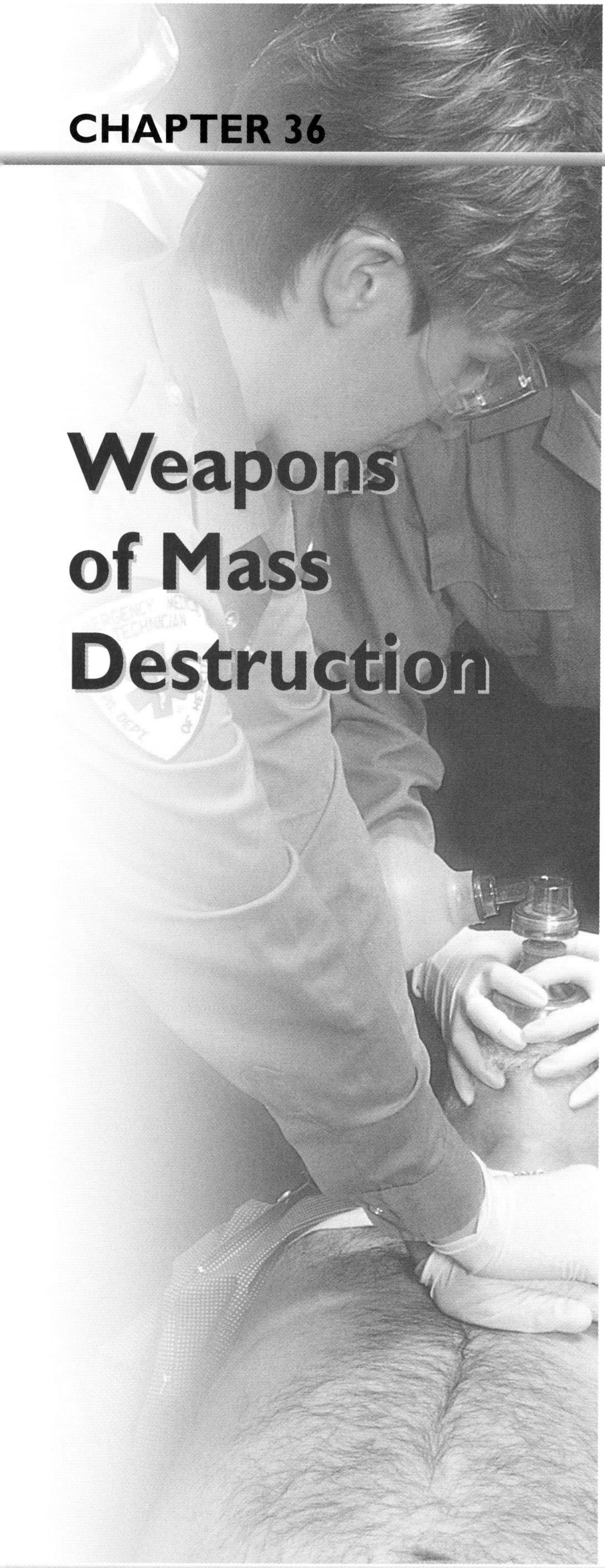

## CHAPTER OUTLINE

I. Terrorism
II. Agents of Terrorism
   A. Chemical Weapons
      1. Nerve agents
      2. Vesicants (blister agents)
      3. Chemical asphyxiants
      4. Lung irritants
      5. Riot control agents
   B. Biologic Weapons
      1. Microbes and toxins
      2. Neurologic conditions
      3. Hemorrhagic viral diseases
      4. Gastroenteritis-causing diseases
      5. Infectious skin diseases
   C. Radiologic Devices
III. Common Management Strategies

## MATCHING I

*Match the terms in Column 1 with the correct definition in Column 2.*

**Column 1**

1. ______ Off-gassing
2. ______ Petechiae
3. ______ Terrorism

**Column 2**

a. Unlawful use of force to achieve political or social objectives
b. Pinpoint, round, red spots that indicate bleeding under the skin
c. The secondary release of nerve agents from a contaminated person

## REVIEW QUESTIONS

1. ______ Organophosphate agents are classified as:
   a. Biologic agents
   b. Radiologic agents
   c. Nuclear agents
   d. Nerve agents

2. What does the acronym SLUDGE stand for?

   S ______________________________

   L ______________________________

   U ______________________________

   D ______________________________

   G ______________________________

   E ______________________________

3. What are the contents of a Mark I kit?

   ______________________________

   ______________________________

4. What other medications in addition to the Mark I kit may be necessary for nerve agent exposure?

   ______________________________

   ______________________________

5. How will the EMS provider note that a biologic weapons event has occurred?

   ______________________________

   ______________________________

6. The most effective way to spread a biologic agent is through ______________________________ of microbes or toxins.

7. List three biologic agents that would present as pneumonia in adults.

   a. ______________________________

   b. ______________________________

   c. ______________________________

8. Nuclear explosions primarily kill by:

   ______________________________

   ______________________________

# DIVISION SEVEN

## Operations



## DIVISION TEST

**Directions:** *Place the letter of the correct answer in the space provided.*

1. ______ Which of the following pieces of equipment should be available for EMT–Basics when responding to emergency calls?
   a. Esophageal airways
   b. Splinting supplies
   c. Intravenous solutions
   d. Cardiac medications

2. ______ Which of the following procedures should be routine when en route to the call?
   a. Seatbelts should be secured.
   b. Red lights and sirens should be used.
   c. Review the specifics of the previous call.
   d. All of the above are correct.

3. ______ Which of the following methods of parking the unit at the scene is acceptable?
   a. Park downhill from hazards.
   b. Park downwind from hazards.
   c. Park 15 m from any wreckage.
   d. Use emergency lights.

4. ______ On arrival at the scene, what should be done?
   a. Notify dispatch of arrival on scene.
   b. Size-up scene.
   c. Call for additional help if necessary.
   d. All the above are correct.

5. ______ Which of the following should be performed while en route to the receiving facility?
   a. Begin to care for life-threatening injuries.
   b. Provide ongoing assessment of the patient.
   c. Provide initial assessment of the patient.
   d. Ask patient for insurance and billing information.

6. ______ When is the verbal patient report given over the radio to the physician or nurse at the receiving facility?
   a. From the scene
   b. While en route to the receiving facility
   c. When arriving at the receiving facility
   d. Report at bedside is sufficient

7. ______ Which of the following pieces of equipment requires high-level disinfection?
   a. Blood pressure cuff
   b. Penlights
   c. Mask of a BVM
   d. Dressings

8. ______ Landing zones for EMS helicopters should be:
   a. Ideally 30 m × 30 m (100 ft × 100 ft)
   b. Ideally 20 m × 20 m (65 ft × 65 ft)
   c. Minimally 30 m × 30 m (100 ft × 100 ft)
   d. Minimally 12 m × 12 m (40 ft × 40 ft)

9. ______ The EMS helicopter:
   a. Should be approached from the rear (6 o'clock position) for safety
   b. Should be approached from the uphill side for safety
   c. Should be used based on time and injury considerations
   d. Is used only for trauma situations

10. ______ Which of the following statements is *true?*
   a. Simple access can still require power tools for patient extrication.
   b. Patient safety precedes the safety of crewmembers once EMT–Basics begin care.
   c. Turnout coats and helmets are required for any rescue situation.
   d. Patients can be removed from a vehicle crash without spinal precautions if they have no neck or back pain.

11. ______ What is the role of the nonrescue EMT–Basic?
   a. Coordinate the efforts of the rescue EMTs.
   b. Extricate the patient using nonpower tools.
   c. Cooperate with other workers without allowing their activities to interfere with patient care.
   d. Provide care while others are extricating the patient.

12. ______ CHEMTREC is:
   a. A manufacturer of chemicals that are not hazardous to people or the environment
   b. A hazardous materials team that responds to major incidents
   c. A reference book listing all chemical placards
   d. A service that provides immediate online advice about hazardous materials

13. ______ EMT–Basics should receive education at least to the ______ level for hazardous materials.
   a. First Responder operations
   b. First Responder awareness
   c. Hazardous materials specialist
   d. Hazardous materials technician

14. ______ Which of the following statements is *true?*
   a. Hazardous materials are not found in homes or offices.
   b. Park the ambulance upwind from hazardous materials.
   c. If no hazardous materials are detected, the scene is safe to enter.
   d. Almost every chemical has an odor or color.

15. ______ Which of the following sectors of an incident command system is responsible for coordinating available resources of receiving hospitals, air medical services, and ambulances?
   a. Transportation sector
   b. Staging sector
   c. Support sector
   d. Supply sector

16. ______ Triage means:
   a. Sorting patients based on their type of injury or illness (respiratory, cardiac, trauma, and so forth)
   b. Categorizing patients based on age
   c. Categorizing patients based on severity of illness or injury
   d. Treating patients based on their injuries

17. ______ During triage, EMT–Basics should:
    a. Splint angulated injuries.
    b. Complete an initial assessment and detailed physical examination.
    c. Categorize patients based on the type of injury.
    d. Correct life-threatening injuries.

18. ______ Patients with no pulse or respirations are categorized as:
    a. Highest priority
    b. Intermediate priority
    c. A higher priority compared with minor burns and cuts
    d. The lowest priority

19. ______ A patient with burns to the face, neck, and throat, with difficulty breathing, would be categorized as:
    a. Highest priority
    b. Second priority
    c. The same priority as a patient with major bone injuries
    d. Lowest priority

## CHAPTER 37

# Advanced Airway Techniques

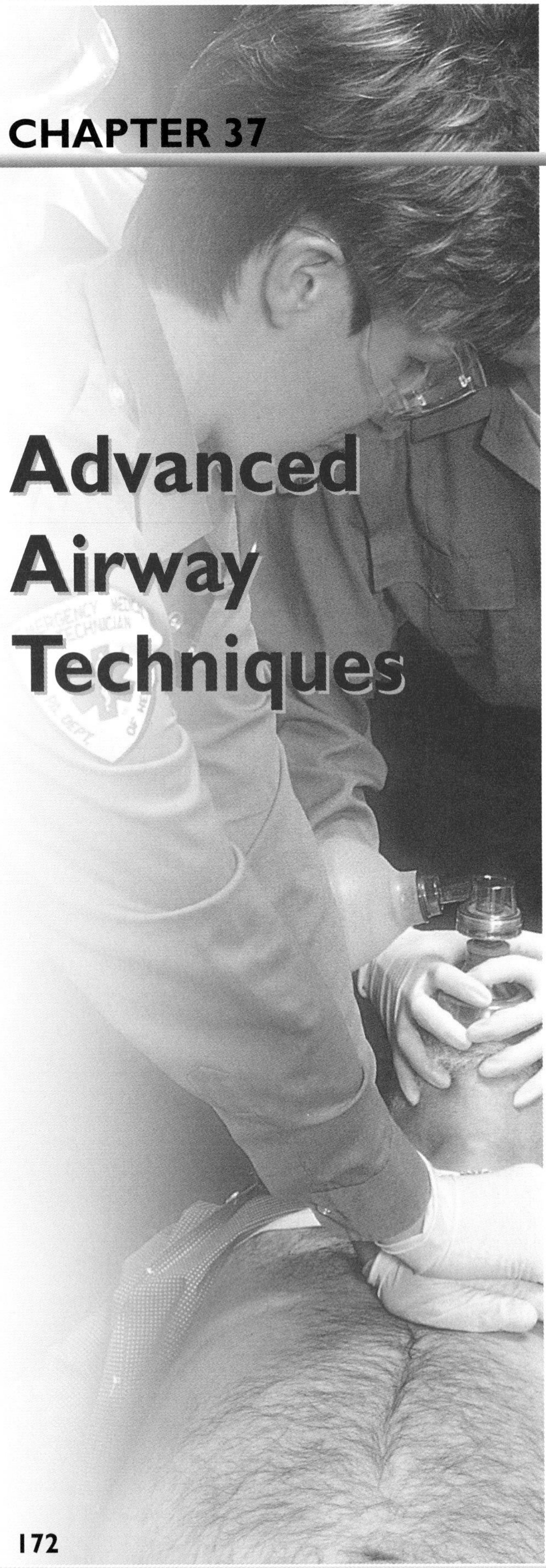

### CHAPTER OUTLINE

I. Sellick Maneuver
   A. Purpose
   B. Anatomic Location
   C. Technique
   D. Special Considerations
II. Advanced Airway Management of Adults
   A. Orotracheal Intubation
      1. Purpose
      2. Indications
      3. Equipment
      4. Techniques of insertion
      5. Complications
   B. Esophageal Tracheal Combitubes
      1. Purpose
      2. Indications
      3. Equipment
      4. Techniques of insertion
      5. Complications
   C. Tracheal Suctioning
III. Advanced Airway Management of Children and Infants
   A. Nasogastric Tubes
   B. Orotracheal Intubation
      1. Anatomic and physiologic considerations
      2. Indications
      3. Equipment
      4. Techniques of insertion
      5. Complications

## MATCHING 1

*Match each term in Column 1 with the correct definition in Column 2.*

**Column 1**

1. ______ Apices of the lungs
2. ______ Bases of the lungs
3. ______ Carina
4. ______ Epigastrium
5. ______ Glottic opening
6. ______ Mainstem bronchi
7. ______ Sternal notch
8. ______ Vallecula

**Column 2**

a. Two branches from the trachea to the lungs
b. Anatomic space between the vocal cords leading to the trachea
c. Bottoms of the lungs, located approximately at the level of the sixth rib
d. Tops of the lungs, located just under the clavicles bilaterally
e. Anatomic location created by the clavicles and the sternum
f. Anatomic space between the base of the tongue and the epiglottis
g. Area over the stomach
h. Point at which the trachea divides into the two mainstem bronchi

## MATCHING 2

*Match each term in Column 1 with the correct definition in Column 2.*

**Column 1**

9. ______ Apneic
10. ______ Compliance
11. ______ Gastric distention
12. ______ Pulse oximetry
13. ______ Self-extubation

**Column 2**

a. Term referring to patients who are not breathing
b. Process of indirectly measuring the amount of oxygen carried in the blood
c. Measure of the elasticity of the lungs
d. Patient's intentional or unintentional removal of a tube
e. Accumulation of air in the stomach, which places pressure on the diaphragm, making artificial ventilation difficult and increasing the possibility of vomiting

## MATCHING 3

*Match each term in Column 1 with the correct definition in Column 2.*

**Column 1**

14. ______ Direct laryngoscopy
15. ______ Endotracheal tube
16. ______ Extubation
17. ______ Laryngoscope
18. ______ Murphy's eye
19. ______ Nasogastric tube
20. ______ Orotracheal intubation
21. ______ Stylet

**Column 2**

a. Process of placing an endotracheal tube into the trachea while visualizing the glottic opening with a laryngoscope
b. Removal of a tube
c. Bendable device placed in the endotracheal tube, giving it rigidity and enabling it to hold a shape
d. Tube placed into the trachea to increase the delivery of oxygen to the lungs and decrease the possibility of aspiration
e. Tube placed through the nose, down the esophagus, and into the stomach
f. Process of inserting an endotracheal tube through the mouth
g. Small hole in the side of an endotracheal tube that provides a passage of air if the tip of the tube becomes clogged
h. Instrument used to visualize the airway during endotracheal intubation

## REVIEW QUESTIONS

1. What is the purpose of the Sellick maneuver?

_______________________________________

_______________________________________

2. ______ The proper place to push on the trachea to perform the Sellick maneuver is the:
   a. Adam's apple
   b. Cricoid ring
   c. Thyroid cartilage
   d. Cricothyroid membrane

3. ______ The Sellick maneuver must be maintained until an endotracheal tube is in position and the position of the tube is confirmed. True (T) or false (F)?

4. List four indications for endotracheal intubation.

   a. _______________________________________

   b. _______________________________________

   c. _______________________________________

   d. _______________________________________

5. Label the parts of the endotracheal tube.

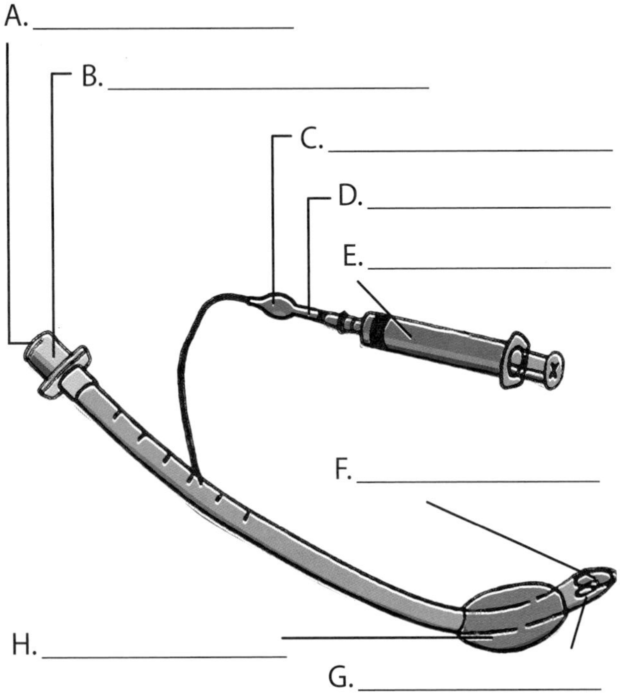


6. ______ Most men require an endotracheal tube between __________, and most women usually require a __________.
   a. 8 and 9; 6 to 8
   b. 8 and 8.5; 7 to 8
   c. 8 and 10; 6.5 to 7.5
   d. 8.5 and 9.5; 7.5 to 8.5

7. List the function of the following:

   Stylet: _______________________________________

   _______________________________________

   Pilot balloon: _______________________________________

   _______________________________________

   Murphy's eye: _______________________________________

   _______________________________________

8. The straight, or ____________________________,

   blade lifts the epiglottis, whereas the curved, or

   ____________________________________, blade

   lifts just in front of the epiglottis to help visualize

   the cords.

9. ______ A commercial device should be used to secure the endotracheal tube in place; tape will not secure the tube adequately. True (T) or false (F)?

10. ______ Which of the following is *true?*
    a. The adult patient's head should be placed in a flexed position when preparing for intubation.
    b. The endotracheal tube should be inserted into an adult patient until Murphy's eye just passes the vocal cords.
    c. Infants may require a towel to be placed under the upper back to elevate the shoulders.
    d. The Sellick maneuver should not be performed on infants before intubation.

11. ______ Gurgling sounds heard over the epigastrium with ventilation mean the tube is in the __________ and must be removed immediately.
   a. Trachea
   b. Right mainstem bronchus
   c. Esophagus
   d. Vallecula

12. ______ The absence of breath sounds on the left side of the chest and presence of breath sounds on the right side of the chest after intubation usually means the tube is in the:
   a. Stomach
   b. Right mainstem bronchus
   c. Esophagus
   d. Left mainstem bronchus

13. ______ The maximum amount of time that is allowed for an intubation procedure between ventilations is ________ seconds.
   a. 60
   b. 15
   c. 30
   d. 45

14. List five complications of intubation.

   a. ______________________________

   b. ______________________________

   c. ______________________________

   d. ______________________________

   e. ______________________________

15. ______ Which of the following is required for use of the esophageal tracheal combitube?
   a. The head must be in the sniffing position.
   b. You must be able to visualize the vocal cords.
   c. Bleeding cannot be present in the airway.
   d. The patient cannot have a gag reflex.

16. ______ If the esophageal tracheal combitube is placed into the trachea, it must be removed and replaced. True (T) or false (F)?

17. The large cuff of the esophageal tracheal Combitube is designed to hold ____________ ml of air; the small cuff is designed to hold __________ ml of air.

18. ______ You have placed the esophageal tracheal Combitube and are listening over the epigastrium while ventilating through the #1 clear tube. You hear gurgling sounds. You should:
   a. Immediately withdraw the tube.
   b. Continue to ventilate through this port.
   c. Ventilate through the blue port and assess epigastric and breath sounds.
   d. Continue to ventilate through this port while assessing breath sounds.

19. List two indications for tracheal suctioning.

   a. ______________________________

   b. ______________________________

20. ______ A nasogastric tube is indicated for which of the following patients?
   a. A patient with head trauma and without spontaneous respirations
   b. A patient who is apneic with a palpable central pulse
   c. A patient who is alert and responsive with abdominal pain
   d. A patient you are unable to ventilate because of gastric distention

21. List four indications for endotracheal intubation in an infant or child.

   a. ______________________________

   b. ______________________________

   c. ______________________________

   d. ______________________________

22. ______ The formula used to select an endotracheal tube size for children is:
    a. (16 + age in years) ÷ 4
    b. (16 + age in months) ÷ 4
    c. (4 + age in years) ÷ 16
    d. (4+ age in months) ÷ 16

23. What two anatomic structures can be used as alternate methods to determine the size of a child's airway?

    a. ______________________________

    b. ______________________________

24. ______ A slow heart rate in a child is an indication that the patient is receiving adequate amounts of oxygen. True (T) or false (F)?

25. ______ Which of the following complications is of greater risk in the infant and child than the adult?
    a. Self-extubation
    b. Mainstem intubation
    c. Esophageal intubation
    d. The risks are the same

26. Your crew is working a cardiac arrest. The automated external defibrillator (AED) has been applied, and shocks have been delivered. Medical direction advises you to intubate the patient's trachea.

    a. Why is endotracheal intubation indicated, and what are the advantages?

    ______________________________

    ______________________________

    b. List the equipment required for intubation.

    ______________________________

    ______________________________

    c. After intubating the patient's trachea, your partner notes diminished lung sounds on the left side. What does this sign indicate, and what should you do to correct it?

    ______________________________

    ______________________________

# DIVISION EIGHT

## Advanced Airway

Chapter 37 Advanced Airway Techniques

## DIVISION TEST

**Directions:** *Place the letter of the correct answer in the space provided.*

1. ______ What is the name of the maneuver performed to prevent passive regurgitation?
   a. Sellick maneuver
   b. Trendelenburg maneuver
   c. Thyroid maneuver
   d. Gastric pressure

2. ______ Which of the following statements best defines the anatomic location of the cricoid ring?
   a. Superior to the cricothyroid membrane
   b. Inferior to the cricothyroid membrane
   c. Superior to the thyroid membrane
   d. Medial to the cricothyroid membrane

3. ______ Which of the following methods would the EMT–Basic use when intubating?
   a. Blind intubation
   b. Retrograde intubation
   c. Digital intubation
   d. Orotracheal intubation

4. ______ Which of the following patients meets the criteria for intubation by an EMT–Basic?
   a. Responsive patient with acute pulmonary edema
   b. Patient who is unresponsive to verbal stimulus but has a gag reflex
   c. An apneic patient who cannot be ventilated with a BVM
   d. Responsive patient with difficulty breathing

5. ______ What size endotracheal tube should be used as a rule for emergency intubation of all adult patients?
   a. 7.0-mm internal diameter
   b. 7.5-mm internal diameter
   c. 8.0-mm internal diameter
   d. 8.5--mm internal diameter

6. ______ When using the curved blade, what anatomic landmark should be used for its placement?
   a. Vocal cords
   b. Epiglottis
   c. Vallecula
   d. Glottic opening

7. ______ What should be used to lubricate the endotracheal tube?
   a. Water
   b. Vaseline
   c. Water-soluble gel
   d. Tubes should not be lubricated

8. ______ How far into the endotracheal tube should a stylet be inserted?
   a. Approximately 1 inch from the end of the tube
   b. 0.25 inches from the cuff or proximal end of Murphy's eye
   c. Stylets should not be used for intubation
   d. To the tip of the endotracheal tube

9. ______ Which of the following statements best describes how the blade is inserted into the patient's mouth?
   a. Hold the laryngoscope in your left hand, insert laryngoscope blade into the right corner of the patient's mouth, and lift and sweep the tongue to the left.
   b. Hold the laryngoscope in your right hand, insert laryngoscope blade into the left corner of the patient's mouth, and lift and sweep the tongue to the right.
   c. Hold the laryngoscope in your left hand, insert laryngoscope blade into the left corner of the patient's mouth, and lift and sweep the tongue to the left.
   d. Hold the laryngoscope in your left hand, insert laryngoscope blade into the middle of the patient's mouth, and lift and sweep the tongue to the left or right.

10. ______ How much air should be inserted in the cuff of the endotracheal tube in the adult patient?
   a. 3 to 5 ml
   b. 5 to 10 ml
   c. 10 to 20 ml
   d. 30 ml

11. ______ What location should be auscultated first following insertion of the endotracheal tube?
   a. Left base
   b. Right base
   c. Sternal notch
   d. Epigastrium

12. ______ If no sounds are heard over the lung fields and gurgling is heard over the stomach, the EMT–Basic should:
   a. Ventilate the patient 12 times per minute.
   b. Put more air in the cuff of the endotracheal tube and listen again.
   c. Deflate the cuff and remove the tube.
   d. Pull back on the endotracheal tube until breath sounds are heard.

13. ______ If the tube is placed in the right mainstem bronchus, what action should the EMT–Basic take?
   a. Deflate the cuff and slowly pull the tube back until breath sounds are heard in all lung fields.
   b. Put more air in the cuff of the endotracheal tube and listen again.
   c. Deflate the cuff, remove the tube, hyperventilate the patient for 2 to 3 minutes, and attempt to intubate again.
   d. Remove the tube, ventilate the patient, and do not attempt to reintubate the patient.

14. ______ Where should the cuff of a properly placed endotracheal tube lie?
   a. At the carina
   b. Superior to the epiglottis
   c. Just past the vocal cords
   d. At the sternal notch

15. ______ Which of the following is a complication of intubation?
   a. Airway protection
   b. Bradycardia
   c. Increased risk of aspiration
   d. Hypoxia

16. ______ Which catheter should be used to suction the nasopharynx or inside the endotracheal tube?
   a. Rigid catheter
   b. Tonsil tip catheter
   c. Only the suction tube with no catheter
   d. Soft catheter

17. ______ Which of the following devices is used to decompress the stomach?
   a. Endotracheal tube
   b. Foley tube
   c. Nasogastric tube
   d. Nasopharyngeal tube

18. ______ Which laryngoscope blade is preferred when intubating an infant?
   a. A curved blade
   b. A MacIntosh blade
   c. A straight blade
   d. No particular blade is preferred

19. ______ What formula is used to determine the tube size for an infant or child patient?
   a. (16+ age in years) ÷ 4
   b. (18+ age in years) ÷ 4
   c. (16+ age in months) ÷ 6
   d. (4+ age in years) ÷ 4

20. ______ Which of the following features is unique to pediatric endotracheal tubes?
   a. The size is not indicated.
   b. One or more black rings are on the distal end.
   c. Infant tubes take more air in the cuff.
   d. Murphy's hole is in the other side of the tube.

# Answer Key

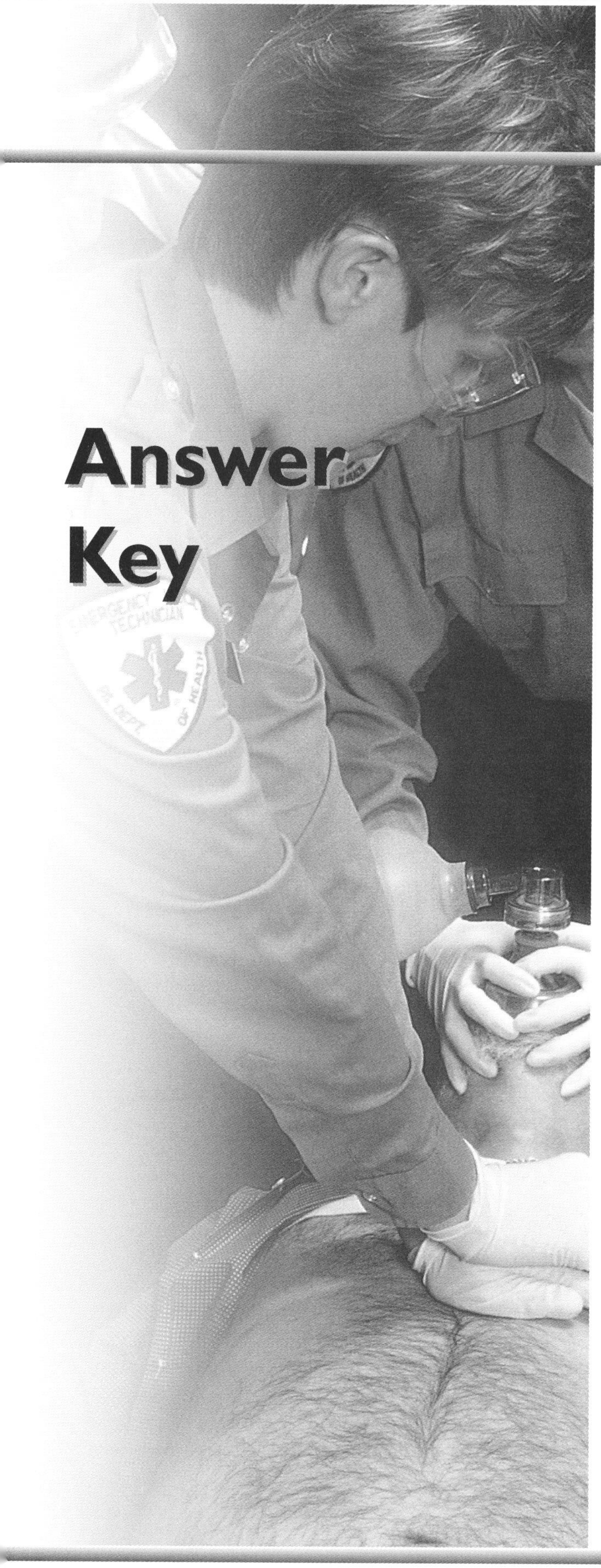

## CHAPTER 1

### INTRODUCTION TO EMERGENCY MEDICAL CARE

#### Matching 1

1. e
2. a
3. d
4. b
5. f
6. c

#### Matching 2

7. b
8. a
9. f
10. e
11. c
12. d

#### Review Questions

1. **True.** Public information and education and resource management are two of NHTSA's 10 standards for EMS. The other eight standards are regulation and policy, human resources and education, transportation, facilities, communications, medical direction, trauma systems, and evaluation.
2. **a.** The NHTSA standard that ensures adequate funding for EMS is the regulation and policy standard.
3. **True.** The facilities standard helps EMS systems make decisions about what is the closest appropriate facility for any particular patient, such as a children's hospital for a pediatric patient.
4. **False.** Not every area in the United States has the ability to reach EMS, police, or fire by dialing 911. EMTs should help educate the public about how to access EMS in their area.

5. **d.** First Responders should provide initial stabilization until additional EMS resources arrive. The First Responder course is designed for people who are likely to encounter an ill or injured patient in their job but who are not educated for ambulance service. First Responders generally stabilize the patient until more help arrives. EMT–Intermediates and EMT–Paramedics are often taught advanced care for trauma patients and to establish intravenous access and administer medications.
6. **c.** The EMT–Basic course prepares people to manage life-threatening injuries and illnesses.
7. Personal safety can be ensured in many ways, including maintaining a healthy body, remaining physically fit, using BSI precautions, and sizing up the scene for potential hazards.
8. **False.** EMT–Basics are responsible for their own personal safety, the safety of their crew members, the patient, and bystanders. EMT–Basics may work with other EMS personnel to ensure the safety of the scene and everyone involved.
9. Roles and responsibilities of the EMT–Basic include personal safety; safety of the crew, patient, and bystanders; patient assessment and care; lifting and moving patients; transport and transfer of care; and patient advocacy.
10. **c.** A medical director is a physician who monitors the care given to patients by EMT–Basics. Medical directors function online and offline.
11. **True.** Direct, or online, medical direction refers to physicians talking with EMT–Basics in the field, face-to-face, or over the radio or telephone.
12. Quality improvement is a system of internal and external reviews and audits of all aspects of an EMS system to identify aspects needing improvement.
13. **c.** Medical direction is the physician monitoring of care that EMTs provide. Medical direction can be direct or indirect and includes the development of protocols and education requirements of EMTs. Medical direction is recommended for EMT–Basics.
14. **a.** Roles and responsibilities of the EMT–Basic include personal safety; safety of the crew, patient, and bystanders; patient assessment; patient care based on assessment findings; lifting and moving patients safely; transport and transfer of care; record keeping and data collection; and patient advocacy (patient rights). **b.** An EMS response includes emergency recognition; system access; EMS personnel dispatch and response; care provided to the patient at the scene; medical direction when necessary; and patient stabilization, transportation, and delivery to the hospital. **c.** By dialing 911 or a 7- or 10-digit telephone number (in areas that do not have 911 access). Talk to your instructor or local EMS provider to find out if EMS providers in your area have any special responsibilities. Be sure you know the correct number for the community to dial to access EMS.

## Chapter 2

## WELL-BEING OF THE EMT–BASIC

### Matching

1. d
2. b
3. c
4. e
5. a

### Review Questions

1. 2—anger; 3—bargaining; 1—denial; 5—acceptance; 4—depression.
2. 3—the patient; 1—personal safety; 4—bystander safety; 2—other crew members.
3. **False.** People move through the stages of death and dying at their own rate. Some people skip stages, and some people never work through all of the stages.
4. EMT–Basics can help a patient who is dying or family members of a dying patient by listening to their concerns without falsely assuring them that the patient will get better. Tell the family members that everything possible is being done. Allow family members to stay with the patient if possible, and allow them to express their emotions. Treat the patient with respect, and protect their privacy.
5. **a.** To reduce stress, change your diet, stop smoking, get regular exercise, learn to relax, balance work, enjoy recreation and family, change your work schedule, and seek professional help.

6. Any situation can cause stress for an EMT–Basic. Situations that are likely to cause stress include mass casualty incidents; infant and child trauma; traumatic amputation; infant or child, spouse, or elder abuse; death or injury of a co-worker or other public safety personnel; and emergency response to the illness or injury of a friend or family member.
7. Stress can be caused by *physical, chemical,* or *emotional* factors.
8. Warning signs of stress include irritability with co-workers, family, friends, and patients; inability to concentrate; physical exhaustion; difficulty sleeping or nightmares; anxiety; indecisiveness; guilt; loss of appetite; loss of interest in sexual activities; isolation; loss of interest in work; increased substance use or abuse; and depression.
9. **True.** Stress can build up over time or occur as a result of a single critical incident.
10. **True.** CISD allows people to talk over their fears and feelings, helping to speed up the recovery process.
11. **False.** Family members of EMT–Basics often face stress related to the EMS profession. Stress is caused by not understanding the profession; by the inability to plan family events because of on-call shifts, rotating shifts, and late ambulance calls; and by the fear of injury on the job.
12. **a.** Critical incident stress occurs when the EMT–Basic is unable to function in the job because of unusually strong emotional reactions. The other three signs listed are associated with stress, but the EMT–Basic is not necessarily unable to function in the job because of them.
13. **d.** Following a debriefing, referrals for additional help should be available. Debriefings should occur 24 to 72 hours after the event, should include everyone associated with the event, and should be an opportunity to discuss the events without placing blame or determining fault.
14. Comprehensive critical incident stress management is a complete program for dealing with the effects of stress before stressful events occur through education, during times of great stress with support services for workers and families, and after the events are over through follow-up debriefings.
15. **False.** Scene safety is the highest priority for an EMT–Basic in every situation and should be assessed before entering the scene or beginning any patient care.
16. **c.** Hand washing is the single most important measure in the prevention of spreading disease.
17. **a.** Gloves are the only BSI precaution needed when minimal bleeding is present. A mask, protective eyewear, and gown may be necessary anytime the bleeding becomes more severe. Many EMS professionals make a habit of always taking BSI precautions, including wearing protective eyewear.
18. **True.** Anytime a chance of splashing fluids exists, the eyes, nose, and mouth should be covered.
19. **c.** EMT–Basics should not enter hazardous materials scenes or treat contaminated patients unless they have undergone specialized hazardous materials education or a specialized hazardous materials crew has made the scene safe.
20. **b.** Rescue situations require EMT–Basics to wear protective clothing to prevent injury from sharp metal and glass. Hazardous materials require varying levels of protective clothing. This type of protective clothing is not required for routine emergency calls.
21. **a.** The stages of death and dying are denial, anger, bargaining, depression, and acceptance. Not all people will go through all the stages or go through them in order. **b.** The wife is in the bargaining stage. **c.** Listen to their concerns, but do not falsely assure them. Let them know that everything possible is being done to help. Allow the family members to remain with the patient and to express their feelings and provide comfort measures.
22. **a.** Warning signs of stress include irritability with co-workers, family, friends, or patients; inability to concentrate; physical exhaustion; difficulty sleeping or having nightmares; anxiety; indecisiveness; guilt; loss of appetite; loss of interest in sexual activities; isolation; loss of interest in work; increased substance use or abuse; and depression. **b.** Stress-reduction techniques include changing your diet; quitting smoking; getting regular exercise; learning to relax; balancing work, recreation, and family; changing your work schedule; and seeking professional help. **c.** Any situation can cause stress. The following is a list of situations that commonly cause stress: mass casualty incidents; infant and child trauma; traumatic amputation; infant, child, or elder abuse; death or injury of a co-worker or other public safety personnel; and an emergency response to the illness or injury of a friend or family member.

## Chapter 3

# MEDICOLEGAL AND ETHICAL ISSUES

### Matching 1

1. b
2. d
3. c
4. e
5. a
6. f

### Matching 2

7. e
8. f
9. d
10. c
11. b
12. a

### Review Questions

1. **a.** In most states, the Department of Transportation National Highway Traffic Safety Administration's National Standard Curriculum is the basis for the scope of practice for EMT–Basics. Medical directors and state legislation may have the ability to limit or expand the scope of practice but generally do not create the basis for the scope of practice.
2. **False.** Protocols and standing orders are used to expand the EMT–Basic's scope of practice and to allow for greater flexibility in the treatment of patients.
3. Duty to act means that an EMT–Basic has a legal responsibility to provide emergency medical care when called on or presented with an opportunity to do so. Duty to act can involve a legal consideration (either formal or implied) or an informal obligation. In some states, being licensed or certified means that you have been educated to assist in an emergency and will do so when necessary.
4. Four criteria must be met for negligence to be proven. The EMT–Basic must have a duty to act, and a breach of that duty to act must occur; damage must occur to the patient; and the damage that occurs must be the result of the EMT–Basic's actions or inactions, known as proximate cause.
5. **b.** EMT–Basics must ensure that the patient's care is continued at the same level or at a higher level to avoid abandonment. An EMT–Basic releasing a patient to hospital staff is the only example listed of care being transferred to a higher level.
6. The term that describes permission to be treated is called *consent.* All competent patients must give consent before an EMT–Basic can begin treatment.
7. To give expressed consent, the patient must be of legal age, able to make a rational decision, and understand the risks of treatment or refusing treatment.
8. **False.** Parents, as their children's legal guardians, have the right to accept or refuse care on behalf of the child, regardless of the child's wishes.
9. An emancipated minor is a person who is not yet of legal age but is in the military, married, pregnant, or out on his or her own and able to provide for him or herself. The specific statutes pertaining to emancipation vary from state to state.
10. EMT–Basics should try to persuade a patient who is refusing care to accept treatment or at least transport for evaluation at the receiving facility. EMT–Basics must inform the patient of the risks associated with refusing treatment and transport. After ensuring that the patient is competent to refuse, contact medical direction and then properly document the patient's refusal. Be sure to inform the patient that you will be willing to return if the patient changes his or her mind, which should also be documented.
11. **c.** Assault occurs when someone is threatened with offensive physical contact. Battery occurs when someone is actually touched without consent. Assault and battery are often used interchangeably, but they do have separate definitions. Negligence occurs when an EMT–Basic fails to act as a reasonable, prudent EMT–Basic would under similar circumstances.
12. **True.** Advance directives allow a patient's wishes to be known concerning medical treatment in specific situations if the patient is unable to speak for him or herself.
13. **b.** If a DNR order has not been given, the EMTs have no choice but to begin resuscitation.
14. Patient confidentiality is an important concept for EMT–Basics to understand and comply with to protect a patient's right to privacy. EMT–Basics can release confidential information when giving a report to other health care workers who will be taking care of the patient, when a reportable situation (e.g., suspected child abuse, gunshot wounds) exists, for third-party payment for service, and when subpoenaed for information by a court of law.

15. **a.** Gunshot wounds, neglect, rape, stab wounds, animal bites, and certain infectious diseases routinely require reporting.
16. HIPAA, the Health Insurance Portability and Accountability Act, is in place to protect the privacy of patients and to keep their protected health information confidential.
17. **False.** Patients must sign a legal document stating that they wish to donate their organs on dying. EMT–Basics will treat organ donor patients with the same lifesaving measures as they would any other patient.
18. **False.** Although EMT–Basics should disturb as little as possible at the crime scene, treating the patient properly may be impossible without disturbing the scene. The EMT–Basic should provide all treatments necessary and note any movement of evidence.
19. **a.** The standard of care is the minimum acceptable level of care normally provided in the area. **b.** Negligence occurs when a patient suffers damage or injury because an EMT fails to perform to the accepted standard of care. **c.** For negligence to be proven, four criteria must be met: (1) a duty to act exists, (2) a breach of duty has occurred, (3) damage has occurred, and (4) a proximate cause exists.
20. **a.** Because the patient is unresponsive and unable to give expressed consent, permission to treat would be implied in the scenario. **b.** Implied consent assumes that all unresponsive patients with an immediately life-threatening or disabling injury or illness would want to receive treatment and would provide expressed consent if they were able to do so. **c.** Expressed consent means the patient directly agrees to accept your treatment and gives permission to proceed with care. The patient must be of legal age and able to make a rational decision and must understand the procedure and any associated risks.
21. **a.** A living will is a type of advance directive that describes the kind of lifesaving treatment that a patient wants (or does not want) if the patient becomes unable to request or refuse that treatment. **b.** Durable power of attorney is a written document identifying a guardian to make medical decisions for the patient when the patient can no longer make these decisions. **c.** You should continue with life-support measures, ask the son to produce the written documents, and consult with medical direction. The documents should bear the patient's and witnesses' signatures and should be notarized.

# Chapter 4

## THE HUMAN BODY

### Matching 1

1. b
2. a
3. e
4. d
5. c

### Matching 2

6. c
7. f
8. b
9. g
10. e
11. d
12. a

### Matching 3

13. a
14. d
15. c
16. b
17. e

### Matching 4

18. a
19. d
20. b
21. e
22. c
23. f

### Labeling

1. **a.** Lateral; **b.** posterior; **c.** midaxillary line; **d.** superior; **e.** anterior; **f.** inferior; **g.** medial; **h.** midline.
2. **a.** Vertebral column; **b.** ribs; **c.** radius; **d.** skull; **e.** mandible; **f.** clavicle; **g.** sternum; **h.** humerus; **i.** pelvis; **j.** femur; **k.** patella; **l.** tibia.

### Review Questions

1. **a.** The midaxillary line runs through the armpits and ankles, dividing the body into front and back halves, or anterior and posterior planes.
2. The sole of the foot is called the plantar surface.
3. **a.** A patient lying supine is lying on his or her back. Patients lying with their head elevated are in a Fowler's position, with feet elevated is in a shock position, and facedown is prone.

4. **d.** The oropharynx is directly behind the mouth. The nasopharynx is directly behind the nose. The epiglottis is a leaflike flap that prevents food from entering the trachea. The larynx is just below the epiglottis, at the opening of the trachea.
5. **a.** The trachea is also known as the windpipe.
6. **c.** The diaphragm and the intercostal muscles are used during normal breathing. The diaphragm flattens and lowers when the muscle fibers contract, causing air to be pulled into the lungs. Intercostal muscles contract, causing the ribs to move upward and outward.
7. **b.** When the muscle fibers in the diaphragm contract, the dome of the diaphragm flattens and lowers, drawing air into the lungs.
8. **b.** Blood returned to the lungs from the body is high in carbon dioxide and low in oxygen. Gas exchange takes place in the alveoli, and oxygenated blood is returned to the body.
9. **b.** The normal adult respiratory rate is between 12 and 20 breaths per minute.
10. **b.** The trachea of small child is soft and easily obstructed.
11. **b.** The heart consists of four chambers—two atria and two ventricles.
12. **b.** Oxygen-poor blood enters the right atrium and is pumped into the right ventricle. The blood is then pumped to the lungs where it is oxygenated. Blood returns from the lungs into the left atrium, to the left ventricle, and is then pumped to the body.
13. **d.** Arteries carry blood away from the heart, and veins return blood to the heart. The aorta is an example of an artery. Venules are tiny veins, and capillaries are the smallest blood vessels in the body.
14. **b.** The average adult man has 5 to 6 L of blood in his body.
15. **c.** Plasma is the fluid component of blood. Red blood cells carry oxygen, white blood cells are important in the body's defense system, and platelets play a role in blood clotting.
16. **a.** The first number recorded in the blood pressure is the systolic pressure, which is the pressure in the arteries when the heart contracts. The second number is the diastolic pressure, which is the pressure in the arteries when the heart is at rest.
17. **d.** The zygomatic bones form the cheekbones.
18. **a.** The cervical vertebrae are in the neck, the thoracic vertebrae attach to the ribs, the lumbar vertebrae are in the lower back, and the sacral vertebrae form the pelvis.
19. **d.** The superior portion of the breastbone (or sternum) is called the manubrium. The xiphoid process is the distal tip of the breastbone.
20. **a.** The shoulder is an example of a ball and socket joint.
21. **a.** The central nervous system consists of the brain and spinal cord. The peripheral nervous system consists of the sensory and motor nerves.
22. **True.** The peripheral nerves carry sensory and motor information between the spinal column and the other parts of the body, relaying information from the environment to the brain and commands from the brain to the body.
23. **True.** Signals are sent to the motor nerves from the brain. The motor nerves cause the skeletal muscles to react and are responsible for the movement of the body.
24. **b.** The epidermis is the outermost layer; the dermis is the deeper layer containing the sweat glands, hair follicles, blood vessels and nerve endings; and the subcutaneous layer is the deepest layer, which stores fat and serves as insulation for the body.
25. The digestive system breaks down food so that it can be absorbed into the blood and delivered to the cells as nutrients, vitamins, and minerals.
26. Chemicals released from glands within the body are called *hormones.* Hormones are chemicals released into the bloodstream that regulate many of the body's activities.
27. **a.** The trachea splits into two mainstem bronchi. The bronchi subdivide into smaller and smaller air passages until they end at the alveoli. **b.** The process of ventilation uses two main sets of muscles: the diaphragm and intercostal muscles, which increase the size of the thoracic cavity, pulling air into the lungs. Exhalation begins with relaxation of these muscles, which decreases the size of the thoracic cavity, forcing air out through the nose and mouth. **c.** As oxygen-rich air enters the alveoli, blood with low levels of oxygen and high levels of carbon dioxide is flowing through the capillaries surrounding the alveoli. Gases move from areas of greater concentration to areas of lesser concentration, and therefore oxygen enters the blood and carbon dioxide is removed.

28. **a.** Blood pressure is the measurement of the pressure exerted against the walls of the arteries, measured in millimeters of mercury (mm Hg). **b.** The top number is known as the systolic reading, which is the measurement of the pressure pushing against the arterial walls when the heart contracts. The bottom number is the diastolic reading, which is the measurement of the pressure against the arterial walls when the heart relaxes. **c.** You should advise the woman that age and various individual factors can affect blood . pressure readings. You also should tell her that the measurement of 184/96 mm Hg is considered higher than average but may be normal for her. She should make an appointment with her private physician to have her blood pressure evaluated more thoroughly.
29. **a.** What are skeletal muscles? **b.** What is the peripheral nervous system? **c.** What is the dermis?

## Chapter 5

## BASELINE VITAL SIGNS AND SAMPLE HISTORY

### Matching 1

1. d
2. a
3. i
4. h
5. b
6. c
7. f
8. e
9. g

### Matching 2

10. a
11. e
12. c
13. d
14. b
15. f

### Matching 3

16. a
17. b
18. d
19. c

### Review Questions

1. When assessing breathing, assess the *rate* and *quality* of the patient's respirations. Rate, how often the patient breathes, is expressed in breaths per minute. Quality is measured by assessing depth, use of accessory muscles, and any noises from the airway.
2. **d.** The average respiratory rate for an adult is 12 to 20 breaths per minute, for children is 15 to 30 breaths per minute, and for infants is 25 to 50 breaths per minute.
3. The respiratory rate is determined by counting the number of breaths in 30 seconds and multiplying by two. If the breathing is irregular, you may need to assess for a full minute.
4. **False.** The noise made by the tongue partially blocking the airway is called *snoring.* Crowing is a long, high-pitched sound when breathing in. Both cases indicate a respiratory problem.
5. **d.** Wheezing is a high-pitched whistling sound that is usually caused by constriction of smaller airways or bronchioles. Snoring is a sign that the patient cannot keep the airway fully open. Gurgling indicates liquid in the airway. Grunting is the sound created when the patient forcefully exhales against a closed glottic opening, which traps air and keeps the alveoli open.
6. **False.** Pulses can be felt in the arteries when the heart contracts but not in the veins. Assess pulses in areas when the arteries pass over a bone and close to the skin.
7. When assessing the pulse, note the *rate* and *quality.* The rate is determined by counting the beats in 30 seconds and multiplying by two. Assessing quality includes determining the regularity and strength of the beats.
8. **a.** The average resting pulse rate for an adult should be 60 to 80 beats per minute. This number is only an average, and rates outside of the average may be normal for a patient.
9. A regular pulse means that the length of time between each beat is constant. An irregular pulse means that the time between beats is not constant. A weak pulse means that the heart is not pumping effectively or that blood volume is low.
10. **c.** When assessing the skin, assess the color, temperature, and condition of the skin. Capillary refill may be assessed in infants and children.

11. The skin color is assessed in the nail beds, oral mucosa, or conjunctiva, where the normal color is pink for patients with light or dark skin. The level of oxygen in the blood is easy to assess because the capillary beds run close to the surface of the skin.
12. Abnormal skin colors include *flushed* or red, *cyanotic* or blue-gray, *jaundiced* or yellow, and pale.
13. To identify skin temperature, the skin of the *trunk* is more reliable than the skin of the extremities. The extremities will become cool faster than the rest of the body and may not provide an accurate assessment.
14. Abnormal skin temperatures include hot (which may be caused by fever or exposure to heat), cool (which may be caused by poor perfusion or exposure to cold), and cold (when the patient is exposed to extreme cold).
15. The normal skin condition is dry. Abnormal skin conditions include moist, wet, and extremely dry. Cool and moist skin is called clammy skin.
16. **b.** Capillary refill in infants and children should take less than 2 seconds. A longer time may indicate poor perfusion.
17. *Dilated* pupils are big, and *constricted* pupils are small.
18. Equal and reactive to light means that both pupils constrict when a light is shined into them and that they constrict and dilate equally in relationship to one another.
19. **c.** When pupils react normally to light, they should constrict equally.
20. If the light in a room is too bright, the pupils may not react when a light is shined into them. In this case, cover the eyes from light and then expose them to light again to measure the reaction.
21. **True.** Blood pressure is a measure of the force exerted against the walls of the arteries, when the heart is both contracting (systolic pressure) and at rest (diastolic pressure).
22. Blood pressure can be measured by listening using a stethoscope, called *auscultation,* or by feeling for the return of a pulse, called *palpation.*
23. **d.** Stable patients should be reassessed every 15 minutes, and unstable patients should be reassessed every 5 minutes. Be sure to record this information and include the information in the report to the receiving facility.
24. **True.** SAMPLE stands for signs and symptoms, allergies, medications, past pertinent history, last oral intake, and events leading to the illness or injury.
25. **False.** When assessing a patient's SAMPLE history, assess only the patient's past pertinent medical history.
26. **False.** A medical identification tag may alert you to information regarding the patient's history, medications, or allergies that would cause you to care for the patient differently. When patients are unable to give you information about themselves, always look for medical identification tags.
27. Accurately recording the vital signs and patient history is important because trends in the patient's condition may be noted by comparing sets of vital signs. The patient's condition may cause medical direction to direct you to change your care. The history and vital signs also will be valuable information for the personnel at the receiving facility when they begin to decide how they will treat the patient.
28. Pertinent negatives are clinical signs and symptoms that assist in determining a clear field impression. The absence of these pertinent negatives may help you distinguish specific clinical conditions.
29. **a.** 30 to 40 breaths per minute; **b.** 80 to 120 beats per minute; **c.** 94/54 mm Hg.
30. **a.** Evaluate the rate and quality of the patient's respirations. **b.** Intercostal muscles, neck muscles, chest muscles, abdominal muscles, and upper and lower back muscles are often used as accessory muscles. **c.** Wheezing is a high-pitched whistling sound that is usually caused by constriction of smaller airways.

# Chapter 6

## LIFTING AND MOVING PATIENTS

### Matching I

1. d
2. a
3. c
4. f
5. b
6. e

### Matching II

7. b
8. a
9. c
10. e
11. d

### Review Questions

1. **False.** Knowing both your and your partner's lifting capabilities is important. Call for additional help when necessary.

2. To lift safely, keep your back straight and use your legs, not your back, to lift the patient. Keep the weight close to your body. Call for additional help if necessary. Do not twist your torso when lifting, and keep your feet shoulder-width apart.
3. **False.** When possible, roll rather than carry a patient. Sometimes, however, carrying the patient is preferable, such as when the terrain is uneven.
4. **False.** One-handed carrying techniques allow more rescuers to carry the weight and allow for better balance of the weight.
5. When transporting a patient down stairs is necessary, use the stair chair whenever possible. The stair chair is more maneuverable and was designed to carry patients down stairs. The stair chair cannot be used if the patient is unresponsive or has a suspected spinal injury.
6. **b.** When possible, do not reach far in front of you or reach for long periods. When reaching, keep your back in a locked position, avoid leaning back over your hips, and avoid twisting your back.
7. When performing a log roll, keep your back straight while leaning over the patient, lean from the hips, and use your shoulder muscles to help with the roll.
8. **a.** When possible, push the weight rather than pull. Pushing causes less strain on your body than pulling.
9. Although time to immobilize the patient is insufficient when an emergency move is required, the *spine* can be protected by pulling against the long axis of the body.
10. **b.** Emergency moves are used when a danger to the patient or the rescue crew exists.
11. **True.** Although the patient should be moved rapidly during an urgent move, take time to protect the spine if injury is suspected.
12. **a.** A pregnant patient should be rolled onto her left side to prevent the fetus from compressing the vena cava.
13. **False.** Any patient with a suspected spinal injury should be fully immobilized on a long backboard.
14. **c.** A patient with signs and symptoms of shock should be transported in the shock position, on his or her back, with the legs elevated 8 to 12 inches.
15. **a.** All patients (except those who are unresponsive or have suspected spinal injuries) should be transported in the position of comfort.
16. **a.** A stair chair is the best method to use when you must carry a responsive patient down steep stairs. **b.** A stair chair should not be used for any patient with a possible spinal injury or who is unresponsive. **c.** A patient with a possible spinal injury should be transported down stairs immobilized on a long spine board.
17. Yes. He is unresponsive, has inadequate breathing, and needs lifesaving care.

## Chapter 7

## ASSISTING THE ALS PROVIDER

### Matching

1. e
2. j
3. f
4. k
5. d
6. h
7. g
8. b
9. a
10. i
11. c

### Review Questions

1. The right arm lead is white, the left arm lead is black, and the left leg lead is brown.
2. Before applying ECG electrodes, you may need to remove excess moisture or excess hair from the skin.
3. Discard IV fluid if the bag is expired, it is discolored, or any fluid is leaking.
4. **a.** A macrodrip administration set delivers 1 ml of fluid for each 10 or 15 drops, depending on the set. A microdrip administration set delivers 1 ml of fluid for each 60 drops.
5. b. When preparing an administration set, clamp the tubing and insert the spike into the fluid bag. Squeeze the drip chamber, open the clamp, and then run fluids through the line.
6. Tape a small loop of IV tubing onto the patient's skin while securing the IV site to help prevent dislodgement of the catheter from the insertion site.
7. **a.** Direct laryngoscopy is the most common method of endotracheal intubation.

8. A straight laryngoscope blade is called a *Miller blade.* A curved laryngoscope blade is called a MacIntosh blade.
9. To assist the ALS provider with preparing the endotracheal tube, the EMT can check the distal cuff by inflating and deflating the cuff, insert a stylet, and lubricate the tube.
10. Endotracheal tube placement can be confirmed by listening to breath sounds, the use of an end-tidal carbon dioxide detector or esophageal detector device, the absence of epigastric sounds, symmetrical chest rise and fall, and improved skin color.

## Division One Examination

1. **d.** EMT–Basics provide primary care for life-threatening illnesses and injuries before the patient reaches the hospital. First Responders stabilize the patient until the ambulance arrives. EMT–Paramedics are advanced-level prehospital care providers. Definitive care for trauma patients cannot be provided in the prehospital setting.
2. b. The NHTSA standard for EMS that ensures that everyone has access to basic emergency medical care is resource management.
3. c. The standard for the education of prehospital emergency care providers is set by the National EMS Education and Practice Blueprint.
4. **b.** In most states, EMT-Basic is the minimum acceptable education level for ambulance staff.
5. **b.** One role of the EMT–Basic is to be concerned about patients' rights or be an advocate for patients. EMT–Basics often work with other public safety personnel, including firefighters and police officers. EMT–Basics should be concerned with personal safety first, then the safety of crew members, followed by safety of the patient and then of bystanders. All health care providers require continuing education to keep their skills current and stay informed about the latest changes in health care.
6. **a.** EMT–Basics have many roles and responsibilities, including personal safety, safety of the crew, patient, and bystanders, patient assessment, patient care based on assessment findings, lifting and moving patients safely, transport and transfer of care, record keeping and data collection, and patient advocacy (patient rights).
7. **a.** Scene and personal safety must be the first priority during any emergency call. None of the other aspects of patient care can occur if the EMT–Basic is injured.
8. **c.** Direct medical direction means that direct communication is taking place between the physician, medical directors, and the EMT in the field. Development of protocols, teaching in primary and continuing education courses, and quality improvement following EMS responses are all indirect medical direction.
9. **a.** Dying patients or their families may experience denial, anger, bargaining, depression, and acceptance. Not all patients and their families go through all of the stages, or the order of stages may vary.
10. **a.** Respect the patient's needs for dignity, sharing, communications, privacy and control. Do not lie or falsely assure the patient or the family for any reason. Be honest and direct when answering their questions. When appropriate, a reassuring touch can console and comfort the patient and the family members. Allow the patient to remain near family members when possible.
11. **d.** CISD is an acronym for critical incident stress debriefing, which is a process to help emergency workers deal with emotions and stresses caused by on-the-job responsibilities.
12. **a.** Critical incident stress debriefing includes preincident stress education, on-scene peer support, support for families of emergency workers, and follow-up care for emergency workers.
13. **c.** Surgical masks (worn by the patient or the EMT–Basic) or high-efficiency particulate air respirators (worn by the EMT–Basic) can be used by EMT–Basics when necessary as part of their BSI precautions. Some masks have eye-protection shields attached. Self-contained breathing apparatus may be used in some situations but are not routinely included in BSI precautions from blood and other body fluids. Industrial grade goggles and helmets with chinstraps are used for rescue operations.
14. **b.** Negligence occurs when a patient suffers damages or injury because of the EMT–Basics actions or inactions. Abandonment occurs when care is not continued at the same or higher level. Assault or battery (or both) occurs when a patient is treated without his or her consent or after refusing treatment.
15. **b.** Abandonment occurs when care is discontinued without the patient's consent and without ensuring that care is being continued at the same or a higher level. Assault is the threat of harm, and battery is unlawfully touching a person without consent.

16. **a.** When a contract exists between an ambulance service and a municipality, EMTs have a legal duty to act. Even when no legal duty to act has been established, an ethical duty to act may exist.
17. **c.** Patients under the influence of alcohol or drugs cannot make rational decisions about their care and can be treated under implied consent.
18. **b.** Patients who are unresponsive can be treated under the terms of implied consent. A patient must be responsive to give expressed consent. Parents have the right to refuse care for their children, and EMT–Basics must honor this refusal. Patients have the right to change their mind and refuse care even after initially giving consent.
19. **d.** When you are not sure if a patient should be treated or not, err on the side of treatment. When a patient refuses care, the EMT–Basic must explain why care is needed and explain the potential risks involved with refusing treatment. Contact medical direction and have the patient and a witness sign a refusal form. Patients have the right to refuse or withdraw from treatment any time. Parents can make decisions regarding the care of their child, even if the child refuses.
20. **a.** Patients have the right to decide, along with their physicians, what treatment plan is best for them in the event that they cannot speak for themselves. Some states do not recognize the DNR order as being within the scope of practice for prehospital care providers. The DNR order must be signed by the physician and the patient and must be seen by the EMT–Basic at the scene.
21. **c.** Confidential information can be released when the patient is involved in a reportable situation, such as child abuse. EMT–Basics should take care not to divulge confidential information when using a case for continuing education. EMT–Basics can give confidential information to law enforcement personnel when subpoenaed.
22. **a.** The pharynx is another word for the throat. The olecranon process is part of the upper extremity. The mitral valve is in the heart to prevent the backflow of blood from the left ventricle to the left atrium. Adrenaline is a hormone that helps prepare the body for emergencies.
23. **d.** Gas exchange takes place in the alveoli, the small air sacs that are surrounded by capillaries in the lungs.
24. **a.** Children usually breathe more quickly than adults because children have greater oxygen demands. Normal respiratory rate for an adult is 12 to 20 breaths per minute. Children's normal respiratory rate varies with age.
25. **c.** The trachea of an infant or child is more easily obstructed by swelling or foreign objects because of the smaller size. In general, all of the structures of the respiratory system in children are smaller and more easily obstructed. The tongue is large and often causes obstruction. The trachea is very flexible because it is less developed.
26. **a.** Oxygenated blood is pumped from the lungs into the left atrium, to the left ventricle, and then to the body. The average man has approximately 5 L of blood. Platelets are important for blood clotting. White blood cells are important for fighting infection. The upper chambers of the heart are the atria, and the lower chambers are the ventricles.
27. **b.** The femur is the thigh. The tibia and fibula are both bones in the lower leg. The patella is the kneecap.
28. **c.** The middle layer of the skin is the dermis, the outer layer is the epidermis, and the deeper layer is the subcutaneous level. The central nervous system is composed of the brain and spinal cord. The peripheral nervous system is composed of motor nerves that carry information from the brain to the body and sensory nerves that carry information from the body to the brain. The endocrine system releases hormones in the body.
29. **b.** The average pulse rate range for an adult is 60 to 80 beats per minute. These numbers are only the average. A pulse rate higher or lower can be normal for an individual.
30. **d.** Bilateral chest expansion means that both lungs are expanding equally, which is associated with normal respirations. Increased effort of breathing, grunting and stridor, and use of accessory muscles indicate abnormal breathing.
31. **a.** The skin temperature can be described as hot, warm, cool, or cold. Dry and clammy are skin conditions; pale is a skin color.
32. **b.** Capillary refill is assessed only in patients younger than 6 years of age. Pupils should constrict equally when exposed to light. The diastolic pressure is the measurement of force exerted when the heart is at rest. The systolic pressure is the measurement of the forces exerted when the heart is contracting. Vital signs should be reassessed every 5 minutes for an unstable patient and every 15 minutes for a stable patient.

33. **d.** The acronym *SAMPLE* stands for signs and symptoms, allergies, medications, past pertinent history, last oral intake, and events leading to the illness or injury. A symptom is something the patient must describe to you. A sign is an observable condition. Ask the patient about any allergies, including food, medications, and insects. The patient's pertinent history should be assessed; a complete medical history is unnecessary.
34. **a.** When lifting, be sure to lift with your legs, not your back. Do not twist your body to move the patient. Use as many rescuers as necessary to safely lift or move the patient.
35. **c.** Do not bend at the waist when lifting. Bending at the waist means that you will be lifting with your back, not your legs. Both the power-lift and power-grip will help the EMT–Basic lift safely.
36. **a.** Emergency moves are used when immediate danger is present or when you cannot treat the patient in his or her current position. Spinal protection measures can be taken during urgent moves. A patient with signs and symptoms of shock would require an urgent move.
37. **a.** Unresponsive patients without traumatic injuries should be transported in the recovery position to help maintain an open airway.
38. **d.** Responsive patients without traumatic injuries should be transported in the position of comfort.
39. **b.** A 12-lead ECG system uses six electrodes placed on the patient's chest and four electrodes placed on the extremities.
40. **c.** A macrodrip administration set delivers 10 or 15 drops of fluid per milliliter. A microdrip administration set delivers 60 drops of fluid per milliliter.

# Chapter 8

## THE AIRWAY

### Matching 1

1. b
2. d
3. c
4. e
5. a
6. f

### Matching 2

7. e
8. b
9. f
10. d
11. c
12. a

### Matching 3

13. c
14. b
15. a
16. d
17. f
18. e

### Matching 4

19. a
20. b
21. d
22. e
23. c
24. f

### Labeling

1. **a.** Nasopharynx; **b.** oropharynx; **c.** epiglottis; **d.** larynx; **e.** right bronchus; **f.** diaphragm; **g.** left bronchus.
2. **a.** One-way valve; **b.** self-inflating bag; **c.** oxygen reservoir valve; **d.** face mask; **e.** oxygen supply; **f.** oxygen reservoir.

### Review Questions

1. **True.** When the diaphragm contracts, it flattens and increases the size of the chest, pulling air into the nose and mouth.
2. **False.** Exhalation is normally a passive process but can be an active process if the patient has respiratory compromise.
3. **c.** The normal respiratory rate for an adult is 12 to 20 breaths per minute. This range is only an average; a patient may be breathing faster or slower and still be within his or her normal limits.
4. Signs and symptoms of inadequate breathing include difficulty breathing or shortness of breath; a rate that is too fast or too slow; an irregular rhythm; diminished or absent breath sounds; unequal or inadequate chest expansion; increased effort of breathing; inadequate tidal volume (shallow breathing); cyanotic, pale, or cool and clammy skin; and use of accessory muscles. Signs of adequate breathing include adequate rate and depth, regular rhythm, bilateral chest expansion, quiet breathing, and no visible labor associated with breathing.

5. Children rely most heavily on their diaphragm for respiration; their chest muscles are less developed and not as efficient as the muscles of an adult.
6. To deliver oxygen to a patient, you will need an oxygen source, such as an oxygen cylinder, a regulator (to get the oxygen at an appropriate rate and pressure), and a delivery device, such as a nonrebreather mask, nasal cannula, or ventilation device.
7. EMT–Basics commonly use nonrebreather masks and nasal cannulas. EMT–Basics use nonrebreather masks in most cases. If a patient will not tolerate a mask, a nasal cannula may be used.
8. **c.** Nonrebreather masks can deliver up to 90% oxygen when the flow rate is set at 15 L/minute.
9. **d.** Set the flow rate at 15 L/minute when delivering oxygen by nonrebreather mask.
10. **False.** The nasal cannula is a low-flow device and therefore a poor substitute for a nonrebreather mask. The nasal cannula is used only when the patient will not tolerate a mask.
11. **c.** The oxygen flow rate can be set up to 6 L/minute when using a nasal cannula.
12. The patient loses muscular control of the jaw, the tongue falls posteriorly into the airway, and the epiglottis can block the opening to the trachea.
13. **False.** The head-tilt, chin-lift maneuver is used most commonly to open the airway, unless trauma is suspected. When trauma is suspected, the jaw thrust must be used to open the airway.
14. When performing the head-tilt, chin-lift maneuver, with one hand on the forehead, tilt the head back and use the other hand to lift the chin. The jaw thrust is performed by placing your index fingers at the angles of the jaw and the meaty parts of your thumbs on the maxilla, using your thumb tips to keep the mouth open. Both methods are designed to maintain a patent airway.
15. Oral airways are measured from the corner of the mouth to the *earlobe* or the *angle of the jaw.* The correct size is important to ensure that the tongue is lifted out of the airway.
16. **b.** For infants and children, the preferred method for inserting an oral airway is by using a tongue depressor to lift the tongue out of the airway and then inserting the oral airway right side up.
17. **True.** An oral airway will stimulate the gag reflex of a responsive patient. A nasal airway may be better tolerated.
18. The nasal airway is measured from the tip of the nose to the *earlobe.* The airway is inserted with the bevel toward the *septum* of the nose.
19. Gurgling is one of the most common signs of liquid in the airway, and immediate suction is indicated. Suction must be readily available at all times during patient assessment and care.
20. **b.** You should insert the suction catheter only as far as you can see. Rigid suction catheters are easy to control and can be used on responsive and unresponsive patients.
21. **a.** Bulb syringes are used to suction the mouth and nose of infants and children as old as 3 or 4 months of age; the syringes must be compressed before being placed into the mouth or nose.
22. **a.** Suctioning should not last more than 15 seconds before delivering more oxygen to the patient.
23. When performing mouth-to-mouth ventilation, open the airway, take a deep breath, pinch the patient's nostrils closed, make a seal with your mouth on the patient's lips, exhale until the chest rises over 1 second, and ventilate once every 5 seconds for adults and every 3 to 5 seconds for infants and children.
24. **c.** Mouth-to-mask is the preferred ventilation technique because it provides excellent ventilatory volumes, requires only one person, allows for a two-hand mask seal, and can be attached to supplemental oxygen.
25. **b.** When using the two-person technique, one person maintains the mask seal with both hands, and the second person squeezes the bag. Two people are preferred when maintaining a mask seal is difficult for one person. In either technique, ventilate the patient once every 5 seconds for adult patients and once every 3 seconds for infants and children.
26. **d.** The flow-restricted, oxygen-powered ventilation device delivers 100% oxygen when the trigger is pushed at a maximum flow rate of 40 L/minute. The EMT–Basic must maintain an open airway and a good mask seal. This device is not recommended for infants and children because it may cause lung tissue damage and cause air to enter the stomach.
27. **b.** The EMT–Basic who is maintaining the mask seal also can perform the jaw thrust. The head-tilt, chin-lift maneuver is not recommended for trauma patients. The mask seal is not changed, and the patient should be ventilated once every 5 seconds for adult patients and once every 3 seconds for infants and children.

28. Signs of adequate ventilation include chest rises and falls with each ventilation, heart rate returns to the normal age-appropriate rate, and skin color improves. Signs and symptoms of inadequate ventilation include failure of the chest to rise and fall with ventilation, a rate that is too fast or too slow, gastric distention, a heart rate that does not return to normal, and cyanosis that is present or worsens.
29. When chest rise during ventilation is poor, (1) reposition the jaw or head, (2) check the mask seal, (3) try a different technique, and (4) check for an obstruction.
30. You can usually ventilate a patient with a tracheal stoma with a mask directly through the stoma. Create a seal with the mask, and ventilate as usual using a BVM or mouth-to-mask technique. The head does not need to be positioned because you are ventilating below the level of the tongue and epiglottis.
31. **False.** An oral airway can be used for an unresponsive trauma patient to help maintain an open airway.
32. **True.** Dentures and other dental appliances help create a mask seal by giving structure to the face. They should be left in place unless they are so loose that they may cause an obstruction.
33. **a.** The airway structures of infants and children are smaller than those in adults. The tongue takes up proportionately more space, and the trachea is very narrow and easily obstructed by small amounts of fluid or swelling. **b.** Signs and symptoms of inadequate breathing include difficulty breathing, shortness of breath, fast or slow rate, irregular rhythm, diminished or absent breath sounds, unequal or inadequate chest expansion, increased breathing effort, inadequate tidal volume, shallow breathing, use of accessory muscles, cyanosis, pallor, and cool, clammy skin. **c.** Tidal volume is the amount of air that a person exchanges in one breath. The easiest way to evaluate tidal volume is to watch the chest rise and fall with each ventilation. If the chest is moving only slightly, tidal volume is inadequate.
34. **a.** When ventilating a patient, you should observe the chest rise and fall with each ventilation, the heart rate should return to normal, and the skin color should improve. **b.** Other methods of ventilation include mouth-to-mask ventilation and the flow-restricted, oxygen-powered ventilation device. **c.** The patient's airway may be obstructed causing poor ventilation. You should consider performing abdominal thrusts or suctioning the patient's airway.

## Division Two Examination

1. **c.** The chest expands during inhalation. As the diaphragm contracts and lowers, the ribs move upward and outward, increasing the size of the thoracic cavity; air is then pulled into the lungs.
2. **b.** The normal respiratory rate in children is between 15 to 30 breaths per minute. Always remember that this range is only an average. A faster or slower rate may still be normal for the child.
3. **d.** When a patient is breathing adequately, the chest expands equally, a normal rate and adequate tidal volume occur, and breathing is regular and relaxed. Signs and symptoms of inadequate breathing include difficulty breathing or shortness or breath; a rate that is too fast or too slow; a rhythm that is irregular; diminished or absent breath sounds; unequal or inadequate chest expansion; increased effort of breathing; inadequate tidal volume; cyanotic, pale, or cool and clammy skin; and the use of accessory muscles.
4. **d.** The airways of infants or children are easily kinked with improper positioning. The tongue takes up more room in the mouth than an adult's tongue. The trachea is narrow and easily blocked. The cricoid ring is undeveloped and pliable.
5. **d.** This patient is presenting in respiratory distress with signs and symptoms of poor oxygenation. He should receive high-concentration oxygen from a nonrebreather mask. The flow rate should be set at 15 L/minute.
6. **b.** The maximum oxygen flow rate for the nasal cannula is 6 L/minute.
7. **c.** The jaw thrust will keep the head in neutral alignment. All of the other techniques listed will move the head, potentially causing damage to the spinal cord.

8. **d.** Oral airways may be inserted using a tongue depressor, or you may insert the oral airway upside down until resistance is met, then rotate the airway 180 degrees until the flange rests against the patient's teeth. The oral airway is measured from the corner of the patient's mouth to the angle of the jaw or the earlobe. Oral airways can be used only on patients who do not have a gag reflex.
9. a. Nasal airways are inserted after lubricating with water-soluble lubricant. Insert the airway with the bevel facing the septum in adult or pediatric patients who require assistance in airway management.
10. **d.** Insert the suction catheter only as far as you can see. For rigid or soft catheters, the suction catheter should never be inserted any further than you can see, usually to approximately the base of the tongue.
11. **a.** If large amounts of material are in the airway, log-roll the patient and clear the airway. After rolling the patient back, suction may be used if necessary. The patient should not be continuously suctioned without ventilation. You should suction the patient first before you attempt to ventilate to avoid pushing emesis or secretions into the airway.
12. **c.** Suction the patient for no longer than 15 seconds before providing oxygen.
13. The preferred order for ventilation devices for EMT–Basics set forth in the National Standard Curriculum are (1) mouth-to-mask, (2) two-person BVM, (3) flow-restricted, oxygen-powered ventilation device, and (4) one-person BVM.
14. **a.** BVMs should not have pop-off valves. Pop-off valves may lead to ventilating with too little air. The BVM should have a self-refilling bag that is either disposable or easily cleaned and sterilized, an oxygen inlet and standardized fittings, and a one-way valve. The BVM should work in all temperatures and come in a variety of sizes.
15. **c.** When ventilating using a flow-restricted, oxygen-powered ventilation device, the alarm should sound when the relief valve pressure exceeds 60 ml of water. Flow-restricted, oxygen-powered ventilation devices can deliver up to 100% oxygen at a peak flow rate of 40 L/minute. The device allows the EMT–Basic to use both hands to ventilate the patient.
16. **c.** The one-person BVM technique is difficult to perform and requires extensive practice.
17. **a.** The neck and head must remain in the neutral position so that they are stabilized before ventilation. Any procedure that tilts the head should not be used when cervical spine trauma is suspected. The ventilation rate of once every 5 seconds for adults and once every 3 seconds for infants and children does not change for trauma patients.
18. **d.** If you cannot ventilate a patient through the tracheal stoma, seal the stoma and ventilate through the patient's mouth and nose as usual.
19. **b.** EMT–Basics need to avoid excessive bag pressure when ventilating an infant or child because gastric distention is more likely and causes problems when ventilating. Pop-off valves should not be used because ventilation may occur with too little volume. The head should be in a neutral position for infants and tilted slightly further back for children, avoiding kinking the trachea.
20. **b.** If dentures or other dental appliances become dislodged, they may become an airway obstruction and should be removed.

## Chapter 9

## SCENE SIZE-UP

### Matching

1. e
2. d
3. g
4. c
5. a
6. b
7. f

### Review Questions

1. **True.** Personal protection includes BSI precautions to prevent exposure to blood and other body fluids and protective clothing such as turnout gear and helmets. Personal protective equipment will vary with each situation.
2. Take BSI precautions, assess for scene safety, determine the MOI or NOI, assess the number of patients and need for additional help.
3. **a.** Patient assessment does not occur during the scene size-up. The scene size-up occurs before you enter the scene and is designed to protect you and your crew from injury and to help identify any need for additional resources. You will determine the number of patients after ensuring scene safety.

4. Many hazards may be present at an automobile crash. Some of these hazards include broken glass, torn metal, gasoline, angry bystanders, and traffic hazards. Each scene has its own potential hazards; therefore keep alert and look for danger.
5. Although hazards at the scene of a medical call are not as common or obvious as at the scene of a trauma call, the EMT–Basic still must be alert and look for hazards. Hazards may include people (for example, a violent person on scene or a mentally unstable patient), animals (a protective dog), the environment (for example, extreme heat or cold or carbon monoxide or natural gas in the air), and exposure to blood or other body fluids.
6. You must use your senses to evaluate the scene and determine if any hazards are present. Look at, listen to, and smell the environment to determine if any unsafe situations exist or substances are present.
7. If the scene is not safe and you cannot make it safe, do not enter the scene. EMT–Basics will not be able to help the patient if they are injured themselves.
8. **a.** The nature of illness is also called the chief complaint. The chief complaint usually describes the reason for calling EMS.
9. **True.** You can usually determine many of the factors of the mechanism of injury by observing the patient's surroundings, but you cannot always discover every factor that may have caused injury to the patient.
10. Identifying the mechanism of injury will help you determine if any hidden internal injuries are present, in addition to the external ones you can see.
11. Taking time to determine the total number of patients at the scene early in the scene size-up will allow you to request additional resources if patients outnumber the personnel on scene. While determining the number of patients, age- or gender-specific articles (e.g., a baby car seat, a woman's purse) may indicate the presence of an unseen patient.
12. Additional help should be requested for lifting assistance for a large patient, to control traffic, to deal with hazardous materials, for fire suppression or exposed electrical lines, to provide rescue equipment, or if patients outnumber the available personnel.
13. **a.** Consider the need for BSI precautions and don protective gear. Because shots have been fired, a potential exists for contact with blood and other body fluids. **b.** Ensure your own safety before addressing the safety of the patient or bystanders. Once you are sure the scene is safe, proceed with patient care. **c.** The scene has become unsafe, and you should move to a safe area.
14. **a.** During the scene size-up, you should check for scene safety, determine the mechanism of injury, determine how many patients are involved, and evaluate the need for additional help. **b.** Look for the presence of broken glass, torn metal, hazardous fluids, and bystanders. Take note of any unusual odors (e.g., gasoline). Listen for expected and unexpected sounds (e.g., an engine running, arcing wires). **c.** Protect the patient from metal, flying glass, or sparks created by extrication tools. Provide protection from the environment, such as extreme heat or cold.

## Chapter 10

## INITIAL ASSESSMENT

### Matching

1. d
2. c
3. a
4. b

### Review Questions

1. EMT–Basics form a general impression to determine the patient's priority of care and to form a plan of action for continuing to assess the patient and provide care.
2. **c.** The general impression is formed in seconds by simply looking at and listening to your patient. The patient's name is not necessary to form your general impression, although you may ask the patient his or her name early in your interaction to establish rapport. The patient's medical history and allergies will be assessed later. While forming a general impression, determine the nature of illness or mechanism of injury; the patient's age, race and gender; and if the patient has any life-threatening injuries.

3. **False.** You will assess the mental status of a child in different ways based on the child's age. Older children should be able to answer simple questions. Young children may only be able to tell you their name. Children of all ages prefer to be with their parents rather than strangers. A child who does not respond when removed from the parents is not alert. Children will try to locate their parents' voices or will be startled by loud verbal stimuli. Assess response to pain in the same manner as you would an adult, with a mildly painful stimulus.
4. An alert patient will look at you or talk to you without prompting. If a patient is not alert, talk to the patient to determine if he or she is responsive to verbal stimuli. If the patient does not respond, test for response to a painful stimulus. A painful stimulus should be strong enough to cause a reaction from the patient but not strong enough to injure the patient. A pinch on the shoulder, the fingers, or the foot is sufficient to elicit a painful response. If the patient does not respond to painful stimuli, he or she is unresponsive.
5. **False.** Mental status changes are one of the most sensitive indicators of changes in the patient's condition. Patients often become restless or confused very early when they are becoming hypoxic or going into shock.
6. **c.** The head-tilt, chin-lift maneuver is the most common way to open the airway of a medical patient. However, the maneuver will cause a change in the alignment of the spine and should not be used for trauma patients. The jaw thrust should be used for trauma patients because the head will remain in the neutral position.
7. The head of a trauma patient is stabilized in the neutral position to prevent any movement of the head, which will, in turn, move the spine. Minimizing movements of the spine is important to protect the patient from further injury. The jaw thrust is used for trauma patients because the head-tilt, chin-lift maneuver also will move the spine.
8. EMT–Basics should administer oxygen to an adult patient breathing less than eight times per minute or greater than 24 times per minute. Patients breathing less than eight times per minute may require positive-pressure ventilations.
9. You can determine if a patient is breathing by opening the airway and watching the rise and fall of the chest and listening for airflow. You would assess the respiratory efforts by checking the rate and quality.
10. **False.** EMT–Basics should assess the rate and quality of breathing of an infant or child the same way as they would for an adult. The normal range of respiratory rates of infants and children is higher than those for adults but should still be evaluated. A slow respiratory rate for an infant or child can be a sign of a serious respiratory problem.
11. **False.** Life-threatening conditions should be cared for as they are found. Do not wait to begin to correct a life-threatening condition such as an airway obstruction or major bleeding.
12. **a.** Initially assess the adult or child patient's pulse by palpating the radial artery. If the radial pulse cannot be felt, palpate the carotid pulse. For infants, begin by assessing the brachial pulse.
13. The EMT–Basic first assesses for external bleeding during the *general impression* and again when evaluating the patient's *circulation.* You may need to remove clothing from a trauma patient to properly evaluate for external bleeding. Any major bleeding should be considered a life threat and should be controlled immediately.
14. Normal skin color is pink when evaluated at the nail beds, inside of the lips, or inside the eyelids. Abnormal skin colors include pale (poor perfusion), cyanotic (inadequate oxygenation), flushed (hot or exposed to carbon monoxide), or jaundiced (poor liver function). The skin is normally warm. Abnormal skin temperatures include hot (exposure to heat or fever), cool (exposure to cold or poor perfusion), cold (exposure to extreme cold), or clammy (cold and moist, a sign of hypoperfusion). The skin condition is normally dry. Abnormal skin conditions include moist (possible sign of shock), wet (possible sign of shock), and extremely dry (dehydration).
15. **True.** Capillary refill should take less than 2 seconds to return to normal. Assess capillary refill by pushing on the nail bed until it blanches and then count the time taken for the color to return to normal. Assess capillary refill on patients younger than 6 years of age.
16. **b.** Patients with severe pain anywhere are considered to be priority patients. Other priority patients include any patient who has a poor general impression, is unresponsive with no gag reflex or cough, is responsive but unable to follow commands, has difficulty breathing, has signs and symptoms of shock, has complicated childbirth, has chest pain and a blood pressure of less than 100 mm Hg systolic, and has uncontrolled bleeding.

17. During the initial assessment, determine the patient's priority for care so that priority patients can be rapidly transported to the receiving facility. Time should not be wasted on scene with further assessment of these patients. All further assessments can take place in the back of the ambulance en route to the closest appropriate receiving facility.
18. **a.** During the initial assessment, form a general impression; assess mental status; assess the airway; assess breathing, rate, and quality; assess circulation; identify any life-threatening injuries and provide appropriate care; and make an initial decision. **b.** Initiate spinal precautions, position the patient, and open his airway. The blood, vomit, and teeth must be cleared before performing any other assessments or care. **c.** Using the AVPU categories, the patient is "P" (painful) because he responds only to painful stimulus.
19. **a.** The 27-year-old patient shot in the chest has a potential for displaying the signs and symptoms of shock. **b.** Contact dispatch and request advanced life support (ALS) intercept or ALS backup; notify dispatch to send additional crew members to the scene. **c.** Priority patients are those who have poor general impression, are unresponsive with no gag reflex or cough, are responsive but unable to follow commands, have difficulty breathing, have signs and symptoms of shock, have complicated childbirth, have chest pain and a blood pressure less than 100 mm Hg systolic, have uncontrolled bleeding, and have severe pain anywhere.

## Chapter 11

## FOCUSED HISTORY AND PHYSICAL EXAMINATION FOR TRAUMA PATIENTS

### Matching

1. c
2. g
3. e
4. f
5. h
6. b
7. a
8. i
9. d

### Review Questions

1. If you are unsure if the patient has a medical condition or a traumatic injury, you should assess the patient using the focused history and physical examination for trauma patients.
2. The mechanism of injury will help guide the EMT–Basic toward the patient's injuries. A serious mechanism of injury will help the EMT–Basic in the search for hidden injuries or maintain a high index of suspicion when a patient appears to be only slightly injured.
3. Significant mechanisms of injury include falls of greater than 20 feet, the ejection of driver or passenger from a vehicle, being in a car where another person died, vehicle roll-over, high-speed vehicle collision, vehicle-pedestrian collision, motorcycle crash, patients who are unresponsive or who have an altered mental status, and penetrating trauma to the head, chest, or abdomen.
4. **True.** Older patients and very young patients are more easily injured than healthy adults. A less serious mechanism of injury may result in a serious injury to these patients.
5. D—deformities; C—contusions; A—abrasions; P—penetrations; B—burns; T—tenderness; L—lacerations; S—swelling.
6. The rapid trauma assessment should take approximately *60 to 90* seconds. With practice, you should be able to complete the rapid trauma assessment in less than 90 seconds.
7. Anytime a life-threatening condition is discovered, the assessment should be stopped long enough to care for the condition, and then you should continue the assessment.
8. **b.** Auscultate the bases of the lungs at the midaxillary line and the apices at the midclavicular line to determine if breath sounds are present and equal.
9. **a.** Most patients will have a soft abdomen at rest. A firm or rigid abdomen can be a sign of injury to the abdomen or blood accumulating in the abdomen. When palpating the abdomen, gently push against all four quadrants, feeling for rigidity and noticing if the palpation causes the patient any pain.
10. **c.** When evaluating the pelvis, flex the pelvis by pushing posteriorly on the iliac wings and then compress by pushing toward the midline. Do not assess the pelvis if the patient has any pain in the pelvic region or if the mechanism of injury suggests that the patient may have injured the pelvis. If the pelvis is painful or unstable during the first examination of the pelvis, do not repeat this step of the examination.

11. When evaluating the extremities, assess for DCAP-BTLS and distal pulse, motor function, and sensation. Ask patients if they can feel you touching their extremity and if they can move their fingers and toes slightly.
12. **False.** If the patient has a serious mechanism of injury, you should perform the rapid trauma assessment, even if the patient complains only of an isolated injury. Patients are often not aware of their most serious injury, only the most painful injury.
13. **False.** Not every patient will require a rapid trauma assessment. If the patient has no serious mechanism of injury and complains only of an isolated injury, you can direct your assessment toward the injury. A patient who dropped a heavy object on his or her foot will not require a head-to-toe trauma assessment.
14. **False.** Patients are often aware of only the most painful injury, not necessarily the most serious. The mechanism of injury and the information obtained during the rest of the focused history and physical examination will help you determine if the patient should receive a rapid trauma assessment.
15. F. This injury is an isolated injury with no serious mechanism of injury.
16. F. This patient has an isolated injury to her ankle and no serious mechanism of injury.
17. R. This patient has sustained a serious mechanism of injury. Even though he complains only of arm pain, a trauma assessment is needed.
18. **a.** Yes. Falls of greater than 20 feet are considered to be high risk for hidden injury. **b.** Because the patient is responsive, you can obtain a SAMPLE history, including the cause of the event, during the initial assessment. This information would include the reason for the fall (e.g., loss of balance) and whether an associated loss of responsiveness occurred before or after the fall. You also might ask the patient to describe any pain or discomfort that resulted from the fall. **c.** A patient who has sustained a significant mechanism of injury should be prepared for transport with full spinal precautions.
19. **a.** Your first priority is to secure the patient's airway. This process includes positioning the patient and opening her airway while maintaining spinal precautions. Suction the airway as needed. **b.** Before beginning the assessment, control the airway and manually stabilize the head and spine. **c.** You would assess this patient for deformities, contusions, abrasions, penetrations or punctures, burns, tenderness, lacerations, and swelling. Based on the mechanism of injury, this patient may have sustained trauma to every body system; thus the rapid trauma assessment is indicated.

## Chapter 12

## FOCUSED HISTORY AND PHYSICAL EXAMINATION FOR MEDICAL PATIENTS

### Matching

1. e
2. a
3. f
4. c
5. b
6. d
7. g

### Review Questions

1. **False.** A responsive medical patient receives a focused history and physical examination based on the chief complaint. An unresponsive medical patient receives the rapid trauma assessment to evaluate for trauma and to complete a head-to-toe assessment.
2. O—onset; P—provocation; Q—quality; R—radiation; S—severity; T—time.
3. P. "What position makes you feel better?" Provocation or palliation means what makes the pain worse or better.
4. O. "How long have you had cardiac problems?" Onset refers to the beginning of the patient's condition.
5. T. "How long have you had this pain?" Time refers to the time when this specific episode began.
6. S. "Is this the worst pain you've ever had?" Severity is often scored on a scale from 1 to 10, with 10 being the worst pain the patient ever felt.

7. **P.** "What makes the pain worse?" Provocation is what makes the pain worse.
8. **R.** "Does the pain spread or move?" Radiation refers to any movement of the pain.
9. **Q.** "Can you describe the pain you are feeling?" Quality of pain is how the patient describes the feeling. Let the patient describe the pain in his or her own words.
10. **False.** You need not wait until you have heard the entire history of a medical problem before you begin treatment. For example, if the patient has chest pain, you should apply oxygen before you complete the focused assessment.
11. **True.** The EMT–Basic should always ask patients about information regarding their history. Valuable information can be gained and forwarded to the referring facility.
12. S—signs and symptoms; A—allergies; M—current medications; P—past medical history; L—last food or drink; E—events leading to this illness.
13. The focused history and physical examination for the medical patient is guided by the patient's *chief complaint.* The EMT–Basic generally has no reason to perform a head-to-toe assessment on a responsive medical patient with no history of trauma.
14. If the patient has a known medical condition, the way the EMT–Basic cares for that patient may change. For example, if the patient has a history of cardiac disease, the patient's physician may have prescribed the medication nitroglycerin. If the patient has nitroglycerin, the EMT–Basic can, in some instances, assist the patient with administration of the medication.
15. **True.** To help determine what may be wrong with the unresponsive medical patient, EMT–Basics should perform a focused history and physical examination the same as they would for the trauma patient. A head-to-toe rapid trauma assessment should be performed.
16. When a medical patient is unresponsive and cannot provide a SAMPLE history, information can be obtained from *family members or bystanders.* If no family members are present, ask bystanders to describe what they witnessed.
17. **c.** Place unresponsive medical patients with no history of trauma in the recovery position to help maintain a patent airway.
18. **a.** The "O" signifies onset or origin of the patient's medical problem. Questions to ask this patient include, "Do you have a history of cardiac diseases?" and "How long have you had a cardiac condition?" **b.** The "Q" signifies the quality of the pain. Questions to ask this patient include, "Can you describe the discomfort you are feeling?" **c.** The "T" signifies duration of time since the patient recognized the necessity to call EMS. Questions to ask include, "How long have you been experiencing this chest discomfort?" and "What happened to make you call EMS?"
19. **a.** After ensuring scene safety, assessment and control of the airway with spinal precautions is your first priority. **b.** Because the patient is unresponsive and cannot direct you toward her illness or injury, the focused history and physical examination for a trauma patient would be indicated. You would perform a rapid trauma assessment on this patient. **c.** If you can be certain that no trauma is involved, transport the patient in the recovery position to allow secretions to drain from her mouth and to help maintain an open airway. Otherwise, immobilize the patient to a long spine board.

# Chapter 13

## DETAILED PHYSICAL EXAMINATION

### Matching

1. d
2. f
3. h
4. e
5. a
6. g
7. b
8. c

### Review Questions

1. **True.** The rapid trauma assessment is generally performed quickly on scene (within 60 to 90 seconds), where lighting may or may not be ideal. The detailed physical examination is slower and occurs in the back of the ambulance, where the lighting may be better.

2. **False.** Not every trauma patient will receive a detailed physical examination. Patients with isolated trauma and with no significant mechanism of injury will not require a detailed physical examination. Some trauma patients may be so severely injured that the EMT–Basics spend all of their time evaluating and managing airway, breathing, and circulation and never have time to complete a detailed physical examination.
3. **True.** This patient was involved in a crash with serious mechanism of injury and should receive a detailed physical examination.
4. EMT–Basics will perform a detailed physical examination for medical patients who are unresponsive. Because the patient cannot direct you toward a specific chief complaint, a head-to-toe examination may help you determine the cause of the unresponsiveness or help you determine if the patient has any traumatic injuries. For medical patients with a specific chief complaint, examining the specific involved body area may be all that is necessary.
5. D—deformities; C—contusions; A—abrasions; P—penetrations; B—burns; T—tenderness; L—lacerations; S—swelling.
6. **False.** When evaluating the ears, nose, and mouth during the detailed physical examination, use a penlight to look for drainage or trauma. During the rapid trauma assessment, the ears, nose, and mouth are examined quickly. Performing the detailed physical examination gives you the opportunity to examine these areas carefully.
7. When evaluating the neck, you should assess for DCAP-BTLS and *jugular vein distension (JVD).* If the cervical spine immobilization device has already been applied, it may need to be removed for this examination.
8. The patient's pelvis should be examined unless he or she has complaints of pain or if the mechanism of injury suggests a pelvic injury. Do not reevaluate the patient's pelvis if it was unstable or painful during the first assessment. In all other cases, the pelvis should be evaluated by flexing and compressing the pelvic girdle to determine stability.
9. **c.** The detailed assessment should ideally be performed in the back of the ambulance en route to the receiving facility. If no means of transporting the patient is available, the detailed physical examination can be performed on the scene.
10. **a.** Yes. All patients with a significant mechanism of injury should receive a detailed physical examination. **b.** DCAP-BTLS—deformities, contusions, abrasions, penetrations or punctures, burns, tenderness, lacerations, swelling. **c.** Because of the fall, you would suspect a possible spine injury. Have your partner manually stabilize the patient's neck for DCAP-BTLS, jugular vein distension, and crepitation. Then, apply a cervical spine immobilization device and secure the patient to a long backboard.
11. **a.** No. The detailed physical examination is indicated for trauma patients and unresponsive patients who may have hidden injuries that are not revealed in the initial assessment. Your initial assessment of this patient identified the nature of his injury. **b.** Assessment of the injury would be limited to DCAP-BTLS on the injured body surface. **c.** Yes. The patient's condition allows for assessment of blood pressure, pulse, and respirations.

## Chapter 14

### ONGOING ASSESSMENT

#### Review Questions

1. The ongoing assessment allows the EMT–Basic to reevaluate the patient's condition, to check the effectiveness of the interventions, and to document trends in the patient's condition. Trends or changes in the patient's condition can provide valuable clues to the receiving facility about the patient's status and can help hospital personnel make decisions about the patient's care.
2. The initial assessment includes checking the mental status; evaluating the airway patency; assessing breathing rate and quality; assessing pulse rate and quality; assessing skin color, temperature, condition, and perfusion; and reestablishing patient priority.
3. Stable patients are reassessed every 15 minutes. Unstable patients are reassessed every 5 minutes. Anytime a patient's condition changes, be sure to reevaluate the patient, and change the status to unstable if appropriate.
4. 5—assess skin color, temperature, condition, perfusion; 1—assess mental status; 4—assess pulse; 2—assess airway patency; 3—assess breathing rate and quality; 6—reassess patient priority.

5. **False.** The EMT–Basic should reevaluate the patient's chief complaint during the ongoing assessment. Although chief complaints do not usually change, the patient may be more descriptive about the illness or injury.
6. An isolated set of vital signs does not provide the EMT–Basic with much information. Successive sets of vital signs show changes in the patient's condition over time and allow the EMT–Basic to establish a baseline for the patient. Comparing successive sets of vital signs over time is called *trending*.
7. The EMT–Basic should check any intervention that was performed to make sure it is still functioning properly. Examples of interventions to check include the oxygen supply and delivery system, the adequacy of artificial ventilations, dressings are still controlling bleeding, splints are still immobilizing extremities without being too tight, and straps on the backboard are still immobilizing the patient. Interventions that are inadequate should be corrected immediately.
8. **a.** This patient is unstable. The ongoing assessment should be repeated every 5 minutes or less. **b.** You should interact constantly with the patient throughout transport. This action allows you to observe the patient's mental status and to note any changes for either better or worse. **c.** If the patient is unresponsive, check the response to verbal and painful stimuli to establish mental status.
9. **a.** Check to ensure the flow rate is set at 15 L/minute. **b.** Ensure that oxygen is adequately flowing, that the mask is a nonrebreather, that the reservoir bag remains inflated, and that enough oxygen remains in the cylinder for the duration of the trip. **c.** If the patient cannot be convinced to keep a nonrebreather mask in place, apply a nasal cannula. Ensure that the prongs are placed correctly in the patient's nose, set the rate at 6 L/minute, and ensure that the oxygen is flowing adequately. The nasal cannula is a low-flow device, which delivers low concentrations of oxygen, and is a poor substitute for the nonrebreather mask.

## Chapter 15

# COMMUNICATIONS

### Matching

1. c
2. a
3. b
4. d

### Review Questions

1. **b.** A base station is a radio at a stationary site with superior transmission and receiving capabilities. A repeater is a remote receiver that receives a transmission from a low-power radio and transmits at a higher power. An encoder is part of a digital system that blocks out radio transmissions not intended for certain units.
2. The agency that regulates and monitors radio transmissions is called the Federal Communications Commission (FCC).
3. Monitor the frequency for 5 seconds before transmitting to ensure that the frequency is clear. Transmitting without monitoring the frequency may result in interruptions of other medical care professionals.
4. **a.** Wait for 1 second after pushing the push-to-talk button to ensure that your entire transmission is heard.
5. The phrase *stand-by* means that you should wait until you are given a go-ahead to begin transmitting.
6. **True.** Everyday language will reduce confusion in radio communications.
7. **False.** Courtesy is always assumed. Continuously saying "please" and "thank you" takes up valuable time on the radio.
8. **c.** EMS channels are considered to be public channels by the FCC and can be monitored by the public over scanners. EMS channels may be taped for legal purposes. EMS channels may be shared between various EMS agencies, but they are dedicated for the use of EMS agencies.
9. **b.** Communicate with dispatch when you receive the call, respond to the call, arrive at the scene, arrive at the patient's side, leave the scene for the receiving facility, arrive at the receiving facility, leave the hospital for the station, and arrive at the station.
10. **c.** If the communication with medical direction is unclear, ask the physician to clarify the information.

11. **b.** The radio report should be concise, organized, and pertinent. Avoid lengthy or comprehensive reports over the radio. A longer and more detailed report can be given at the bedside. All of the pertinent information that the receiving hospital will require is also documented in the written report.
12. The standard medical reporting format includes the patient's age and gender, chief complaint, history of present illness, pertinent medical history, mental status, assessment findings, vital signs, emergency care given, response to emergency care, estimated time to load the patient for transport, estimated travel time from the scene to the hospital, and opportunity for questions from the receiving facility or medical direction physician.
13. Tips for effective communication: verbalize your support, be a good listener, offer a reassuring touch, be respectful, separate personal bias, and be silent when appropriate. Good communicators will evaluate the situation and communicate with the patient and family members based on the situation.
14. **True.** Body language is communicated without words by factors such as posture, facial expression, and tone of voice.
15. **a.** The standard medical reporting format includes the patient's age and gender, chief complaint, history of present illness, pertinent history, mental status, assessment findings, vital signs, emergency care given, response to emergency care, estimated time to load the patient for transport, and estimated travel time to the hospital. **b.** Allow an opportunity for questions from the receiving facility or medical direction physician before ending your report. **c.** Any time you are unclear about an order, ask questions that will help clarify the physician's order.
16. **a.** Use a calm, reassuring voice and age-appropriate language. Be sure to explain everything you are doing, and be honest. **b.** Do not assume that elderly patients cannot hear you. Introduce yourself and assess their ability to hear you, consider how fast you are speaking, slow down and allow the patient to process your questions, and use simple terms. **c.** Use an interpreter, write notes, be patient, and do not show signs of frustration.

## Chapter 16

## DOCUMENTATION

### Matching

1. a
2. b
3. d
4. c

### Review Questions

1. **True.** Trending means comparing *trends* in a patient's condition over time by comparing sets of information.
2. **d.** The time of arrival is part of the administrative information set. All of the other elements are part of the patient care data set.
3. 1:00 AM—0100; 6:30 PM—1830; 12 noon—1200; 4:20 AM—0420; 10:30 PM—2230; 8:25 PM—2025; 2:40 AM—0240; 12:30 AM—0030.
4. **True.** The prehospital care report is used to document what care the EMT–Basic provided for the patient. This document is also a legal record of events at the scene and care provided. EMT–Basics must be careful to document all events that happened at the scene and to be truthful when documenting care given.
5. O—I saw him drinking at that bar; S—The patient was drunk; S—It looked like the car was going over the speed limit; O—Her blood pressure was 120/80 and the pulse was 72; O—The patient's skin is cool, clammy, and moist to the touch.
6. The primary function of the prehospital care report is to document care given to the patient. The prehospital care report is also used as an educational tool, for billing purposes, for research, for evaluation, and for continuous quality improvement.
7. Most prehospital care report forms have a section for writing a patient *narrative,* allowing EMT–Basics to write about the events in the standard medical reporting format. The narrative should describe facts and record observations in an objective manner.
8. Chief complaint—CC; gunshot wound—GSW; every—q; shortness of breath—SOB; history—Hx; immediately—stat; treatment—Rx; alcohol—EtOH.
9. **False.** Errors should be corrected by drawing a single line through the error, initialing beside the error, and then writing in the correct information.

10. Refusal is the right of any *competent* adult. Patients must be informed about their decisions and able to make a rational decision.
11. Special situation reports should be used in the event of an infectious disease exposure, injury to the EMT–Basic or bystanders, equipment damage or malfunction, vehicle crashes involving the response unit, patient refusals, abuse or neglect, crime scenes, and hazardous materials incidents. Individual EMS systems may have additional special reports used in their region or state.
12. **a.** Patient information and administrative information are both part of the minimum data set. **b.** Pertinent information includes age and sex; chief complaint; cause of injury; preexisting conditions; signs and symptoms present; injury description; level of responsiveness (using the AVPU categories); pulse rate; respiratory rate; systolic blood pressure in patients over 3 years of age; skin perfusion; skin color, temperature, and condition; procedures performed on the patient; medications administered; and response to treatment, including medications. **c.** For administrative purposes, gather the following information: incident location, type of location, date and time the incident was reported, date and time the EMS unit was notified, time the unit responded, time of arrival at the scene, time of arrival at the patient, time EMS left the scene, time EMS arrived at destination, time of transfer of patient care, time the EMS unit was back in service, use of lights and sirens, and crew members responding.
13. **a.** Yes. All competent adults have the right to refuse treatment for themselves or others in their care. **b.** Inform the patient why treatment and transport are necessary and what may happen without treatment, contact medical direction, and have a physician speak with the patient. **c.** Document assessment findings; have the patient sign a refusal form; document that you have informed the patient of adverse effects that may result from not accepting care or transportation, including possible death; have a family member, police officer, or bystander sign the form as a witness; before leaving the scene, tell the patient about other ways to receive care; and state and document your willingness to return for treatment and transportation.

## Division Three Examination

1. **b.** BSI precautions are designed to protect the EMT–Basic from blood- and airborne pathogens. Need for BSI precautions should be determined in the scene size-up. BSI precautions should be used anytime a chance exists of contact with any body fluid, not just blood.
2. **b.** The EMT–Basic should always be concerned with his or her own safety first. If the EMT–Basic is injured, he or she will not be able to help anyone at the scene. After personal safety, priorities include safety of other crew members, patient safety, and bystander safety.
3. **a.** During the scene size-up, the EMT–Basic will determine scene safety, the mechanism of injury or nature of illness, the number of patients, and the need for additional help. No patient information will be obtained during the scene size-up.
4. **a.** During the scene size-up, EMT–Basics should check for scene safety, determine the nature of illness or mechanism of injury, determine the number of patients present, and call for additional help if necessary. If the scene has too many patients for the EMT–Basics to treat, call for additional help and begin treating the most seriously injured patients. No patient care takes place during the scene size-up.
5. **b.** The best source of information about a responsive medical patient is usually the patient. Pay attention to the patient's description of the nature of illness and the circumstances surrounding his or her illness.
6. **a.** The first phase of the initial assessment is to form a general impression.
7. **c.** During the general impression, the EMT–Basic determines the patient's age, gender, and race; mechanism of injury or nature of illness; and if any life threats are present. Form a general impression in the first few seconds, before any additional patient assessment is performed.
8. **b.** The AVPU acronym stands for alert, responsive to verbal stimuli, responsive to painful stimuli, or unresponsive. AVPU is used to categorize a patient's mental status.
9. **c.** A slow respiratory rate is a threat to life and should be treated immediately. Have your partner ventilate the patient using a pocket mask, one- or two-person BVM, or a flow-restricted, oxygen-powered ventilation device.

10. **b.** For alert adult or child patients, assess the radial pulse first. If the adult or child patient is unresponsive, or if you cannot feel a radial pulse, evaluate the carotid pulse. Evaluate the brachial pulse for infants.
11. **a.** To assess perfusion, the EMT–Basic should look at the skin color of the nail beds, the inside of the lips, or the inside the eyelids. The normal skin color in these areas is pink, regardless of race.
12. **d.** A radial pulse that is weaker than the carotid pulse may be a sign of hypoperfusion. Skin color should be assessed at the nail beds, inside the lips, or inside the eyelids. Temperature should be assessed on the trunk, not the extremities. Capillary refill is an accurate measure of perfusion for children younger than 6 years of age.
13. **a.** A patient who is unresponsive with no gag reflex is a priority patient. Other priority patients include patients who have poor general impression, who are responsive but unable to follow commands, who are experiencing difficulty breathing, who have signs and symptoms of shock, who are having complicated childbirth, who have chest pain and a blood pressure of less than 100 mm Hg systolic, who have uncontrolled bleeding, and who have severe pain anywhere.
14. **a.** If the patient is involved in a crash where another occupant in the same vehicle compartment died, the patient may have sustained a significant mechanism of injury. Other significant mechanisms of injury include ejection of driver or passenger from a vehicle, a fall of more than 6 m (20 feet), vehicle roll-over, high-speed vehicle collision, vehicle-pedestrian collision, motorcycle crash, unresponsive patients or patients with an altered mental status, and patients with penetrating trauma to the head, chest, or abdomen.
15. **c.** The rapid trauma assessment should take 60 to 90 seconds for most patients. EMT–Basics will be able to perform the trauma assessment rapidly with practice.
16. **a.** The acronym DCAP-BTLS stands for deformities, contusions, abrasions, penetrations, burns, tenderness, lacerations, and swelling.
17. **c.** The abdomen should be evaluated for DCAP-BTLS and softness, tenderness, and distention.
18. **c.** If the patient has an isolated injury and no serious mechanism of injury, the EMT–Basic may choose to evaluate the isolated injury only. If any doubt exists about the seriousness of the injury, a complete rapid trauma assessment should be performed.
19. **c.** The acronym OPQRST is used to remember what questions to ask during the focused history and physical examination for medical patients when evaluating their chief complaint. The acronym stands for onset, provocation, quality, radiation, severity, and time.
20. a. The "R" in the OPQRST assessment stands for radiation.
21. **a.** Emergency care for patients is based on the assessment findings of the focused history and physical examination and advice from medical direction. Unresponsive medical patients are treated much like unresponsive trauma patients. Unresponsive medical patients with no suspected trauma should be placed in the recovery position. All patients receive an initial assessment, including an evaluation of their airway, breathing, and circulation.
22. **a.** The "S" in the SAMPLE history stands for signs and symptoms, the "A" for allergies, the "M" for medications, the "P" for past pertinent history, the "L" for last oral intake, and the "E" for events leading to the illness or injury.
23. **c.** The rapid assessment for a medical patient is directed toward the patient's chief complaint. The clothing may be removed in the area assessed, but all of the patient's clothes do not need to be removed. A head-to-toe assessment may be indicated if the patient is unresponsive. The rapid assessment will help identify trauma but cannot rule it out.
24. **d.** The rapid trauma assessment should be performed on unresponsive medical patients to try to find signs of trauma or medical conditions. The trauma assessment should be performed if trauma is suspected. The patient should be immobilized unless you can be sure the patient has no spinal injury.
25. **b.** The detailed physical examination is designed for trauma patients who have been seriously injured and who may have hidden injuries. The examination is slower and more methodical than the focused history and physical examination. The detailed physical examination ideally should be performed en route to the receiving facility. The detailed physical examination can be performed on medical patients but is primarily for trauma patients.

26. c. Medical patients who are unresponsive should receive a detailed physical examination to try to find clues about their condition. Responsive medical patients without injuries do not routinely receive a detailed physical examination. Patients with an isolated injury do not require a detailed physical examination.
27. a. While performing the detailed physical examination of the head, evaluate the ears and nose for drainage, the eyes for discoloration, and the mouth for foreign bodies. The pupils and stability of the face are assessed the first time during the focused history and physical examination, and the mouth is examined for any airway obstructions during the initial assessment. These steps are repeated in the detailed physical examination.
28. d. The neck should be assessed for trauma and jugular vein distention. Breath sounds are assessed in four places: bilaterally at the apices and the bases of the lungs. The abdomen is assessed in all four quadrants. The pelvis should not be evaluated if any sign of injury is present or if the patient complains of pain in the pelvis.
29. b. When assessing the extremities, in addition to DCAP-BTLS, assess for distal pulse, motor function, and sensation.
30. d. The ongoing assessment allows the EMT–Basic to document trends in the patient's condition. Vital signs are evaluated every time the ongoing assessment is repeated. The initial assessment is repeated during the ongoing assessment. The ongoing assessment is repeated based on the patient's condition.
31. c. The ongoing assessment is repeated every 15 minutes for stable patients and every 5 minutes for unstable patients.
32. b. The ongoing assessment should be repeated one last time approximately 5 minutes away from the receiving facility, enabling you to report a recent assessment at bedside. If an intervention is inadequate, it should be corrected immediately. Pupil size and mental status are assessment criteria, not interventions. Whether the patient is responsive or unresponsive, the entire ongoing assessment should be repeated, including the focused history and physical examination.
33. c. The Federal Communications Commission (FCC) regulates radio frequencies and is responsible for assigning radio channels, licensing radio operators, and routinely monitoring radio transmissions.
34. a. To ensure clear communications, hold the radio microphone 2 to 3 inches from your mouth.
35. a. The medical direction physician with whom you talk may be at the receiving facility or at another location. Orders from medical direction should be repeated back to the physician word for word to check accuracy. If the order is unclear, ask questions until you are sure of the order. Reports to medical direction should be concise and organized, enabling the patient's condition to be understood quickly.
36. c. Everyday language is less confusing than codes and should be used for radio communications. Pause briefly before speaking to allow your entire transmission to be heard. Speak clearly and slowly to minimize confusion. Words that are difficult to hear such as "yes" and "no" should be avoided.
37. b. A repeater is a remote receiver that receives a transmission from a low-power portable receiver and transmits the signal at a higher power. A base station is a stationary radio with superior transmitting and receiving capabilities. Encoders and decoders can be used to block out radio transmissions not intended for a particular unit.
38. c. EMT–Basics should notify dispatch when receiving the call, responding to the call, arriving at the scene, arriving at the patient's side, leaving the scene for the receiving facility, arriving at the receiving facility, leaving the hospital for the station, and arriving at the station. Information regarding the patient's status is not routinely communicated with dispatch. Notify dispatch when arriving at the receiving facility, not after giving bedside report.
39. b. Administrative information includes the incident location, the type of location, the date the incident was reported, the time the incident was reported, the date the EMS unit was notified, the time the EMS unit was notified, the time the unit responded, the time of arrival at the scene, the time of arrival at the patient, the time the EMS unit left the scene, the time of the EMS arrival at the destination, the time of transfer of patient care, the time the EMS unit was back in service, the use of lights and siren to and from the scene, and the crew members responding to the scene.
40. c. The patient information includes age and gender; chief complaint; cause of injury; preexisting conditions; signs and symptoms present; injury description; level of responsiveness; pulse rate; respiratory rate; systolic blood pressure in patients 3 years of age and older; skin perfusion; skin color, temperature, and condition; procedures performed on the patient; medications administered; and response to treatment.

41. **c.** The prehospital care report can be used for case reviews or continuing education if the patient's confidentiality is protected. Care reports can be released for billing purposes to other health care professionals assuming care for the patient. The prehospital care report should contain only objective information. EMT–Basics should treat the patient based on signs and symptoms present and not make a diagnosis.
42. **c.** The correct abbreviation for nothing by mouth is NPO. For a list of common medical abbreviations, refer to *Mosby's EMT–Basic Textbook.*
43. **d.** Situations such as infectious disease exposure, injury to EMT–Basics or bystanders, equipment damage or malfunction, vehicle crashes involving the response unit, patient refusals, abuse or neglect, crime scenes, or hazardous materials incidents should be documented on a special report form. Documentation errors should have a single line drawn through them, with the correct information printed beside the incorrect information. Initial beside the correction. Refusals should be carefully documented, with a witness other than your partner signing the refusal form. Be careful to document only the care that was given, even if you know you left out important care.
44. **c.** If a patient refuses care, you should document your assessment findings and the emergency medical care given, and then have the patient sign a refusal form. In addition, document that you have informed the patient of the adverse effects that may result from not accepting care or being transported, or both, including possible death. Having a family member sign as a witness is not recommended. Have a police officer or bystander sign the form as a witness. If the patient refuses to sign the refusal form, have a police officer or bystander sign the form saying that the patient refused to sign.

# Chapter 17

## GENERAL PHARMACOLOGY

### Matching 1

1. d
2. b
3. c
4. f
5. a
6. e

### Matching 2

7. a
8. d
9. b
10. e
11. c

### Matching 3

12. c
13. b
14. d
15. a

### Review Questions

1. **False.** Pharmacology is the science of drugs and includes the study of their origin, ingredients, uses, and actions on the body. A medication is any substance that alters the body's functions when taken into the body. Medication and drug are two words often used interchangeably.
2. EMT–Basics carry the medications, *oxygen, activated charcoal,* and *oral glucose* on the EMS unit.
3. EMT–Basics may assist patients with their physician-prescribed nitroglycerin, prescribed inhaler, or epinephrine autoinjector.
4. **a.** The manufacturer assigns the medication its trade name. The generic name is usually a simple form of the chemical name listed in the *U.S. Pharmacopeia.*
5. **True.** Because more than one company may manufacture a drug, it may have more than one trade name.
6. EMT–Basics will commonly deal with medications in the form of a suspension, gel, gas, fine powder for inhalation, compressed powders or tablets, sublingual spray, and liquid for injection. The route of administration will affect the speed of absorption of the drug.
7. **True.** A contraindication is any factor that makes a medication unsafe to administer or a procedure unsafe to perform. Contraindications apply to a situation when a medication should not be used because it will be of little benefit or potential harm.
8. **a.** The dose of a medication may depend on the patient's age and weight, or one standard dose may be meant for all patients. Factors such as gender, race, and height do not affect the medication dose.

9. **False.** Oral medications cannot be delivered to unresponsive patients because the patient must be alert enough to swallow. Oral medications administered to an unresponsive patient may cause an airway obstruction.
10. **False.** Medications delivered via the oral route must travel through the digestive tract to the site where it will be absorbed; thus the onset of action for these medications is relatively slow.
11. EMTs may assist with the administration of activated charcoal and oral glucose by the oral route.
12. **b.** When medications are administered sublingually, the medication is absorbed by the capillaries under the tongue, bypassing the digestive tract.
13. **False.** Sublingual drugs are dissolved and absorbed into the capillaries under the tongue.
14. EMTs may assist with the administration of nitroglycerin by the sublingual route.
15. EMTs may assist with administration of medications in prescribed inhalers and oxygen by the inhalation route.
16. **False.** Inhaled medications usually have a rapid onset of action.
17. **d.** Epinephrine autoinjectors deliver medication through the intramuscular route. The medication is absorbed into the tissues and then into the bloodstream.
18. The undesirable actions of a medication are called *side effects.* The known side effects of a medication should be anticipated when the EMT–Basic administers the drug.
19. **True.** Many medications have predictable side effects. By knowing the pharmacology of a medication, EMT–Basics are better able to anticipate side effects and be prepared for them.
20. After administering a medication, carefully monitor the patient for *desired effects* and *side effects.* Report any findings to the receiving facility and document them in your prehospital care report.
21. **a.** EMT–Basics typically carry the medications oral glucose, activated charcoal, and oxygen. **b.** EMT–Basics can assist a patient with his or her prescribed inhaler, nitroglycerin, and epinephrine autoinjector. **c.** An indication is the most common use of a medication for treating a specific illness or condition—signs and symptoms for when a medication is used. A contraindication is a situation in which a medication should not be used. A dose is the amount of the medication that should be administered.

# Chapter 18

## RESPIRATORY EMERGENCIES

### Review Questions

1. **a.** Pharynx; **b.** nasopharynx; **c.** oropharynx; **d.** epiglottis; **e.** larynx; **f.** trachea; **g.** right bronchus; **h.** diaphragm; **i.** left bronchus.
2. When air enters the nose and mouth, it is warmed, filtered and humidified.
3. **b.** The firm cartilage ring forming the lower portion of the larynx is the cricoid cartilage.
4. **d.** The intercostal muscles move the ribs up and out during inhalation, increasing the size of the chest cavity.
5. **True.** Carbon dioxide is given up from the body and oxygen is absorbed into the body through the alveoli.
6. **a.** Inhaled air contains high concentrations of oxygen, whereas exhaled air contains high concentrations of carbon dioxide.
7. **c.** The normal respiratory rate for a child is 15 to 30 breaths per minute. The normal rate for an adult is 12 to 20 breaths per minute and for an infant is 25 to 50 breaths per minute. These respiratory rates are averages. A patient may be breathing slower or faster and still be within his or her normal limits.
8. Adequate breathing means the patient has a normal rate, rhythm, chest expansion, and tidal volume.
9. **False.** A rate that is too fast or too slow may cause the patient to receive less oxygen than the body needs.
10. **c.** Shallow respirations indicate respiratory distress because the patient may not be getting enough oxygen.
11. **False.** Normal breathing should be silent. Noises made during breathing can be signs of respiratory difficulty.
12. General signs and symptoms of difficulty breathing include shortness of breath, restlessness or anxiety, patient position, altered mental status, abdominal breathing, increased or decreased breathing rate, and increased pulse rate. Visual signs and symptoms of difficulty breathing include changes in skin color, temperature, or condition; unusual anatomy; and retractions or use of accessory muscles. Auditory signs and symptoms of breathing difficulty include noisy breathing, inability to speak as a result of breathing efforts, coughing, irregular breathing rhythm, and unequal breath sounds.

13. **False.** Changes in a patient's anatomy, such as a barrel chest, can occur over long periods of respiratory problems.
14. **d.** Patients in respiratory distress tend to sit straight up and will feel increased difficulty breathing when lying down.
15. Three diseases associated with chronic obstructive pulmonary disease are asthma, bronchitis and emphysema.
16. **c.** Cigarette smoke is the leading cause of emphysema in the United States.
17. The acronym OPQRST is used during the focused history and physical examination and stands for onset, provocation, quality, radiation, severity, and time.
18. **False.** Children will feel more comfortable and safe with their parents than they will alone. Removing a child from his or her parents may increase the child's anxiety and increase the respiratory distress. Allow the parents and child to remain together.
19. The first medication to administer to a patient in respiratory distress is oxygen.
20. **False.** EMTs can assist patients with their prescribed inhaler only if these patients have their own medication prescribed to them by a physician.
21. **b.** Inhalers are used to dilate bronchioles and decrease resistance inside the airways. Decreased resistance makes breathing easier for the patient.
22. Albuterol and isoetharine are *generic* names for the medication in an inhaler.
23. To use an inhaler, patients must (1) have signs and symptoms of difficulty breathing and (2) have their own physician-prescribed inhaler, and (3) the EMT must obtain permission from medical direction to help with the administration of the medication.
24. Contraindications for the use of a prescribed inhaler include a patient who is not oriented enough to use the device properly, a patient using an inhaler that was prescribed for someone else, the patient has already taken the maximum recommended dose, or medical direction has not granted permission.
25. **False.** A spacer is a device used to help a patient get the maximum effect from the medication. If the patient has a spacer, it should be used.
26. **False.** Infants and very young children generally lack the coordination to use an inhaler.
27. **a.** Possible side effects of prescribed inhalers include increased pulse rate, tremors, nervousness, and sometimes nausea.
28. 6—hold breath as long as comfortable; 1—check expiration date; 3—remove oxygen mask, patient exhales deeply; 2—shake vigorously; 5—begin inhalation, depress inhaler; 4—place mouth over inhaler mouthpiece.
29. **a.** General signs and symptoms of difficulty breathing include shortness of breath, restlessness or anxiety, patient position, altered mental status, use of accessory muscles, abdominal breathing, increased or decreased breathing rate, and increased pulse rate. **b.** Using OPQRST, you would attempt to ascertain if a history of respiratory problems is indicated, what makes it better or worse, is associated pain occurring, severity of distress, when it started and how long it lasted, and if the patient takes any medication for breathing problems. Additionally, SAMPLE history should include signs and symptoms, allergies, medications, past pertinent history, last oral intake, and events leading to the event. **c.** Allow the patient to assume a position of comfort. Most patients will prefer to sit upright to make breathing easier.
30. **a.** Common trade names include Proventil, Ventolin, Bronkosol, Bronkometer, Alupent, and Metaprel. **b.** The medication is absorbed into the tissues of the lungs, generally dilating the bronchioles to decrease resistance inside the airways. **c.** You should obtain a brief pertinent history of past and present illness and how many doses of the inhaler the child took before you arrived. **d.** (1) The patient must have signs and symptoms of a respiratory emergency. (2) The patient must have his or her own physician-prescribed inhaler. (3) You must obtain specific authorization from medical direction to aid the patient in inhaled medication administration through either on- or offline medical direction.

# Chapter 19

## CARDIOVASCULAR EMERGENCIES

### Matching I

1. i
2. f
3. a
4. b
5. g
6. h
7. d
8. c
9. e

### Matching 2

10. e
11. c
12. d
13. h
14. f
15. b
16. g
17. a

### Labeling

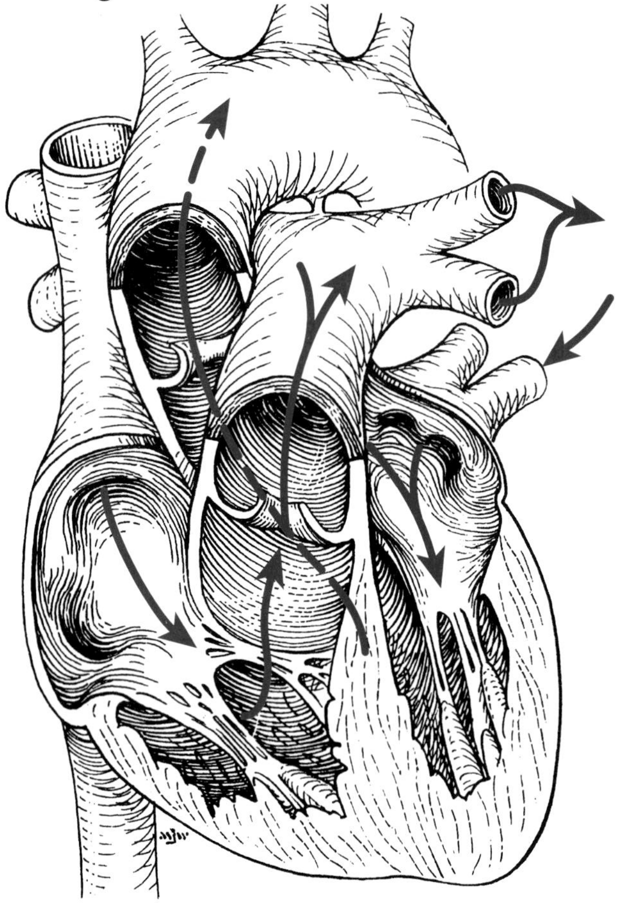

### Review Questions

1. **True.** The two upper chambers of the heart are called the atria, and the two lower chambers are called the ventricles; valves between the chambers prevent the backflow of blood.
2. **a.** Blood from the vena cava enters the right atrium, then the right ventricle, to be pumped to the lungs to be reoxygenated.
3. The tiny blood vessels that connect arterioles to venules are called *capillaries.*
4. b. Platelets are essential for the formation of blood clots.
5. **True.** The contraction of the ventricles causes a wave of blood to be sent through the body, generating a pulse.
6. Central pulses can be palpated at the carotid and femoral arteries. Peripheral pulses can be located at the radial, brachial, dorsalis pedis, and posterior tibial arteries.
7. The first number in a blood pressure is the *systolic* value, measuring the pressure in the arteries when the heart contracts, and the second number is the *diastolic* value, measuring the pressure in the arteries when the heart relaxes.
8. Another term used to describe shock is *hypoperfusion.*
9. **d.** Anxiety is an indicator of shock. Other signs and symptoms of shock (hypoperfusion) include rapid and weak pulse; pale or cyanotic skin; cool, clammy skin; rapid and shallow breathing; restlessness; mental dullness, confusion; nausea, vomiting, and thirst; low or decreasing blood pressure (usually a late sign); and subnormal temperature.
10. Chest pressure or discomfort that usually goes away with rest is called *angina.*
11. **b.** When muscles can no longer get oxygen, they become ischemic, which causes pain.
12. Respiratory pain is often *sharp or stabbing* and *increases* with breathing. Cardiac pain is usually *crushing, dull, or pressure* and *does not change* with movement.
13. Cardiac pain can radiate anywhere in the body but commonly radiates to the shoulder, neck, or jaw.
14. Severity can be measured on a scale of 1 to 10, with 10 being the worst pain.
15. The acronym OPQRST can be used to evaluate a patient's signs and symptoms. O stands for onset, P for provocation, Q for quality, R for radiation, S for severity, and T for time.
16. The first medication delivered to the cardiac patient is *oxygen.*
17. **d.** Responsive medical patients should be transported in the position of comfort. Most patients prefer to sit up when they are experiencing chest pain or difficulty breathing.
18. **False.** Nitroglycerin can be administered only after an initial assessment and focused history and physical examination and with permission from medical direction.
19. **b.** Nitroglycerin dilates blood vessels, allowing more blood to flow through them. Nitroglycerin may cause a drop in blood pressure.

20. Nitroglycerin is contraindicated when (1) the patient's blood pressure is less than 100 mm Hg, (2) the patient does not have his or her own physician-prescribed nitroglycerin, (3) the patient has a head injury or is not alert, (4) the patient is an infant or child, (5) patient has taken Viagra in the last 24 hours, or (6) the patient has received the maximum dose.
21. **a.** Nitroglycerin does not commonly cause muscle tremors. Common side effects include lower blood pressure, headache, pulse rate changes, and a burning sensation under the tongue.
22. The primary intervention that makes the most difference in survival from cardiac arrest is *early defibrillation.*
23. **c.** Ventricular fibrillation is the condition in which the heart is not contracting effectively and is quivering.
24. **c.** The AED should be placed only on patients who are in cardiac arrest. The EMT should confirm that the patient is pulseless, apneic, and unresponsive.
25. **True.** The EMT performing the defibrillation must make sure that no one is in contact with the patient or the stretcher before delivering the shock.
26. **False.** AEDs can be used routinely on patients older than 8 years of age. AEDs may be used on patients between 1 and 8 years of age, but you should consult medical direction first.
27. **False.** Check the pulse periodically while performing CPR.
28. **a.** Angina is the discomfort felt when the heart does not receive enough oxygen. Angina is commonly experienced after exertion, and the patient usually feels better with rest. **b.** The indications for nitroglycerin include signs and symptoms of cardiac chest pain and patient has physician-prescribed sublingual tablets or spray. The EMT–Basic must have approval from medical direction. **c.** Nitroglycerin administration is contraindicated when the patient has a systolic blood pressure of less than 100 mm Hg, does not have his or her own nitroglycerin that is prescribed by a physician, has a head injury or is not mentally alert, is an infant or child, or has already taken the maximum prescribed dosage before EMS arrival.
29. **a.** Common signs and symptoms for cardiac compromise include squeezing, dull pressure or pain in the chest that radiates to the arms, neck, jaw, or upper back; sudden onset of sweating; difficulty breathing; anxiety or irritability; feeling of impending doom; abnormal and sometimes irregular pulse rate; abnormal blood pressure; epigastric pain; and nausea or vomiting. **b.** No. The medication was not prescribed for this patient.
30. **a.** AEDs will recognize ventricular fibrillation and ventricular tachycardia as shockable rhythms. **b.** One electrode is placed to the right of the upper portion of the sternum below the clavicle. The other electrode is placed over the ribs to the left of the nipple with the center in the midaxillary line.

# Chapter 20

## DIABETES AND ALTERED MENTAL STATUS

### Matching

1. f
2. d
3. e
4. a
5. b
6. c

### Review Questions

1. **False.** You can treat the patient with altered mental status by caring for airway, breathing, and circulation, even if you do not know the cause of the altered mental status.
2. **False.** Altered mental status can be caused by medical conditions such as hypoglycemia and seizures and by trauma, such as trauma to the head.
3. Signs and symptoms of hypoglycemia include slurred speech, unresponsiveness, appearance of intoxication or taking drugs, increased heart rate, cool, clammy skin, and combativeness.
4. **True.** Not all seizures cause the body to convulse.
5. Common causes of seizures include fever, infection, poisoning, intoxication, hypoglycemia, head trauma, decreased levels of oxygen, epilepsy uncontrolled by medication, or no known cause.
6. **False.** Not all seizures are life threatening.

7. One of the most common causes of seizures in children is a *fever.*
8. The time following a seizure when the patient may be disoriented is called the *postictal* period.
9. a. Most strokes are caused by blood clots in the arteries leading to the brain, called ischemic strokes.
10. Common signs and symptoms of stroke include sudden weakness or numbness (often on one side of the body), confusion, trouble speaking, or seeing. Additionally, these patients may complain of headache and difficulty walking. You should always be concerned about the possibility of a stroke when assessing a patient with difficulty speaking, confusion, or altered mental status.
11. c. Positive findings on the Cincinnati stroke scale include slurred speech, facial droop, and arm drifting away or to the floor when held out in front of the patient.
12. Common causes of altered mental status include low blood sugar, seizure, poisoning, intoxication, infection, head trauma, decreased oxygen levels, and hypothermia or hyperthermia.
13. The primary goal of emergency treatment for patients with altered mental status is maintaining an *open airway.*
14. Major points to assess during the focused history and physical examination of a patient with altered mental status include the onset, duration, associated signs and symptoms, evidence of trauma, seizures, and fever.
15. **True.** Evaluating the scene can reveal signs of trauma or evidence of a medical condition (such as a Medic Alert bracelet or medications).
16. **c.** Patients with altered mental status are considered unstable, and their vital signs should be reevaluated every 5 minutes.
17. Ask patients with a history of diabetes when they ate their last meal and whether they have taken their medications.
18. **False.** Oral glucose is indicated only for patients with an altered mental status and a history of diabetes. The patient must be alert enough to swallow so the glucose does not cause an airway obstruction.
19. **True.** The patient must be alert enough to swallow so the oral glucose does not cause airway compromise.
20. **a.** Oral glucose is a generic name. Trade names include Insta-Glucose and Glutose.
21. **False.** The medication should be administered by a tongue depressor placed between the patient's cheek and gums to be absorbed.
22. Absence of a *gag reflex* is a contraindication for administration of oral glucose.
23. Oral glucose improves the patient's condition by increasing *blood sugar.*
24. **True.** Medical direction must be involved with the administration of any medication to a patient, including oral glucose.
25. **a.** Hypoglycemia. If your partner takes her insulin but does not eat, the insulin will draw on other stores of sugar in the body tissues. **b.** Altered mental status, cold and clammy skin, hostility or agitation, anxiety, combative behavior (in extreme cases), and seizures are signs and symptoms of a diabetic emergency. **c.** Request the dispatcher to send out another EMS unit to the crash scene. Contact medical direction to obtain an order for oral glucose. As long as she remains responsive, you may administer the full tube of glucose between your partner's cheek and gum, allowing the mucous membrane to absorb the glucose.
26. **a.** You should perform an initial assessment that includes assessing the level of responsiveness, positioning the patient (with spinal precautions), and checking the airway, breathing, and circulation. **b.** Common causes of altered mental status include low blood sugar, seizure, poisoning, intoxication, infection, head trauma, decreased oxygen levels, and hypothermia or hyperthermia. **c.** Assess the scene for additional clues, obtain baseline vital signs and monitor them every 5 minutes, check the patient for medical identification tags, maintain airway and ventilation, and rapidly transport for physician evaluation.

## Chapter 21

## ALLERGIC REACTIONS

### Review Questions

1. **d.** Allergic reactions are exaggerated immune responses to an allergen. Reactions can be severe, causing hypoperfusion and respiratory difficulty, or minor, producing only a local reaction.
2. **False.** Some allergic reactions are mild; others can be life threatening. The type of reaction depends on the allergen involved and the individual patient.
3. Common allergens include food (shellfish, crustaceans, peanuts), plants (poison ivy), medications (penicillin, aspirin), and environmental particles (dust, pollen).

4. Common signs and symptoms of an allergic reaction include itchy, watery eyes; coughing or stridor; wheezing; rapid, labored breathing; headache; runny nose; tightness in the throat; increased heart rate; decreased blood pressure; itchy, red, or flushed skin; hives; and swelling.
5. Itchy, watery eyes, a runny nose, and a headache are signs and symptoms of a *mild* allergic reaction.
6. The first sign of hypoperfusion may be a change in *mental status.*
7. *Anaphylaxis* is the term used to describe a significant allergic reaction.
8. **b.** Signs and symptoms of hypoperfusion (including low blood pressure) and respiratory compromise are signs of a true medical emergency.
9. **b.** The epinephrine autoinjector is used for patients with severe allergic reactions, characterized by hypoperfusion and respiratory compromise.
10. A patient with an allergic reaction and signs of respiratory compromise should be reassessed every 5 minutes.
11. **a.** Epinephrine works by dilating the bronchioles, making breathing easier, and constricting the blood vessels, increasing blood pressure.
12. To use an autoinjector, the patient must have a severe allergic reaction (with respiratory distress or hypoperfusion, or both) and have medication prescribed by the patient's own physician; medical direction must authorize the use.
13. **False.** When the patient is experiencing a life-threatening reaction, no contraindications exist to the use of the autoinjector. All of the indications listed in question 12 must be met.
14. **True.** An autoinjector is designed for people who are not familiar with calculating drug doses and giving injections. The medication is automatically injected at the right dose when the needle is depressed against the thigh.
15. **c.** Epinephrine does not typically cause sleepiness. Common side effects of epinephrine include increased heart rate, pale skin, dizziness, chest pain, headache, nausea and vomiting, excitability, and anxiousness.
16. **False.** Airway management is always a priority in patient care.
17. **a.** Signs and symptoms of allergic reactions include itchy, watery eyes; coughing or stridor; wheezing; rapid labored respirations; headache; runny nose; tightness in the throat; increased heart rate; decreased blood pressure; itchy, red, or flushed skin; hives; and swelling. **b.** To use the epinephrine autoinjector, you will need assessment findings of a severe allergic reaction, the patient must have his or her own physician-prescribed medication, and you will need authorization from medical direction. **c.** To administer the autoinjector, remove the safety cap on the autoinjector; place the tip of the autoinjector at a 90-degree angle against the lateral portion of the patient's thigh midway between the waist and the knee; push the injector firmly against the thigh and hold the injector in place for at least 10 seconds or until the medication is injected; dispose of the injector in a biohazard container.
18. **a.** Insect bites, foods, plants, medications, chemicals, dust, and pollen can cause mild allergic reactions. **b.** Any assessment findings that reveal (a) hypoperfusion, such as cool, clammy skin, an elevated heart rate, or decreased blood pressure, or (b) respiratory distress, such as coughing or stridor, tightness in the throat, or rapid labored breathing, would indicate a severe allergic reaction. **c.** No. She has no physician-prescribed autoinjector. The patient is not wheezing and has no signs of respiratory compromise or hypoperfusion.

## Chapter 22

## POISONING AND OVERDOSE

### Matching

1. c
2. f
3. d
4. e
5. b
6. a

### Review Questions

1. **True.** Any medication can cause a poisoning if a larger dose than recommended is taken.
2. Ongoing assessments are performed every 5 minutes for unstable patients and every 15 minutes for stable patients.

3. When assessing the poisoning or overdose patient, ask the following questions in addition to the questions you would normally ask during the focused history and physical examination for medical patients: What substance was involved? When did you ingest or become exposed to the substance? If you ingested the poison, how much did you ingest? Over what time period did the poisoning occur? What has happened since the poisoning? How much do you weigh?
4. **False.** Poisoning from medications that are chronic (occurring over weeks or months) may be treated differently than poisoning from a single ingestion. Ask the patient over what time period the poisoning occurred.
5. **False.** Over-the-counter treatments may not be appropriate, depending on the type of poison involved. When contacting medical direction, inform them that the patient has taken home remedies.
6. **b.** Ingested toxins commonly cause nausea, vomiting, and diarrhea but can also cause altered mental status, abdominal pain, chemical burns around the mouth, and particular breath odors.
7. Any pills or tablets in the mouth should be removed so that no further medication is absorbed and to prevent airway compromise. The EMT–Basic should use gloved hands to remove the pills from the mouth of an unresponsive patient and insert a bite block in the patient's mouth so the EMT–Basic is not bitten.
8. Inhaled toxins typically affect the brain, lungs and respiratory system.
9. Inhaled toxins can cause difficulty breathing, chest pain, coughing, hoarseness, dizziness, headache, confusion, seizures, and altered mental status.
10. The primary treatment for inhaled poisoning is *oxygen.* After ensuring that the scene is safe for you and the patient, begin to administer oxygen at 15 L/minute via a nonrebreather mask.
11. Injected toxins can reach the body by bites or stings or by intravenous, intramuscular, or subcutaneous injection.
12. **False.** In the case of injection poisonings, the animal that caused the bite or sting can also be dangerous to the rescuer, and you should not attempt to capture the animal.
13. The rate of absorption of the toxin depends on many factors, including location of the injection site, the type of insect or creature that caused the injury, and the blood flow to the bitten area.
14. **c.** Absorbed toxins are substances that come in contact with the skin and are absorbed into the body.
15. **a.** Dry substances should be brushed away from the skin, liquid substances irrigated for at least 20 minutes. Contact medical direction or consult the container for directions for dealing with accidental skin contact.
16. **b.** Activated charcoal is an oral medication and is effective only for ingested toxins.
17. Activated charcoal works by *binding* to the toxin in the *stomach.* The medication is therefore not absorbed into the bloodstream through the digestive system.
18. **a.** Activated charcoal is the generic name, and LiquiChar and InstaChar are examples of trade names for the drug.
19. Contraindications to the use of activated charcoal include (1) a patient with an altered mental status, (2) suspected ingestion of an acid or alkali substance, (3) inability to swallow, or (4) seizures.
20. **False.** Activated charcoal is designed to bind to toxins in the stomach. If the patient vomits, medical direction may order another dose of activated charcoal.
21. **a.** The normal dose of activated charcoal for infants and children is 1 g/kilogram of body weight, or 12.5 to 25.0 g. **b.** The indication for activated charcoal is a patient with clinical signs and symptoms of ingested poisonings. Contraindications are an altered mental status, suspected ingestion of an acid or alkali substance, inability to swallow, and seizures. **c.** Contact medical direction. The physician may order that the dose be repeated one time.
22. **a.** After controlling the airway, oxygen is the first treatment. **b.** Carbon monoxide is an invisible, odorless, and tasteless gas. General symptoms of exposure may include weakness, sleepiness, headache, dizziness, and confusion. **c.** Carbon monoxide poisoning is a serious possibility with fire victims.

## Chapter 23

## ENVIRONMENTAL EMERGENCIES

### Matching

1. d
2. e
3. f
4. b
5. g
6. c
7. a

### Review Questions

1. **True.** Any significant changes in body temperature can affect the functioning of the body.
2. The human body loses heat by evaporation, conduction, radiation, *convection*, and *respiration.*
3. When body temperature begins to decrease, the body produces heat by *shivering.*
4. **b.** When the body temperature begins to rise, the blood vessels dilate to allow more blood to reach the skin where it can be cooled.
5. When body temperature begins to increase, the body produces *sweat,* which cools the body by evaporation.
6. **True.** Any drop below the normal temperature is classified as hypothermia.
7. **False.** The most common cause of generalized hypothermia is exposure to cold environment.
8. Predisposing factors for generalized hypothermia include cold environments, immersion in water, age, alcohol, shock, head or spinal cord injury, burns, generalized infection, diabetes, hypoglycemia, and some medications and poisons.
9. Elderly patients are at increased risk of developing hypothermia resulting from loss of insulating body fat, less efficient body warming mechanisms and as a result of some medications.
10. An unreliable sign of hypothermia is cool *extremities.* Blood flow to the extremities is usually limited when the body is trying to preserve heat.
11. Cool abdominal skin is a sign of a generalized cold emergency.
12. **a.** Signs and symptoms of early hypothermia include rapid pulse, normal blood pressure, rapid breathing, red skin, reactive pupils, and shivering.
13. **True.** As the body tries to increase heat production, the heart rate and respiratory rate increase.
14. Allowing the body to produce its own heat while preventing further heat loss is passive rewarming. Adding heat to the body is active rewarming.
15. Heat packs at the axilla and groin are a form of *active* rewarming.
16. **False.** Rewarming a patient in late hypothermia can cause lethal arrhythmias. Simply prevent heat loss in the patient and transport gently to the receiving facility.
17. A pulse check for a severely hypothermic patient should be between 30 and 45 seconds.
18. Five body areas most susceptible to localized cold injuries are the fingers, toes, ears, nose, and face.
19. **c.** A tingling sensation occurs in early local cold injuries. Late local cold injuries usually involve a loss of sensation.
20. **False.** Rubbing and massaging a cold area can cause serious tissue damage.
21. Predisposing factors for heat emergencies include hot, humid weather, vigorous activity, elderly patients, infants and newborns, heart disease, dehydration, obesity, previous history of hyperthermia, fever, fatigue, diabetes, and drugs and medications.
22. Signs and symptoms of generalized heat emergency include muscle cramps; weakness or exhaustion; dizziness or fainting; rapid, pounding heartbeat; altered mental status; moist, pale, cool, or normal skin; nausea and vomiting; and abdominal cramps.
23. **True.** A sign of a severe heat emergency exists anytime the patient has hot skin, either dry or moist.
24. When the patient has hot skin, all measures to cool the body should be used, including fanning the patient and turning up the air conditioning, keeping the skin wet, and applying cold packs.
25. Drowning is defined as death following immersion in water. Near drowning means the patient survived an immersion incident.
26. **True.** Patients found unresponsive in the water should be treated and evaluated for possible spinal injury.
27. **False.** As with any patient, the first priority in the management of a patient with a bite or sting is to assess and manage airway, breathing, and circulation.
28. **b.** Extremities with bite or sting injuries should be positioned slightly below the level of the heart.
29. **True.** Use a credit card or similar material to scrape the stinger out of the skin. Do not squeeze a stinger with tweezers because this may cause additional venom to be injected into the patient.

30. **a.** Predisposing factors for generalized hypothermia include cold environments, immersion in water, extremes of age, alcohol consumption, shock, head or spinal cord injury, burns, generalized infection, diabetes, hypoglycemia, and some medications and poisons. **b.** Hypothermic patients often exhibit poor coordination, memory disturbances, reduced or absent sensation of touch, mood changes, joint or muscle pain, poor judgment, less communicative, dizziness, and speech difficulties. **c.** You should remove the patient from the cold environment and protect the patient from further heat loss. Remove any wet clothing, and cover the patient with a blanket. You should avoid rough handling, administer high-flow oxygen, not allow the patient to eat or drink stimulants, avoid massaging the extremities; and check for a pulse for 30 to 45 seconds before starting CPR.
31. **a.** Immobilize the spine if trauma is suspected; ensure an adequate airway; artificially ventilate the patient with supplemental oxygen; and suction as needed. **b.** Place the patient on the left side (or tilt the long backboard to the left). With suction immediately available, place your hand over the epigastric area and apply firm pressure to relieve the distention. **c.** No. Do not attempt to relieve gastric distention unless it interferes with artificial ventilation. The risk of aspiration is significant.

## Chapter 24

## BEHAVIORAL EMERGENCIES

### Matching

1. d
2. e
3. a
4. b
5. c

### Review Questions

1. The way that people act on a day-to-day basis is called their *behavior.*
2. A person's behavior can be altered by many factors, including situational stress, alcohol, legal and illegal drugs, illness, diabetes, hypoxia, hypoperfusion, thermoregulatory emergencies, and trauma.
3. **b.** Patients who are not thinking rationally should be treated carefully and calmly. Do not excite or agitate these patients.
4. Risk factors for suicide include patients who are older than 40 years of age, are widowed or divorced, are alcoholic, are depressed, have a history of self-destructive behavior, have a serious illness, have an unusual gathering of destructive articles, have suffered the recent loss of a loved one, have recent arrests or imprisonment, and have recently lost a job.
5. **False.** Patients who commit suicide may display no risk factors, and people with many risk factors for suicide may never consider killing themselves.
6. **True.** Scene size-up, including scene safety, is the most important aspect of entering any potentially violent or dangerous scene.
7. Signs of potential violence include sitting on the edge of the chair, clenched fists, yelling and using profanity, throwing things, standing or moving toward the EMT–Basic, holding onto a potentially dangerous object, and behavior that makes the EMT–Basic uneasy.
8. **False.** All patients who are displaying behavioral emergencies should be evaluated to determine if the cause of their problem is medical, trauma, or psychologic.
9. **True.** Do not argue with a patient who is displaying irrational thinking, but do not agree with the patient's disturbed thinking.
10. Patients who do not calm down or are showing signs of destructive behavior may need to be *restrained.*
11. Restraints may help you provide adequate care to the patient, but if used incorrectly, they can cause *injury or harm to the patient.*
12. **False.** The staff at the receiving facility should remove restraints. If a restraint appears to be too tight, loosen but do not remove the restraint.
13. **False.** Never restrain a patient in a prone position.
14. **False.** Patients who are not able to make competent, reasonable decisions can be transported against their will, after consulting medical direction, local law enforcement, or following local protocols.

15. When documenting care for a patient with a behavioral emergency, be sure to include the position in which the patient was found, any aggressive or abnormal actions made by the patient, anything unusual the patient says, aspects of assessment and the findings in detail, restraining procedures used and assessment findings before and after their use, and any persons assisting or witnessing the treatment and transport of the patient.
16. Assistance in determining the need for transport of a patient refusing care should be obtained through *medical direction.*
17. The amount of force required to keep patients from injuring themselves or others is called *reasonable* force.
18. **a.** Assess how the patient actually feels and if the patient expresses suicidal tendencies. Questions to ask this patient include: "What is your name, the date, and your address?" "How do you feel?" "Would you like some help with your problem?" "Do you have history of diabetes or other medical problem that requires medication?" **b.** Ask all questions in a calm and reassuring manner; do not be judgmental; repeat the patient's answers to show that you are listening; always acknowledge how the patient feels; and do not challenge or argue with the patient. **c.** Document the position in which the patient was found, any aggressive or abnormal actions, unusual statements, aspects of assessment and findings, any restraining procedures used and assessment and findings before and after their use, and persons assisting or witnessing the treatment and transport.

# Chapter 25

## OBSTETRICS AND GYNECOLOGY

### Matching 1

1. d
2. a
3. f
4. b
5. e
6. c

### Matching 2

7. c
8. b
9. e
10. d
11. f
12. a

### Matching 3

13. b
14. f
15. d
16. c
17. g
18. e
19. a

### Review Questions

1. The fetus grows and develops in the *uterus.*
2. During pregnancy, the fetus receives nutrition from the mother through the *placenta.*
3. **False.** The placenta is an organ that develops during pregnancy and is expelled from the woman's body after the birth of the baby.
4. **c.** The amniotic sac contains 1 to 2 L of amniotic fluid, surrounding and cushioning the fetus.
5. **b.** The usual length of pregnancy is 40 weeks, or approximately 9 months.
6. During pregnancy a woman's blood volume *increases* to accommodate for the needs of the baby.
7. **True.** The first stage of labor begins with the first contractions and ends when the fetus enters the birth canal. The second stage of labor begins when the fetus enters the birth canal and ends when the baby is delivered. The third stage of labor begins with the delivery of the baby and ends with the delivery of the placenta.
8. **False.** Crowning is a sign that delivery is very close. If crowning is seen in the assessment of the mother, time is insufficient to transport the mother, and delivery will occur on scene.
9. The OB kit contains (1) surgical scissors or a scalpel used to cut the umbilical cord, (2) hemostats or cord clamps used to clamp the umbilical cord, (3) umbilical tape or sterilized cord used to tie the umbilical cord, (4) bulb syringe used to suction the infant's mouth and nose, (5) towels to dry the infant, (6) $2 \times 10$ gauze sponges to wipe the infant's mouth and nose, (7) sterile gloves to wear during delivery, (8) baby blanket to warm the infant, (9) sanitary napkins for the mother after delivery, and (10) a plastic bag to transport the placenta to the hospital.
10. **True.** Pregnant women should be treated based on their signs and symptoms the same as any other patient would be. The care that is best for the mother will also provide the best care for the fetus.

11. Labor pains are associated with the contraction of the *uterus.*
12. **False.** Labor and delivery involve a large amount of blood and body fluids; EMT–Basics will therefore need to wear gloves, eye protection, mask, and gown.
13. A miscarriage usually occurs in the first 3 months of a pregnancy.
14. When deciding whether to transport the mother or to assist in delivery on scene, consider: When is the baby due? Are any contractions or pain occurring? Is any bleeding or discharge occurring? Is the mother feeling an increasing pressure in the vaginal area? Does the mother feel the urge to push? Also assess if crowning is occurring during contractions, and place a gloved hand on the abdomen above the navel to assess contractions.
15. Have the mother lie on her back with her legs flexed and widely separated. Create a sterile field around the vaginal opening with towels or paper barriers, and place towels across her thighs and abdomen.
16. **b.** Gentle pressure should be applied to the perineum to prevent an explosive delivery.
17. **a.** Check to ensure that the umbilical cord is not around the baby's neck. If the cord is around the neck, either loosen the cord and slip it over the baby's head or clamp and cut the cord.
18. Suction the baby's mouth and nose with the *bulb syringe* before the delivery of the torso.
19. **a.** The umbilical cord should be cut between the umbilical clamps after pulsations have stopped in the cord. The first clamp is placed approximately four finger-widths away from the baby and the second several inches further from the first clamp.
20. **False.** The placenta should be allowed to deliver on its own; never pull on the umbilical cord to pull out the placenta.
21. **False.** The placenta must be transported along with the mother and baby to the receiving facility where it will be evaluated for completeness.
22. If the mother loses more than 500 ml of blood during the delivery, the EMT–Basic should provide *uterine massage.* If the mother continues to bleed excessively, the uterus should be massaged with both hands fully extended on the lower abdomen above the pubis, which should lessen bleeding. Treat the mother for the signs and symptoms of shock, if necessary. Breast-feeding will also help the uterus contract. Ask the mother if she would like to breast-feed the infant.
23. **d.** The infant is assessed based on appearance, pulse, grimace, activity, and respiratory effort.
24. The heart rate of a newborn should be greater than 100 beats per minute.
25. **c.** If the heart rate is less than 80 beats per minute after ventilations, the EMT–Basic should start chest compressions, following neonatal CPR standards.
26. **b.** Transport the mother with a prolapsed cord in whatever position will relieve the most pressure from the cord, either with her hips elevated or with her head lowered.
27. **a.** Use a gloved hand to make a "V" around the baby's face to prevent suffocation with a breech presentation.
28. **a.** Babies from multiple births are often smaller and born earlier than single births. The infants may need to be treated the same as premature infants are treated. The mother may not know that she is having more than one baby, even if she has had prenatal care. Complication rates are higher for twins; therefore be prepared with extra personnel. Cut the umbilical cord of the first infant born, then prepare for the delivery of the second infant.
29. **True.** When one limb presents, the baby cannot deliver in this position and will require a surgical delivery.
30. **True.** Meconium, or fetal stool, is usually associated with fetal distress and can create an airway problem.
31. Infants born at less than 37 weeks or weighing less than 5.5 pounds are considered to be *premature.*
32. **True.** Premature infants have less developed respiratory and cardiac systems and may require resuscitation.
33. **True.** Discourage the patient from washing, bathing, or going to the bathroom until she has been examined and the evidence is collected.
34. **a.** When is the baby due? Are any contractions or pain present? Is any bleeding or discharge occurring? Is the mother feeling increasing pressure in the vaginal area? Does the mother feel the urge to push? Is crowning during contractions occurring? **b.** Attempt to loosen the cord and slip it over the baby's head. If the cord cannot be removed, clamp the cord in two places, cut the cord between the two clamps, and remove the cord from the baby's neck. **c.** Record the time of delivery. Transport the mother, infant, and placenta to the hospital. Be sure to keep the infant warm.

35. **a.** Provide positive-pressure ventilations with a BVM. **b.** Evaluate the infant's heart rate. If the rate is less than 80 beats per minute and the newborn is not responding to ventilations, start chest compressions. **c.** If the heart rate is above 100 beats per minute and respirations are adequate, administer free-flow oxygen and initiate transport of the mother and infant for physician evaluation.

## Chapter 26

## GERIATRICS

### Matching

1. a
2. c
3. d
4. e
5. b

### Review Questions

1. People in the United States are living longer owing to better nutrition, improving health care, vaccinations from potentially fatal disease, and an increase in public health.
2. A generalized decline in body function begins as early as age 30.
3. **False.** From 30 to 80 years of age, the respiratory system shows a 50% decrease in vital capacity.
4. An elderly patient having a myocardial infarction (MI) may have atypical symptoms such as syncope, difficulty breathing, abdominal or epigastric pain, simple fatigue, and shortness of breath.
5. Almost one half of elderly patients with acute MI present with shortness of breath instead of chest pain.
6. Decreasing renal function in the elderly can lead to problems with *water balance.*
7. The two major cardiovascular diseases are heart attack and stroke.
8. **a.** Another word for ministroke is TIA, or transischemic attack.
9. **a.** Patients experiencing vertigo report feeling a spinning or whirling sensation.
10. **False.** Dementia is more common in the elderly but is not a normal process of aging.
11. **d.** Delirium is a syndrome (not a final diagnosis) this is separate from dementia. Delirium has a significant mortality rate, as high as 20%.
12. **a.** Patients commonly have a decrease in height of 2 to 3 inches.
13. Physiologic reasons for the elderly patient's poor tolerance to temperature extremes include vasodilation, use of medications that interfere with heat transfer and sweating, inability to concentrate urine, central nervous system disorders, endocrine disorders, and other chronic illnesses. Social factors usually revolve around fixed incomes and inability to control environmental temperatures.
14. **a.** Organic brain syndromes and mood disorders are the most prevalent psychiatric disorders in older adults.
15. **True.** The elderly have a much higher risk of death and disability from trauma, especially multisystem trauma, than do younger individuals.
16. **False.** Elderly patients do not commonly make suicidal gestures. In many cases, when elderly patients attempt suicide, they are successful.
17. When immobilizing elderly patients, you should pad over bony prominences such as the sacrum and elbows; you may need to pad the head of the board if the patient cannot lie flat; you should pad the extremities for comfort.
18. b. If an elderly patient with difficulty hearing cannot understand your speech, you should consider writing notes. Shouting will distort the sounds and will not help the patient understand you. Make every attempt to talk with the patient.
19. **b.** Elder abuse knows no socioeconomic bounds and becomes a problem when an older person loses his or her independence. Elder abuse usually manifests as neglect. Most states have statutes requiring reporting of elder abuse.
20. EMS providers can intervene in home safety, give influenza vaccines, and be aware of the potential for help from outside agencies.

## Division Four Examination

1. **b.** EMT–Basics carry activated charcoal, oral glucose, and oxygen on the EMS unit. EMT–Basics can assist patients with their own physician-prescribed nitroglycerin, epinephrine autoinjectors, and inhalers.

2. **b.** The generic name is listed in the *U.S. Pharmacopeia,* which is a government publication listing all medications used in the United States. The chemical name is a precise description of the chemical composition of the drug. The trade name is assigned by the manufacturer to market the drug.
3. **b.** A contraindication is a situation in which a medication should not be used. The medication will not be helpful to the patient and may be harmful. An indication is a common use of a medication for treating an illness or condition.
4. **c.** Activated charcoal is a suspension and must be shaken thoroughly to keep the contents mixed.
5. **c.** Oral medications have a slow onset of action because they must be absorbed in the digestive system. Oral medications should not be given to unresponsive patients because they will be unable to swallow the medication. Oral medications are good for responsive cooperative children. A medication sprayed under the tongue is being administered by the sublingual route.
6. **a.** Knowing the side effects of a drug can help the EMT–Basic anticipate its onset and be prepared to deal with any complications. Side effects are the undesirable actions of a drug. The mechanism of action describes how a drug affects the body. EMT–Basics should not help a patient with any medication unless doing so is approved by medical direction and unless the EMT–Basic is thoroughly familiar with the drug.
7. **d.** The larynx is also known as the voice box. The oropharynx is the part of the throat behind the mouth. The diaphragm is the dome-shaped muscle that separates the thoracic cavity from the abdominal cavity and is used in breathing. The trachea is the windpipe.
8. **c.** Respiratory disease can change the shape of a patient's chest over time. Stridor indicates an upper airway obstruction; gurgling is heard when liquid is in the back of the airway. Agonal respirations are sudden short breaths with long pauses in between, often occurring when the patient is near death. These respirations are not normal in any patient. If a patient is showing signs of hypoxia, the patient should receive high-concentration oxygen, even if the patient normally receives low-concentration oxygen.
9. **d.** A rate of 12 to 20 breaths per minute is normal for an adult patient. Shortness of breath and retractions indicate difficulty breathing in any age group. Other signs of adequate breathing include equal chest expansion, a regular rhythm, and an adequate tidal volume.
10. **b.** Proventil and Ventolin are both examples of trade names for albuterol. A medication can have more than one trade name if it is marketed by different manufacturers.
11. **c.** To assist a patient with a prescribed inhaler, the patient must have signs and symptoms of respiratory distress and his or her own prescribed inhaler, and medical direction must authorize its use. If the patient is unresponsive, using an inhaler is contraindicated. EMT–Basics do not carry inhalers on the EMS unit; patients must therefore have their own inhaler.
12. **c.** Common side effects of a prescribed inhaler use include increased pulse rate, tremors, nervousness, and sometimes nausea.
13. **b.** The right ventricle receives oxygen poor blood from the right atrium and then pumps the blood to the lungs via the pulmonary arteries to become saturated with oxygen. The blood then goes to the left atrium, the left ventricle, and the body through the aorta.
14. **d.** The signs and symptoms of shock (hypoperfusion) include a rapid and weak pulse, pale or cyanotic skin, cool and clammy skin, rapid and shallow breathing, restlessness and anxiety, mental dullness, nausea and vomiting, thirst, low blood pressure, and a low temperature.
15. **d.** Position responsive patients with no suspected trauma in a position of comfort. Patients experiencing chest pain or difficulty breathing usually prefer sitting up versus lying flat on their back.
16. **b.** Indications for the use of nitroglycerin or conditions that must be met before nitroglycerin is used include signs and symptoms of cardiac chest pain, the patient has his or her own nitroglycerin, and medical direction authorizes its use. Nitroglycerin should not be used if the patient has already taken the maximum dose, if the patient is not mentally alert, or if the blood pressure is less than 100 mm Hg systolic.
17. **a.** AEDs can be used for patients who are older than 1 year of age. The patient must be unresponsive and have no pulse for the AED to be applied.
18. **d.** Perform CPR for 2 minutes after the AED delivers a shock. After 2 minutes, reanalyze the patient's rhythm and shock again if the AED indicates that this action is necessary.

19. b. Signs and symptoms of a diabetic emergency include an appearance of intoxication, altered mental status, fast heart rate, cool and clammy skin, combativeness, and hunger.
20. b. Common medication names for the control of diabetes include Humulin, Diabinese, Orinase, and Micronase. Ventolin is a respiratory medication, Dilantin is for seizure control, and Procardia is a cardiac medication.
21. b. Common causes of seizures include fever, infection, poisoning, intoxication, hypoglycemia, head trauma, hypoxia, and epilepsy.
22. c. To administer oral glucose, the patient must be alert enough to swallow, have signs and symptoms of altered mental status, and have a known history of diabetes. Oral glucose cannot be administered if the patient is unresponsive or has no known medical history.
23. d. Oral glucose should never be given to an unresponsive patient. Any substance placed in the mouth of an unresponsive patient can cause airway compromise.
24. d. An allergic reaction is an exaggerated immune response to an allergen. Common allergens include food (peanuts, shrimp), medications (penicillin, aspirin), plants (poison ivy), and environmental factors (dust, pollen).
25. b. The SAMPLE history is assessed during the focused history and physical examination for the medical patient. The assessment should be focused on the patient's chief complaint.
26. b. The adult autoinjector contains 0.3 mg of epinephrine. The child autoinjector generally contains one half of the adult dose.
27. c. The autoinjector is placed against the lateral thigh, midway between the waist and knee. Hold the injector firmly in place until the injector activates. Leave the needle in place for at least 10 seconds.
28. c. The autoinjector has a sharp needle that has been in direct contact with the patient's body fluid. Dispose of the entire autoinjector in a biohazard container designed for sharps.
29. a. Common side effects of epinephrine include increased heart rate, pale skin, dizziness, nausea and vomiting, excitability, and anxiousness.
30. c. When questioning a patient who has overdosed or was poisoned, ask the following questions: "When did you ingest or become exposed to the substance?" "How much poison did you ingest?" "Over what time period did the poisoning occur?" "What has happened since the poisoning?" "How much do you weigh?" Do not question the patient's motives or accuse the patient of intentional overdose. Cases of suspected negligence or child abuse should be reported to the proper authorities after the call is over.
31. b. Ingested toxins often cause nausea and vomiting or diarrhea, altered mental status, abdominal pain, chemical burns around the mouth, and particular breath odors.
32. d. Activated charcoal binds to toxins in the patient's stomach; therefore it is useful only for patients who have ingested the toxin.
33. b. The usual dose of activated charcoal for both adult and child patients is 1 g of activated charcoal per kilogram of body weight.
34. b. Common side effects of activated charcoal include vomiting and black stools. Be prepared to suction if the patient vomits. Medical direction may order the administration of a second dose of activated charcoal if the patient vomits.
35. c. The body loses heat by conduction (direct transfer of heat), convection (through moving air or liquids), evaporation (when a liquid changes to a gas), radiation (infrared energy), and respiration (exhaling warm air). Shivering raises the body temperature.
36. c. The skin should be evaluated on the patient's trunk, abdomen, or back. The skin of the extremities is unreliable because blood flow is normally decreased to the extremities to conserve heat. Skin on exposed areas such as the face and hands is also unreliable.
37. a. Signs and symptoms of early generalized hypothermia include rapid pulse, normal blood pressure, rapid breathing, red skin, and reactive pupils. Late signs and symptoms include slow, barely palpable, or irregular pulse; low or absent blood pressure; shallow or absent breathing; pale, cyanotic, or stiff skin; and sluggish pupils.
38. c. Hot skin, whether moist or dry, indicates that the body no longer has the ability to lose heat. This sign indicates an emergency, and the patient should be cooled as quickly as possible.

39. **b.** The incidence of spinal injuries is high in water-related emergencies; therefore be prepared to immobilize the patient if trauma is indicated. Drowning means that the patient has died following an immersion incident; near drowning means the patient has survived. Gastric distention should be relieved only if it interferes with ventilation. Immersion in cold water increases the likelihood of resuscitation after long immersion.
40. **c.** Use the edge of a card to scrape the stinger out of the skin. Tweezers may squeeze the venom out of the venom sac. Using your finger may expose you to the poison or venom. The stinger should be removed so as to prevent further exposure.
41. **d.** Patients considered to be at risk for suicide include those who are more than 40 years of age, are widowed or divorced, are alcoholic, are depressed, have spoken of taking their own lives, have a history of self-destructive behavior, have recently been diagnosed with a serious illness, live in an environment where an unusual gathering of destructive articles are present, have recently lost a loved one, were recently imprisoned, and have recently lost their job.
42. **a.** To calm a patient, be sure to tell the patient what you are doing, and answer honestly any questions the patient may have. Repeat the patient's answers to your questions to show that you are listening. Do not be judgmental toward the patient. Include family members and friends in your assessment of the patient.
43. **c.** EMT–Basics should use wide, soft restraints to avoid cutting off distal circulation to an extremity. Behavioral emergency patients should be assessed for illness or injury. Ask patients about their medical history to search for clues relating to their behavioral emergency. Same-sex attendants should be used whenever possible, and EMT–Basics should have witnesses with them when caring for a patient with a behavioral emergency.
44. **c.** When restraining a patient, use only the amount of force necessary to keep the patient from injuring him or herself or others. This amount is known as reasonable force.
45. **b.** The uterus is the organ in which a growing fetus develops. The uterus contracts during labor to push the baby out of the birth canal. The amniotic sac surrounds the fetus with 1 to 2 L of amniotic fluid and helps cushion the fetus from injury. The birth canal is the lower part of the uterus and the vagina. The perineum is the area of skin between the vagina and anus.
46. **a.** The first stage of labor begins with regular contractions of the uterus and ends when the baby enters the birth canal. The second stage of labor begins with the baby entering the birth canal and ends when the baby is delivered. The third stage of labor begins when the baby is delivered and ends when the placenta is delivered.
47. **b.** The OB kit routinely contains surgical scissors or a scalpel, hemostats or cord clamps, umbilical tape or sterilized cord, a bulb syringe, towels, $2 \times 10$ gauze sponges, sterile gloves, a baby blanket, sanitary napkins, and a plastic bag.
48. **b.** The mother should not be allowed to use the toilet because the baby may deliver while she is trying to have a bowel movement. If contractions are less than 2 minutes apart, the mother feels a strong need to push, or if the baby is crowning, prepare for delivery on scene.
49. **b.** The umbilical cord should be cut approximately four finger-widths from the baby after being clamped.
50. **c.** Uterine massage will help slow bleeding. Losing up to 500 ml of blood is normal for delivery.
51. **b.** Prolapsed cord is when the umbilical cord is the presenting part. Breech delivery means the buttocks or both legs deliver first. Meconium is fetal stool that may be present in the amniotic fluid, indicating fetal distress.
52. **a.** The leading cause of death in the elderly population is cardiovascular disease.
53. **c.** Nitroglycerin in effective in relieving pain from angina.
54. **a.** An ischemic stroke means that brain damage results from narrowing blood vessels in the brain.
55. **d.** Dementia is diagnosed by excluding other diseases.

## Chapter 27

## BLEEDING AND SHOCK

### Matching

1. a
2. g
3. e
4. h
5. c
6. d
7. i
8. f
9. b

## Review Questions

1. The cardiovascular system delivers *blood* through a system of *arteries, veins,* and capillaries.
2. **c.** The average adult has approximately 6 L of blood in the body.
3. **False.** Not every part of the body needs to be perfused equally at all times. For example, the muscles in your thighs require more blood flow when you are jogging than when you are lying down.
4. **a.** The systolic pressure is a measure of the pressure against the arteries when the heart contracts; the diastolic pressure is a measure of the pressure against the arteries when the heart is at rest.
5. Good perfusion of the body requires an adequate *blood pressure.*
6. A decrease in perfusion to the cells in the body results in hypoperfusion or *shock.*
7. When tissues are not adequately perfused they are damaged by lack of *oxygen* and a build-up of *waste products.*
8. The four major organs easily damaged by hypoperfusion are the brain, heart, lungs, and kidneys.
9. Some of the causes of hypovolemic shock include dehydration, vomiting, diarrhea, internal blood loss, and external blood loss.
10. **b.** Changes in mental status are some of the most sensitive indicators or hypoperfusion. These mental status changes can include restlessness, anxiety, and combativeness.
11. **False.** Vasoconstriction means that the blood vessels constrict, allowing less blood to be delivered to an area of the body. Because less blood is directed toward an area, the skin becomes pale, cool, and clammy.
12. **True.** As the body tries to adjust for lowering blood pressures, less blood is directed toward the nonessential areas of the body, such as the extremities, allowing more blood to be directed toward the heart, lungs, and brain. Less blood flow causes weaker pulses.
13. **a.** Capillary refill should return the pink color to the skin in less than 2 seconds in adequately perfusing patients. Capillary refill is measured only in children younger than 6 years of age.
14. **c.** The heart rate will increase to try to meet the body's demands for more oxygen.
15. A late sign of shock is *decreased* blood pressure.
16. The first priority with any patient is to ensure an *open airway.*
17. The legs can be elevated in the shock position, as long as no injuries or suspected injuries have occurred to the (a) spine, (c) pelvis, (d) lower extremities, (e) head, (f) chest, or (g) abdomen. Lifting the legs would aggravate an injury to any of these areas of the body.
18. **True.** Always practice proper BSI precautions when external trauma is present.
19. A sudden loss of 1 L of blood for an adult patient is considered to be a serious blood loss.
20. **c.** Blood coming from an artery is under high pressure and will spurt with each heartbeat.
21. **d.** Blood coming from a vein is under lower pressure than blood from an artery and will flow from the injury site.
22. Bleeding from capillaries is usually minimal and will *ooze* from the injury site.
23. **b.** Concentrated direct pressure will put the maximum amount of pressure on the isolated injury site.
24. In the absence of one, isolated point of bleeding, diffuse direct pressure is the best method to control bleeding. Pressure points, extremity elevation, and splinting will also be effective in controlling bleeding.
25. *Elevating* an injury above the level of the heart may help decrease blood flow to that area and therefore decrease bleeding. An extremity cannot be elevated if it is injured.
26. **c.** By placing pressure against a pressure point, you can minimize the amount of blood flowing to the injury site. Because most areas of the body are perfused by more than one artery, pressure will slow bleeding but not stop it entirely.
27. **True.** Splinting an injury will help minimize bleeding by reducing the motion of sharp bone ends.
28. **True.** Using PASG when a patient has a chest injury may make breathing more difficult for the patient and may cause respiratory compromise.
29. The last resort for bleeding control is applying a *tourniquet.*
30. **a.** Use a tourniquet only after all other methods of bleeding control are exhausted; use a wide device that will not cut or damage tissue; the tourniquet must provide continuous circumferential pressure great enough to stop the bleeding; do not remove or release the tourniquet once it has been applied.
31. If a tourniquet is used, always avoid placing it over a *joint.*

32. Bleeding from the ears and nose can be a sign of a *skull fracture* in a trauma patient.
33. **False.** Applying direct pressure to the site of bleeding from the ears and nose is difficult. For nosebleeds, pinch the fleshy part of the nostrils together. Cover the ears with sterile gauze if bleeding comes from the ears.
34. If a patient has signs and symptoms of shock (hypoperfusion) and a serious mechanism of injury with no obvious bleeding, you should suspect *internal bleeding*.
35. Signs and symptoms of internal bleeding include signs and symptoms of shock, bleeding from any body orifice, blood-tinged vomit or feces, coffee-ground vomit, dark tarry stool, abdominal rigidity or tenderness, and distended abdomen.
36. If you suspect a patient is bleeding internally, you would follow BSI precautions, maintain an open airway and adequate ventilation, treat the patient for the signs and symptoms of shock, splint the injured femur, apply the PASG (if indicated), and transport immediately.
37. The PASG may be considered if the patient has signs and symptoms of shock, a tender abdomen, and suspected pelvic injury. The PASG should not be used if the patient has a chest injury. Local protocol and the presence or absence of other injuries will determine if the PASG is used.
38. **a.** High-concentration oxygen will decrease cell death from the hypoxia caused by hypoperfusion. **b.** The next steps to take in controlling bleeding are extremity elevation and pressure points. Because the patient has an open injury to this lower extremity, elevation would be not be appropriate. Attempt to control the bleeding by applying pressure to the patient's femoral artery. **c.** The PASG is helpful for immobilizing injuries to the lower extremity and in controlling bleeding in the lower extremities.
39. **a.** Bright-red bloody stools indicate bleeding in the lower gastrointestinal tract. **b.** A lowered blood pressure, an increased pulse rate, and increased respirations are classic signs of hypoperfusion caused by hypovolemia. **c.** To treat this patient, use appropriate BSI precautions, maintain an open airway, provide 100% oxygen, elevate the patent's legs 8 to 12 inches, prevent heat loss, and transport immediately.

## Chapter 28

## SOFT TISSUE INJURIES

### Matching 1

1. a
2. e
3. c
4. g
5. b
6. h
7. d
8. f

### Matching 2

9. c
10. a
11. b
12. e
13. g
14. f
15. d

### Review Questions

1. The skin serves as a barrier from infection, regulates body temperature, and contains nerve endings to transmit information to the brain.
2. **b.** Nerve endings are found in the dermis, along with sweat and sebaceous glands, hair follicles, and small blood vessels.
3. A closed injury is defined as an injury in which the skin remains intact and no external bleeding is present.
4. **a.** A contusion or bruise is discoloration of the skin caused by trauma.
5. **b.** A hematoma is a large collection of blood under the skin, producing pain and discoloration.
6. An open injury occurs when the skin is broken and external bleeding occurs.
7. **b.** Abrasions occur when the outermost layers of the skin are scraped away.
8. **c.** Lacerations can be regular or irregular and are caused when an object tears the skin.
9. **a.** Gunshot and stab wounds are examples of penetrations and punctures.
10. **d.** An amputation occurs when an appendage, such as a finger or toe, is removed from the body.
11. **True.** Soft-tissue injuries are often bloody, and the EMT–Basic will need to take proper BSI precautions.
12. **False.** An appropriately sized dressing should cover the wound with approximately 1 inch to spare on all sides.

13. Pressure can be applied by applying a bandage tightly to an injury, using gauze rolls to wrap around the injury, or using an air splint.
14. An occlusive dressing taped on *three* sides allows air to *escape* but not *enter* the wound.
15. **False.** Eviscerated abdominal contents should be protected with a moist, sterile dressing to prevent the contents from drying.
16. Impaled objects should be removed when they are in the cheek and causing airway compromise, when they interfere with CPR, or when the patient cannot be transported because of the object.
17. **b.** Because both eyes move together, they should be covered to minimize movement of the injured eye.
18. **False.** Amputated parts should be placed in a sterile dressing and then wrapped in plastic. Keep the part cool but not frozen.
19. The priority for care for all patients is to manage the *airway*. Caring for bleeding, amputations, eviscerations, and burns are all secondary to maintaining a patent airway.
20. **b.** Immobilize a partial amputation to prevent it from becoming a complete amputation. Dress and bandage the injury to minimize bleeding and contamination.
21. Direct pressure can be used on the head only if no evidence of a *skull fracture* is present.
22. **b.** When the patient has injuries involving the mouth, evaluate for the presence of blood and teeth, which may create an airway compromise.
23. To determine the severity of a burn, evaluate the depth of the burn, the total percentage of body surface area burned, the location of the burn, any preexisting medical conditions, and the age of the patient.
24. A sunburn is a type of *superficial* burn.
25. Dry, leathery, charred skin with little or no pain describes a *full-thickness* burn.
26. If blisters form, the burn is considered to be *partial thickness.*
27. In the "rule of nines," the head of an adult is *9%* of the total body surface area and the head of an infant is *18%*.
28. **True.** A circumferential burn of the torso can cause swelling and inhibit the chest rise, causing respiratory compromise.
29. Five critical areas for burns are the face, upper airway, hands, feet, and genitalia.
30. c—partial-thickness burn of the face; mod—child with a partial-thickness burn of less than 10%; min—full-thickness burn of less than 2%; mod—partial-thickness burn covering 27% of the body.
31. Burned patients are at risk for *hypothermia* and *infection* because the skin has been damaged. These patients must be kept warm.
32. **True.** Jewelry and clothing must be removed when treating a burn patient because the burned area is likely to swell, and these items can be constricting.
33. If a patient has suffered a chemical burn from dry powder, first *brush off* the powder, then *flush* with water.
34. When treating a patient with *electrical* burns, be prepared with the AED because cardiac arrest is more likely. Ensure that the patient is no longer in contact with the electrical source before beginning treatment.
35. **a.** To treat soft-tissue injuries, you should ensure a patent airway and provide ventilatory support as needed. If the patient is showing signs and symptoms of shock, administer high-flow oxygen via a nonrebreather mask; expose the wound, control the bleeding, and minimize contamination with a dry sterile dressing; assess for possible spine injury; and splint extremity injuries. **b.** If the dressing becomes saturated, remove the dressing and apply fingertip pressure (with a gloved hand) directly at the site. **c.** If the patient has signs and symptoms of shock, administer high-flow oxygen via a nonrebreather mask at 15 L/minute; place the patient in a supine position; transport the patient as soon as possible; and try to keep the patient calm and quiet.
36. **a.** A partial-thickness burn involves both the epidermis and dermis but not the underlying tissue. A full-thickness burn extends through all layers of the skin to the underlying tissue, including the subcutaneous layer, and may involve the muscle, bone, and other organs. **b.** 45%. Anterior chest and abdomen (18%), right arm (9%), right leg (18%). **c.** When caring for burn patients, use BSI precautions; use room-temperature water or saline to cool the burn; remove jewelry and smoldering clothes; continually monitor the airway; apply high-flow oxygen; cover the burns with dry, clean dressings; and keep the patient warm during transport to the nearest burn facility according to protocol.

## Chapter 29

# MUSCULOSKELETAL CARE

### Matching 1

1. e
2. b
3. f
4. g
5. a
6. c
7. d

### Matching 2

8. e
9. a
10. b
11. d
12. c
13. f

### Matching 3

14. a
15. c
16. b

### Labeling

1. **a.** Vertebral column; **b.** ribs; **c.** radius; **d.** ulna; **e.** clavicle; **f.** sternum; **g.** humerus; **h.** femur; **i.** patella; **j.** tibia; **k.** fibula.
2. **a.** Cervical vertebrae; **b.** thoracic vertebrae; **c.** lumbar vertebrae; **d.** sacral vertebrae; **e.** fused coccyx.

### Review Questions

1. Muscles give shape to the body, protect internal organs, and provide for movement of the body.
2. Skeletal muscles are attached to *bones* and are responsible for *movement.*
3. Muscles over which we have no direct control are called *involuntary* or *smooth* muscles.
4. Automaticity is a characteristic found only in *cardiac* muscle. Automaticity means that the muscle can contract on its own. Voluntary and involuntary muscles must receive an impulse from the brain to contract or relax.
5. The skeletal system gives shape to the body, protects internal organs, and provides for movement of the body.
6. The knee is an example of a *hinge* joint, and a hip is a *ball and socket* joint.
7. The mechanism of injury helps you determine the severity of the injury and find hidden injuries based on the wounding forces.
8. Signs and symptoms of a musculoskeletal injury include deformity or angulation, pain and tenderness, crepitation, swelling, bruising, exposed bone ends, and joints locked into position.
9. **True.** Splinting is performed after the assessment of airway, breathing, and circulation is complete and no immediate threats to life are found.
10. Splinting *minimizes* the amount of movement of sharp bone ends, and therefore *minimizes* damage to surrounding muscles and nerves. Splinting also reduces pain for the patient.
11. Pulse, motor function, and sensation must be evaluated *before* and *after* splinting.
12. If the distal pulse changes after splinting, *loosen* the splint and reassess.
13. **False.** The position of function is the most natural position for the hand or foot, where the least muscle is stretched. The position of function for the hand is with the palms bent and fingers slightly curled.
14. To be effective, the splint must include the joint *above* and *below* a long bone injury.
15. Full body immobilization should be used if *spinal* trauma is suspected.
16. **b.** Traction splints are used only on midshaft femur injuries, with no involvement of the hip, knee, or lower leg.
17. Pneumatic splints are good for *angulated* injuries because they allow the extremity to remain in the position found.
18. Pneumatic splints apply pressure to sites of bleeding, provide uniform contact for the extremity, and are comfortable for the patient.
19. **True.** The PASG can be used to immobilize suspected injuries to the pelvis and femur.
20. Shoulder injuries usually require a *sling and swathe* for stabilization.
21. A splint that is too loose will not keep the extremity immobilized. A splint that is too tight will cut off distal circulation and possibly cause permanent damage. Splints can compress nerves, tissues, and blood vessels. An improperly applied splint can increase bleeding and tissue damage, cause permanent nerve damage or disability, convert a closed injury to an open injury, and increase pain.

22. **a.** Signs and symptoms of a bone or joint injury include deformity or angulation, pain and tenderness, crepitation, swelling, bruising, exposed bone ends, and joints locked into position. **b.** Evaluate the pulse, motor function, and sensation distal to the injury both before and after applying a splint and record findings. **c.** Align the injury with gentle traction before splinting; pad the splint to prevent pressure and discomfort; and immobilize the hand in the position of function by placing a roll of gauze in the palm to support the hand.

## Chapter 30

## INJURIES TO THE HEAD AND SPINE

### Matching 1

1. e
2. f
3. a
4. b
5. c
6. d

### Matching 2

7. b
8. a
9. c

### Review Questions

1. The components of the central nervous system are the *brain* and the *spinal cord.*
2. Cerebral spinal fluid (CSF) surrounds the *brain* and spinal cord and acts as a *cushion.*
3. Sensory nerves carry information *from* the body *to* the brain. Sensory nerves carry information regarding pressure, pain, heat, and so forth from the body to the spinal cord and brain. Motor nerves carry information from the brain to the body.
4. The spinal column contains 33 bones.
5. In the body are 7 cervical vertebrae, 12 thoracic vertebrae, 5 lumbar vertebra, 5 sacral vertebrae, and 4 coccygeal vertebrae.
6. **False.** Cervical spine immobilization devices do not provide enough immobilization for the patient's head. The EMT–Basic must still provide manual stabilization until the head is immobilized to the long backboard.
7. A short backboard is used to immobilize the head, neck, and torso when the patient is in the *seated* position.
8. Long backboards provide *full* body immobilization.
9. **False.** The patient's head must be secured to the long backboard with a cervical spine immobilization device or tape, and straps are required to keep the body secured to the board.
10. Mechanism of injury refers to how the injury occurred and how much force was applied to the patient's body during the incident.
11. **b.** Knowing the mechanism of injury allows you to know what types of forces caused the patient's injuries, which may lead you to discover hidden injuries.
12. Significant mechanisms of injury include motor vehicle crashes; pedestrians injured in vehicle collisions; falls; blunt trauma to the head, chest, abdomen, or pelvis; penetrating trauma to the head, neck, or torso; motorcycle crashes; hanging; diving accidents; and any trauma that results in an unresponsive patient.
13. A whiplash injury occurs when someone is hit from behind in an automobile. The neck first snaps backward then forward.
14. **True.** Do not ask a patient to move an injured area just to see if pain is present. Immobilize the injured area.
15. Injuries to the shoulder and chest can cause trauma to the *spine.* Injuries to the lumbar or thoracic vertebrae are more likely if injury to the shoulder or chest occur.
16. Numbness, tingling, or weakness are possible signs and symptoms of a *spinal injury.* Paralysis is another sign of a spinal injury.
17. Ask responsive trauma patients, "What happened?" "Where does it hurt?" "Does your neck or back hurt?" "Can you move your fingers and toes?" "Where am I touching you now?"
18. DCAP-BTLS is an acronym for deformities, contusions, abrasions, penetrations or punctures, burns, tenderness, lacerations, and swelling.
19. After every intervention, assess *vital signs, motor function,* and *sensory function.*
20. **True.** Documenting any findings or changes in the patient's condition and reporting them to the receiving facility is important.
21. Completing the assessment of the cervical region *before* applying the cervical spine immobilization device may be helpful. If you assess after the device is applied, you will need to remove the device.

22. The patient with spinal cord injury may have difficulty breathing if the nerves that control the diaphragm are injured. EMT–Basics must carefully assess the patient's breathing status and assist with ventilations if indicated.
23. **a.** Cervical spine immobilization devices and complete spinal immobilization are indicated for patients whose mechanism of injury suggests that they may have injured their head, neck, or back. The cervical spine immobilization device needs to be sized appropriately, and the sizing techniques vary with different brands of devices. If moving the patient's head into neutral alignment causes pain, immobilize the head in the position found. Manual stabilization must be maintained until the patient is completely immobilized.
24. **c.** The patient's head should be immobilized to the long backboard after the shoulders and hips are secured. The legs and arms can be secured after the head is immobilized. The EMT–Basic at the head of the patient is responsible for calling patient movements. If the patient is not aligned on the long backboard, move the patient either upward or downward on the board; never push from side to side.
25. 3—secure the torso to the board; 2—place the backboard behind the patient; 7—reassess pulse, motor function, and sensation; 6—secure the arms, legs, and feet; 4—pad the voids behind the patient's head; 1—attach the straps to the board; 5—secure the head to the board.
26. To immobilize a seated patient, you can use a short backboard or a vest-type device.
27. Patients on short spine boards or KEDs must then be secured to a long backboard for transport.
28. Spinal injuries also may involve injuries to the *brain* and *skull.*
29. **False.** Scalp wounds tend to bleed a lot. Bleeding from the scalp can usually be controlled with direct pressure.
30. The best indicator of a traumatic head injury is *altered mental status.*
31. Signs and symptoms of head injury include altered mental status; irregular breathing pattern; mechanism of injury such as deformity of a windshield or helmet; deformity to the skull or a soft area or depression; blood or other fluid leaking from the ears or nose, or both; bruising around the eyes or ears; neurologic disability; nausea or vomiting, or both; unequal pupil size with altered mental status; seizure activity; contusion, lacerations or hematomas on the scalp; penetrating injury; and exposed brain tissue.
32. A patient should be rapidly extricated when (1) the scene is unsafe, (2) the patient's condition is unstable and warrants immediate movement and transport, or (3) when the patient blocks access to another more seriously injured patient.
33. **c.** The helmet should not be removed if it will cause further injury. Helmets should be removed when the patient's airway or breathing cannot be controlled with the helmet in place, if the helmet does not fit properly and allows for excessive motion, or if the head cannot be immobilized to the backboard with the helmet in place.
34. **a.** Sports helmets are typically open in the front, making access to the airway simple. Full face shield helmets will not allow the EMT–Basic to assess the airway and generally should be removed. If the helmet is left in place, a cervical spine immobilization device probably will not provide adequate immobilization, and you will need to use tape, towels, and bulky dressings in addition to the device. Shoulder pads will need to be removed if a football helmet is removed to keep the spine in neutral alignment.
35. **c.** The head is immobilized by placing one hand on the mandible at the angle of the jaw and the other hand posteriorly at the occipital region. EMT–Basics should reposition their hands as necessary to prevent the patient's head from falling back.
36. For an infant or small child, padding may have to be placed under the *shoulder* to *heels* to maintain neutral alignment.
37. **True.** Osteoporosis and arthritis are two examples of diseases that may make immobilizing an older patient difficult.
38. **a.** Airway control with spinal precautions is always the priority. **b.** Bleeding of the scalp should be controlled with direct pressure, unless a skull fracture is suspected. **c.** Signs and symptoms of head injury include altered mental status, irregular breathing patterns, deformity to the skull, blood or other fluid leaking from the ears or nose or both, bruising around the eyes or behind the ears (this is a late sign, occurring 2 to 4 hours after injury), neurologic disability, nausea or vomiting, and unequal pupil size.

## Division Five Examination

1. **c.** Hypovolemic shock occurs when the volume of blood for the heart to pump and circulate is inadequate. All organs do not need to be perfused equally at all times. The heart, lungs, kidneys and brain, for example, need a continuous supply of blood for the body to function and cannot tolerate an interruption in the supply of blood. The average adult has 5 to 6 L of blood in his or her body.
2. **a.** Changes in mental status occur as a result of changes in the perfusion of the brain. Patients experiencing altered mental status may not be getting an adequate supply of blood to the brain. Changes in mental status are an early indication of hypoperfusion, occurring much earlier than changes in blood pressure.
3. **d.** Signs and symptoms of shock include restlessness, anxiety, combativeness, increased heart rate, decreased capillary refill in infants and children (longer than 2 seconds), pale or clammy skin, thirst, decreasing level of responsiveness, breathing changes, nausea and vomiting, decreased blood pressure, cyanosis, and sluggishly reactive pupils.
4. **b.** When treating a patient with signs and symptoms of shock, maintain an open airway, provide 100% oxygen, control bleeding, elevate the patient's legs, and help the patient lay down, keep the patient warm, and transport immediately. Low blood pressure in a patient is a sign of late shock; injuries should therefore be splinted en route to the receiving facility to expedite transport.
5. **a.** Sudden loss of 1 L of blood is considered serious in healthy adult patients. Children bleed at the same rate as adults do thus equal injuries are more serious for children. Geriatric patients cannot compensate for blood loss as well as a healthy adult patient can. Blood loss of as little as 100 ml is considered serious for an infant.
6. **b.** Arterial bleeding is bright red. Under high pressure, it may spurt and is difficult to control. Venous bleeding is a darker red color, under low pressure, and flows in a steady stream. Capillary bleeding is dark red and usually oozes from the site.
7. **a.** If the bleeding is from one main source, concentrated direct pressure applied with your fingertips is preferred to control bleeding.
8. **d.** Tourniquets cause extensive tissue damage, sometimes requiring amputation of tissue distal to the tourniquet. For this reason, tourniquets are used as a last resort. When a tourniquet is used, a wide band that will not cut the patient is needed. Tourniquets are rarely required, even in cases of amputation.
9. **d.** Signs and symptoms of internal bleeding include signs and symptoms of shock, bleeding from any body orifice, blood-tinged vomit or feces, coffee ground vomit, dark and tarry stool, abdominal rigidity or tenderness, and a distended abdomen. When caring for epistaxis (nosebleed), have the patient lean forward so he or she does not swallow blood. Up to 225 ml of blood can be lost in a closed tibia injury.
10. **a.** The outer layer of skin is the epidermis, the middle layer is the dermis, and the tissue underlying the dermis is the subcutaneous layer.
11. **c.** An abrasion is a scrape, generally with capillary bleeding. A contusion is a bruise, an avulsion is a flap of skin torn loose, and a crush injury occurs when force is applied with a blunt instrument.
12. **c.** A contusion and a hematoma are closed injuries. An abrasion, laceration, avulsion, penetration and puncture are open injuries. Crush injuries can be open or closed.
13. **d.** An avulsion involves a piece of skin that is torn loose or completely off.
14. **c.** Extremities that are injured should be splinted, if time allows, to minimize pain and bleeding. Bandages are used to secure dressings in place. An occlusive dressing is nonporous, preventing air from entering a wound. Injuries to joints should be bandaged in the position in which they are found.
15. **a.** An evisceration is an abdominal injury in which the abdominal contents are exposed. The EMT–Basic should cover the organs and wound to prevent the contents from drying.
16. **b.** Impaled objects in the cheek can be removed if they obstruct the airway. Dress the wound on the inside and outside of the mouth.
17. **b.** Amputated body parts should be placed in a plastic bag and kept cool. Do not freeze amputated parts, allow them to become warm, or place them directly on ice or in water.
18. **b.** A partial-thickness burn is intensely painful and causes blisters. A superficial burn causes pain and red skin. A full-thickness burn will appear dry and leathery and produce little or no pain.

19. **c.** Following the "rule of nines," each leg is 14% body surface, and the arm is 9% body surface, totaling 37%.
20. **a.** A partial-thickness burn involving the feet, hands, genitalia, or face is considered a critical burn. Burns caused by dry lime should not be flushed because water will react with the lime and cause more damage. Electrical burns cause extensive internal damage to the body, with minor damage to the skin. Burn patients cannot regulate their body heat and must be kept warm.
21. **c.** Involuntary muscle, or smooth muscle, is located in the walls of the hollow structure of the gastrointestinal tract, in the urinary system, in the blood vessels, and in the lungs. Voluntary muscle, or skeletal muscle, attaches to bones to provide for movement. Cardiac muscle is found in the heart and contracts to make the heartbeat.
22. **a.** A direct injury occurs when a force acts on a body part, such as a baseball bat striking an arm. Indirect injury means the force was applied somewhere on the body and the injury is in a different place. Twisting force is applied when an extremity is pulled or twisted.
23. **b.** Crepitation is the sound heard when bone ends rub together. When crepitation is present, the EMT–Basic may feel grating when palpating the injury.
24. **b.** When splinting a joint injury, immobilize the bone above and below the injury. Assess distal pulse, sensation, and motor function before and after splinting. Remove clothing around an injury so that you can examine the injury and so the clothing does not become constricting if the injury swells. Protruding bone ends should not be replaced when splinting an injury.
25. **b.** If the patient has signs and symptoms of shock, not enough time is available to splint each individual extremity. Align the body in the normal anatomic position and splint the entire body to the long backboard.
26. **a.** Traction splints are used for injuries that are isolated to the midfemur. Do not use a traction splint if the injury involves the pelvis, knee, or the lower extremities.
27. **a.** The central nervous system is composed of the brain and spinal cord. The peripheral nervous system is composed of motor nerves and sensory nerves.
28. **c.** A properly sized cervical spine immobilization device will immobilize the head in the neutral position. The device will not allow the head to move from side to side or up and down excessively. The chin should fit comfortably in the chin rest without slipping out of place. The rescuer holding the head must maintain stabilization until the head is immobilized to the long backboard.
29. **b.** If you do not have the proper size cervical spine immobilization device, use rolled towels on either side of the patient's head and tape them in place. Do not use a device that is too small or too large.
30. **d.** After immobilizing a patient to a short or long backboard, reassess pulse, motor function, and sensation in the extremities. The head should be secured to the long backboard after the body is secured, and a cervical spine immobilization device should always be used. When using a KED, buckle the lower chest straps before the top chest strap.
31. **b.** Compression injuries of the spine occur when the head is pushed downward and the spine is compressed. Distraction occurs when the spine is pulled apart. Flexion and extension can occur when the head snaps forward and backward.
32. **c.** Always reassess pulse, motor function, and sensation after every intervention. Patients who have no pain can still have injuries to the spine. Patients with injuries to their pelvis can have injuries to their lower spine. Manual stabilization of the head should be maintained from the beginning of the initial assessment until the patient is immobilized on the long backboard.
33. **c.** Rapid extrication should be used when immediate danger to the EMT–Basic or the patient exists, when the patient cannot be treated in his or her current position, and if lifesaving care cannot be provided to another patient unless this patient is moved. If the scene is unsafe for the EMT–Basic to enter, no care should be provided until the scene is made safe.
34. **d.** Helmets should be removed if you cannot assess or treat the patient because the helmet is in the way, if the helmet is loose, and if the head cannot be immobilized with the helmet in place.

35. **d.** Children have relatively large heads in proportion to the rest of their body, requiring special immobilization techniques. Pad the patient from the shoulders to the toes to achieve neutral alignment. Make sure the straps are tight so the child feels secure. Geriatric patients may have conditions that will not allow their spines to be straightened; therefore apply extra padding for comfort and to immobilize.

## Chapter 31

### INFANT AND CHILD EMERGENCY CARE

#### Matching 1

1. a
2. e
3. c
4. d
5. b
6. f

#### Matching 2

7. g
8. h
9. b
10. d
11. f
12. i
13. a
14. e
15. c

#### Matching 3

16. b
17. e
18. a
19. c
20. d
21. f

#### Matching 4

22. c
23. b
24. d
25. a

#### Review Questions

1. **True.** These patients have a large body surface area and have immature thermoregulatory systems; they are also unable to put on or remove clothing by themselves. Be sure to cover the patient or replace the patient's clothing after the examination.
2. To get the most information about an infant or newborn, assess the heart and lungs first. If you can assess the heart and lungs, before they get upset, you will obtain more accurate information.
3. Evaluate an infant's respirations by watching the effort of breathing; by watching the chest rise and fall; by looking at the infant's skin color, level of activity, and use of accessory muscles to breathe; and by watching the infant's interactions with caregivers.
4. **False.** Most toddlers do not like to be touched by strangers.
5. **True.** Parents can relay vital information about their child and keep them calm during your evaluation. Allow the parent and child to remain together whenever possible.
6. **d.** Preschool children like to explore new things, such as your medical equipment. They do not like to be separated from their parents, have their clothing removed, or be touched by strangers.
7. **True.** School-age children should be able to explain to you the circumstances surrounding an accident or events before an illness.
8. The most important anatomic and physiologic difference between infants and children and adults involves the *airway.*
9. **b.** The airway is smaller and therefore more easily blocked by fluid, secretions, or swelling.
10. **d.** The large tongue of a child takes up proportionally more room in the mouth and can cause airway compromise.
11. As children work hard to breathe, they will become *fatigued.* The increased work of breathing uses a tremendous amount of energy, and muscles will tire.
12. To prevent occlusion, or kinking, of the airway, the head-tilt, chin-lift maneuver should put the head into a *neutral* position in which the nose points straight up.
13. **True.** Do not insert the suction catheter further than you can see, and be sure to measure the length of the catheter before insertion.
14. Suction should be limited to *10* seconds, and you should always apply *oxygen* before and after suctioning.

15. To insert an oropharyngeal airway in an infant or child, use a tongue depressor to push down the tongue and insert the airway without rotation.
16. Nasopharyngeal airways can be used when the patient has a gag reflex, whereas oropharyngeal airways cannot.
17. **True.** The oxygen is held close to the patient's face without placing a mask on the patient. Infants and children may tolerate this method of oxygen delivery better than a mask.
18. **b.** Adjust the flow rate to 5 L/minute for infants and 10 L/minute for children when applying blow-by oxygen.
19. **b.** Ventilate an infant or child every 3 seconds, or 20 times per minute.
20. Besides the gentle rise in the chest wall, other indicators of adequate ventilation in children are improvement in the heart rate and skin color.
21. With children, consider examining painful areas last. If the painful area is examined first, the child may be unwilling to allow you to complete your assessment.
22. The acronym AVPU stands for alert, responsive to verbal stimuli, responsive to painful stimuli, and unresponsive.
23. p—stridor on inspiration; l—expiratory wheeze; c—unable to cough or speak; l—skin may appear normal or cyanotic; c—skin may appear pale or cyanotic.
24. **b.** The care for responsive children with a foreign body airway obstruction is the same as that for an adult. Unresponsive infants should receive back blows and chest thrusts but never abdominal thrusts. Blind finger sweeps should never be performed on infants—attempt to remove a foreign body only if you see the object.
25. More than 80% of all cardiac arrests in children begin as *respiratory* arrests. Respiratory distress must be recognized early in children to prevent further deterioration into cardiac arrest.
26. Signs of early respiratory distress in children include increased rate of breathing, nasal flaring, intercostal and supraclavicular retractions, mottled skin color, use of abdominal muscles, seesaw respirations, stridor, wheezing, and grunting.
27. Signs of respiratory failure in children include altered mental status, respiratory rate over 60 or under 20 breaths per minute with signs of fatigue, severe retractions, severe use of accessory muscles, decreased muscle tone, cyanosis, and poor peripheral perfusion.
28. A seizure can be caused by a rapid rise in a *fever.* Seizures also can be caused by chronic medical conditions, infection, poisoning, low blood sugar, head injury, hypoxia, and unknown causes.
29. **c.** A nasopharyngeal airway can be a useful adjunct to help control the patient's airway following a seizure. The recovery position should be used only if no known or suspected trauma to the head or spine has occurred. Do not put anything in the patient's mouth while the patient is having a seizure. Seizures are not always dangerous, but long (greater than 10 minutes) or repeated seizures may require the use of antiseizure medication.
30. Common signs and symptoms of shock in infants and children include rapid respiratory rate, pale or mottled skin, cool and clammy skin, rapid pulse, weak or absent peripheral pulse, decreased blood pressure, absence of tears when crying, poor urinary output, and delayed capillary refill.
31. The top priority in the treatment of near-drowning cases is adequate ventilation and oxygen.
32. **a.** SIDS generally occurs in patients younger than 1 year of age. Follow basic life-support procedures and transport the infant to the nearest appropriate facility.
33. Because it is larger and heavier than the other parts of the body, the *head* is the most frequently injured part of a child's body.
34. **c.** Hypothermia is a concern for any burned patient but especially children and older adults. The skin has been injured and cannot regulate body temperature.
35. PASG may be indicated for children who have sustained trauma with signs and symptoms of hypoperfusion and pelvic instability. The PASG should not be used if evidence exists of penetrating chest trauma. Inflation of the abdominal compartment may hinder breathing and must be carefully monitored. Follow local protocol and advice from medical direction regarding the use of PASG for pediatric patients.

36. Signs and symptoms of abuse include multiple bruises in various stages of healing; injury inconsistent with the mechanism described by parent or caretaker; mechanism of injury inconsistent with child's developmental characteristics; repeated calls to the same address; fresh burns, especially on the feet, hands, and back; parents or caretakers who seem inappropriately unconcerned; conflicting histories given by parents or caretakers; and children afraid to discuss how the injury occurred.
37. **True.** When you treat an infant or child, you must also deal with the fears and concerns of the parent.
38. **a.** Has the child had previous seizures? Does the child take antiseizure medications? If she has had previous seizures, is this seizure similar to others? **b.** Common antiseizure medications include phenobarbital, Tegretol, Clonopin, Depakene, and Dilantin. **c.** Ensure a patent airway; have suction available; place the patient in the recovery position and monitor the airway; provide high-concentration oxygen; request advanced life-support resources if the seizure activity resumes; and transport per medical direction.
39. **a.** You suspect internal blood loss from an abdominal injury. **b.** The decreased blood pressure and increased pulse and respiratory rates indicate that the patient's status may be deteriorating. These are signs of hypoperfusion. **c.** With any change in patient condition, contact medical direction and advise them of the change. You should apply continue high-concentration oxygen and repeat the ongoing assessment every 5 minutes. **d.** Have suction available, and turn the spine board on its side.

## Division Six Examination

1. **a.** Newborns and infants generally do not like to be separated from their parents, but they do not mind being assessed by strangers. EMT–Basics should assess the newborn in a way that prevents excessive heat loss.
2. **d.** Adolescents are not quite adults, but they should be treated as adults. Respect their right to modesty and privacy, and assess them apart from parents and other children.
3. **a.** Infants are obligate nose breathers; the nostrils and nasopharynx should therefore be suctioned if necessary to ease breathing. A child's tongue is relatively large in relationship to the mouth and often causes airway compromise. Children compensate for airway compromise by increasing their breathing rate and effort. An infant's airway is less developed and more flexible than that in an adult.
4. **c.** Nasal airways are useful for maintaining an open airway when a patient's muscles relax following a seizure. The nasal airway can be inserted into either nostril, as long as it is inserted without force. Oral airways are more likely than nasal airways to stimulate vomiting. The preferred method for inserting an oral airway in a child patient is by using a tongue depressor.
5. **b.** Parents can be used to help deliver oxygen to pediatric patients; the children are more comfortable in the company of their parents, and the parent will feel useful. Blow-by oxygen means that the oxygen source is approximately 5 cm from the patient's face. Nonrebreather masks can be used for any patient who needs to receive high-concentration oxygen. The flow rate for a nonrebreather mask should be 12 to 15 L/minute to ensure that enough oxygen is being delivered through the mask.
6. **a.** Ventilate the child until you see a gentle chest rise, rather than trying to determine the tidal volume required for each patient. The ventilation rate for children is one breath every 3 seconds, or 20 breaths per minute. The bag used should be at least 450 to 750 ml and should not have a pop-off valve to ensure adequate tidal volumes and ventilation pressure.
7. **b.** Mottled skin is an early finding of inadequate oxygenation in children, often seen before cyanosis. Children are considered to be responsive to verbal stimulus if they recognize their parent's voice because children may be unable to understand and follow commands. Capillary refill should take less than 2 seconds in a patient who is perfusing adequately. When assessing a child, use the trunk-to-head approach to avoid scaring the child.
8. **d.** Assess the pulse of an infant at the femoral or brachial artery. Assess the pulse of children and adults at the radial or carotid artery.
9. **c.** Assess blood pressure for patients older than 3 years of age.
10. **b.** Abdominal thrusts alone are used for children and adults with a foreign body airway obstruction. Back blows and chest thrusts are used for infants with a foreign body airway obstruction.

11. **a.** Complete upper airway obstruction is characterized by a sick general appearance, gasping or no respirations, pale to cyanotic skin color, inability to cough or speak, and a possible history of foreign body obstruction or cold symptoms. Partial upper airway obstruction is characterized by a relatively well to sick general appearance, increased work of breathing, normal to pale skin color, inspiratory stridor or crowing, and a history suggestive of foreign body obstruction. Patients with lower airway disease exhibit signs and symptoms such as a relatively well to very sick appearance, increased work of breathing, normal to cyanotic skin color, expiratory wheezes, and a history of airway disease.
12. **a.** Wheezing is a sign of early respiratory distress, along with increased rate of breathing, nasal flaring, intercostal and supraclavicular retractions, mottled skin color, use of abdominal muscles, see-saw respirations, stridor, and grunting. Signs of respiratory failure include altered mental status, cyanosis, respiratory rate over 60 or under 20 breaths per minute, severe retractions, severe use of accessory muscles, decreased muscle tone, and poor peripheral perfusion.
13. **c.** Altered mental status may be caused by a diabetic emergency, poisoning, seizure, infection, head trauma, hypoxia, and shock. The EMT–Basic should care for the patient having a seizure without trying to diagnose the cause of the seizure. Airway and ventilation are the primary concern for the near-drowning patient. Activated charcoal can be administered to alert responsive children with the consent of medical direction.
14. **d.** SIDS deaths do not have a clear history or a factor that points to the cause of death. Patients who are abused may present to the EMT–Basic as a SIDS death. Do not question the parents at the scene, but do note any signs of abuse or neglect and report them to the appropriate authorities. SIDS is most common in the first year of life. Unless the patient has rigor mortis, attempt to resuscitate the patient with good basic life-support skills.
15. **b.** Blunt trauma is most common in children, but penetrating trauma, burns, and immersion injuries are also common.
16. **a.** Because of its size and weight, the head is the most commonly injured area of a child.
17. **c.** In an unresponsive patient, the tongue commonly falls back into the airway, causing obstruction. The jaw thrust maneuver should be used to open the airway without moving the patient's neck.
18. **c.** Signs of abuse and neglect include multiple bruises in various stages of healing, injury inconsistent with the mechanism described by caretaker, mechanism of injury inconsistent with the child's developmental characteristics, repeated calls for the same child, fresh burns, parents who seem inappropriately unconcerned, conflicting histories given by parents, and the child being afraid to discuss the injury. Do not question the parents at the scene, but report suspicions to the appropriate authorities. Neglect is giving insufficient attention or respect to a child. Abuse occurs when actions harm a child.
19. **c.** The tube placed directly into the stomach to feed a patient is called a gastric tube. Tracheostomy tubes are used for breathing. Central lines provide venous access.
20. **c.** Parents are often anxious because they are worried about the health of their child and they feel helpless. Allow the parents to help care for the child when possible, and answer their questions honestly.

## Chapter 32

## AMBULANCE OPERATIONS

### Matching

1. f
2. c
3. e
4. b
5. a
6. d

### Review Questions

1. Preparation for the call includes checking availability and readiness of *vehicle, medical supplies,* and *personnel.*
2. **True.** Continuing education keeps you up to date on current information and is considered preparation for the call and for treating patients.
3. Personal protective equipment includes gloves, mask, goggles or other eye protection, and gown.

4. **True.** Nonmedical equipment should be stocked and checked at the beginning of every ambulance shift just as you would for medical equipment. Nonmedical equipment includes personal protective equipment, maps, and reference books.
5. **True.** Different systems give you different dispatch information, but you will generally receive information about the location and nature of illness or mechanism of injury, number of patients, severity of injuries or illness, patient age, and scene hazards.
6. **d.** Safe drivers are physically and mentally fit, are able to perform under stress, have a positive attitude, and are tolerant of other drivers, in addition to the items listed in the question.
7. **False.** Drivers are sometimes startled when they see an emergency vehicle and may drive erratically.
8. Factors contributing to emergency vehicle crashes include excessive speed, reckless driving, failing to obey traffic signals or posted speed limits, disregarding traffic rules and regulations, failing to heed traffic warning signals, inadequate dispatch information, escorts, multiple-vehicle response, and failure to anticipate the actions of other drivers.
9. **e.** During the time while en route to the scene, get more information from dispatch if it is available and plan for the equipment and personnel you may need on the scene.
10. The first priority in parking at the scene is *safety.*
11. **c.** When you arrive at the scene, begin the scene size-up and call for additional resources as necessary.
12. **False.** You should drive with lights and sirens to the hospital only when the patient condition warrants it. Not every response is an emergency, and it is not worth the risk of a traffic accident to respond with lights and siren to a nonemergency.
13. **c.** While en route to the receiving facility, complete the detailed physical examination (if necessary) and perform ongoing assessments based on the patient's condition. The initial assessment and focused history and physical examination should occur on scene before the patient is moved. Life-threatening injuries should be treated as soon as they are found.
14. Patient transfer includes putting the patient in the appropriate room and giving the patient report.
15. **False.** Documentation should be completed before leaving the receiving facility so that your prehospital care report will be available if the staff has any questions and so it can become part of the patient's permanent record.
16. **c.** Low-level disinfection is used for routine cleaning when no body fluids are present.
17. **a.** High-level disinfection is used for equipment that is involved in invasive procedures.
18. Restocking and rechecking inventory occur during the *postrun* phase.
19. Mechanism of injury situations for possible air medical transport include vehicle rollover involving unrestrained passengers, pedestrian struck by a car at speeds greater than 10 mph, a fall of greater than 15 feet, motorcycle crashes at speeds greater than 10 miles per hour, collision involving death of other occupants of the same vehicle, and ejection from a vehicle.
20. **True.** The pilot needs to know that you are near the aircraft to avoid injury.
21. **a.** When called to the scene of a cardiac emergency, you should take basic supplies, patient transfer equipment, suction equipment, artificial ventilation devices, oxygen administration equipment, cardiac compression equipment, and AED. **b.** Due regard for others includes adequate notice of approach to prevent a collision and understanding and following state laws and regulations regarding vehicle stopping, procedures at red lights, stop signs, and intersections, speed limits, direction of traffic flow, and specified turns. **c.** When you arrive at the receiving facility, be sure to notify dispatch, transfer the patient to the appropriate room, provide a brief report that contains all pertinent information to the receiving staff, restock the ambulance and complete the prehospital care report to be left with the patient's chart, and wash your hands and perform infection control measures as necessary.

## Chapter 33

## GAINING ACCESS

### Review Questions

1. Extrication is the process of removing a patient from entanglement in a motor vehicle or other situation in a safe and appropriate manner.
2. The role of the incident commander is to *coordinate* efforts of medical and rescue personnel.
3. **True.** Not all extrication will require special equipment to remove the patient, but special protective equipment and knowledge is always needed.
4. In all cases of entrapment, critical patient care precedes extrication.

5. **a.** EMS and rescue personnel should work together to coordinate the safest and most efficient way to remove a patient. EMS personnel are responsible for patient care and critical interventions.
6. At the scene, the EMT should be concerned with (1) personal safety, then (2) safety of the crew, (3) safety of the patient, and (4) bystander safety.
7. Protective gear during a rescue operation should include impact-resistant protective helmet with ear protection and chin strap, protective eyewear, turnout coat, leather gloves, and boots with steel insoles and toes.
8. **b.** Patients are covered during an extrication to protect them from flying debris. A blanket also may be necessary to keep the patient warm.
9. **False.** Every extrication has a potential for hazards. Bystanders will be at potential risk and should be kept clear of the area.
10. Potential hazards at the scene of an automobile crash include hazardous materials, fire, electrical wires, and unstable vehicles.
11. The safety officer is an *objective* observer who helps identify additional *hazards* not readily apparent to the rescuers.
12. Simple access does not require the use of rescue equipment to access the patient. Complex access requires additional education, skills, and rescue equipment.
13. Types of specialized rescues include vehicle rescue, water rescue, trench rescue, and high-angle rescue.
14. **b.** The patient can be moved if he or she is in danger or cannot be treated in his or her current position. EMT–Basics must immobilize the patient before transport, even if the patient has no pain or other complaints.
15. **False.** Two people will not be enough to move the patient safely and maintain spinal alignment. Three or four people are recommended.
16. **a.** Personal safety is the first priority followed by the safety of your crew, the patients, and bystanders. **b.** Personal protective equipment for this scene includes an impact-resistant protective helmet with ear protection and chinstrap, protective eyewear, puncture-resistant turnout coat, leather gloves, and boots with steel insoles and steel toes. **c.** Only utility or rescue workers educated in managing live power lines should approach the lines or secure them. Advise the victims to stay inside the wreckage. Talk to them through a loudspeaker or public address system if necessary. Have the appropriate agency respond to the scene. You cannot make the scene safe, so do not enter.

# Chapter 34

## OVERVIEWS: SPECIAL RESPONSE SITUATIONS

### Matching

1. b
2. h
3. e
4. k
5. a
6. c
7. f
8. d
9. j
10. i
11. g

### Review Questions

1. **False.** Although supplies of hazardous materials are large at most industrial sites, a hazardous materials incident can occur on the street, at a public pool or school, or at home.
2. The primary concern at any hazardous material scene is *safety.*
3. Always approach a hazardous material scene from an *uphill* and *upwind* direction.
4. **c.** The size and shape of a container may give you an idea of the contents.
5. **True.** As always, if the scene is unsafe and you cannot make it safe, do not enter.
6. **a.** Every EMT should be educated to at least the *First Responder awareness* level of hazardous materials knowledge.
7. When approaching a potential hazardous materials situation, (a) approach from an uphill and upwind direction, (b) isolate the area, (c) avoid contact with the area, (d) be alert for unusual odors, clouds, and leakage, (e) remember that some chemicals are odorless, (f) do not drive through leakage or vapor clouds, (g) keep all personnel and bystanders a safe distance from the scene, and (h) approach the scene with extreme caution.
8. Sources of information and assistance for hazardous materials can be found on placards, material safety data sheet, emergency response guidebook, and CHEMTREC.
9. Incident management systems (a) provide a group leader, (b) provide for orderly communications, (d) provide for interactions between many agencies, and (e) help with decision making. Management systems cannot supply unlimited resources.

10. A major incident should be declared when (1) the situation requires great demand on resources, equipment, or personnel, (2) any hazardous materials situation is present, (3) the situation requires any special resources, and (4) you are unsure if an incident management system is needed.
11. The *treatment* sector provides care for patients as they are received from triage and extrication.
12. The *supply* sector provides resources, supplies, personnel, and equipment.
13. Each sector has a *sector officer* who runs the operation of the sector.
14. **d.** If the incident command system is already established when the EMT–Basic arrives on scene, report to the staging area for an assignment. Report to the sector officer to whom you are assigned and ask for specific instructions.
15. A method of categorizing patient treatment and transport needs is called *triage.*
16. Triage tags are used to identify the needs of a large number of patients so that other members of the team can quickly identify illness or injury without completing an assessment.
17. a—severed artery in leg; c—contusion and laceration to forearm; a—circumferential burn to chest; c—absent pulse and respirations; c—deformity to one wrist with contusions; a—burns to arms, hands, and feet; a—cool, clammy skin, low blood pressure, rapid heart rate; b—pain, swelling, and deformity to thigh; b—severe back and neck pain, motor, sensory functions intact.
18. **a.** Major incidents include situations requiring a great demand on resources, equipment, or personnel; any hazardous materials situation; any situation requiring special fire, rescue, law enforcement, or EMS resources; and any situation in which you are unsure whether the incident management system is needed. **b.** EMS sectors include incident command, extrication, treatment, transportation, staging, supply, and triage. **c.** As triage officer, you should move rapidly through the patients, doing an initial assessment and using triage tags to assign patients in treatment categories. As patients are assessed and tagged, they are moved to a treatment area for further evaluation and intervention.

# Chapter 35

## TACTICAL EMERGENCY MEDICAL SUPPORT

### Matching I

1. d
2. e
3. b
4. a
5. c

### Review Questions

1. A medical threat assessment is an operational assessment that provides the tactical commander with medical knowledge pertinent to the planning and implementation of the tactical mission.
2. **False.** The hot, warm and cold zones are not static, and they change as the situation changes.
3. **c.** The "A" in the acronym ACE stands for awareness.
4. **a.** Cover is the ability to maintain concealment while using a physical barrier. **b.** Concealment means hidden from view.
5. Further medical care provided in the warm zone is routinely called tactical field care.
6. TEMS providers working in the cold zone who have multiple patients should use standard triage protocols.
7. START is simple triage and rapid transport, a method of triage.

# Chapter 36

## WEAPONS OF MASS DESTRUCTION

### Matching I

1. c
2. b
3. a

### Review Questions

1. **d.** Organophosphate agents are classified as nerve agents.
2. The acronym SLUDGE stands for:
   S: salivation
   L: lacrimation
   U: urinary incontinence
   D: defecation of fecal incontinence
   G: generalized weakness
   E: emesis

3. A mark I kit contains an atropine autoinjector and a pralidoxime autoinjector.
4. In addition to the atropine and pralidoxime in a mark I kit, a patient exposed to nerve agents may require diazepam.
5. The EMS provider will detect a biologic event by the increase in normal disease or the presence of unusually severe or bizarre disease.
6. The most effective way to spread a biologic agent is through *aerosolization* of microbes or toxins.
7. Anthrax, ricin, T-2 mycotoxin, Staphylococcus enterotoxin B, plague, tularemia, brucella, influenza can present as pneumonia in adults.
8. Nuclear explosions primarily kill by blast effects.

## Division Seven Examination

1. **b.** Splinting supplies are the only basic equipment listed. EMT–Intermediates and –Paramedics who are educated for advanced procedures may use advanced supplies. EMT–Basics should have basic supplies, patient transfer equipment, airway and ventilation equipment, wound care supplies, splinting material, an OB kit, medications (oxygen, activated charcoal, and glucose), and an AED.
2. **a.** When en route to an emergency call, be sure to use safety belts, drive carefully, obey traffic laws, and have due regard for others. Red lights and sirens should be used for true emergencies. Discuss equipment that may be needed for this call, and obtain additional information if it is available.
3. **d.** When parking at the scene of an emergency, park uphill and upwind from any hazardous material, position the unit for rapid departure from the scene, park at least 100 feet (30 meters) from any wreckage, and use emergency lights to notify others of your presence.
4. **d.** When arriving at the scene, notify dispatch and record the time of arrival, perform the scene size-up, and call for additional help if necessary.
5. **b.** Perform ongoing assessments while en route to the receiving facility. Care for life-threatening injuries should be provided immediately when the life threat is found. The initial assessment should be performed when you first arrive at the patient's side. Billing and insurance information can be obtained at the receiving facility.
6. **b.** Give a radio report to the receiving facility staff while en route to the facility to alert them about the patient's condition. Another report should be given at bedside.
7. **c.** Airway equipment and other pieces of equipment that come in contact with mucous membranes require high-level disinfection. Dressings should be disposable and used for only one patient. Items such as blood pressure cuffs and penlights can be cleaned, or they may be disposable.
8. **a.** Landing zones for EMS helicopters ideally should be 100 × 100 feet (30 × 30 meters) and minimally 60 × 60 feet (18 × 18 meters).
9. **c.** The decision to use an EMS helicopter is based on time and distance considerations and illness and injury considerations. Helicopters can be used for critically ill patients, as well as for injured patients. For safety, approach the helicopter from the front so the pilot can see you and from the downhill side for maximal clearance of the rotor blades.
10. **c.** Personal protective equipment such as gloves, boots, eye protection, turnout coats, and helmets should be worn for every rescue situation. Simple access means no special tools are required to extricate the patient. Personal safety is always the priority, followed by safety of other crew members, the patient, and bystanders. Patients should be immobilized if the mechanism of injury suggests spinal trauma, whether the patient has pain or not.
11. **c.** EMT–Basics not involved in rescue activities should work with rescue workers while providing emergency care for patients and protecting them from further injury.
12. **d.** CHEMTREC provides a 24-hour hotline for information about chemicals and advice for emergency personnel working at hazardous materials scenes.
13. **b.** EMT–Basics should be educated to at least the First Responder awareness level for hazardous materials, which is designed for individuals who are likely to encounter a hazardous materials incident.
14. **b.** Park the ambulance uphill and upwind from hazardous materials. Hazardous materials are found in the home, office, recreational areas, and in industry. Some chemicals are odorless and colorless; therefore do not enter the scene until someone with the appropriate education determines that the scene is safe.
15. **a.** The transportation sector coordinates ambulance, hospital, and air medical resources. The staging sector coordinates movement of vehicles from the scene. The support sector or supply sector obtains resources and supplies.

16. **c.** Triage means categorizing patients based on the severity of their illness or injury so that the most critical patients will be treated and transported first.
17. **d.** EMT–Basics should correct only life-threatening injuries during triage. Categorize patients based on severity of injury or illness, not type of injury.
18. **d.** Patients with no pulse or respirations are considered to be the lowest priority.
19. **a.** Patients with airway or breathing difficulties, uncontrolled or severe bleeding, decreased or altered mental status, severe medical problems, signs and symptoms of shock, and severe burns with respiratory compromise are considered to be high priority patients.

## Chapter 37

## ADVANCED AIRWAY TECHNIQUES

### Matching 1

1. d
2. c
3. h
4. g
5. b
6. a
7. e
8. f

### Matching 2

9. a
10. c
11. e
12. b
13. d

### Matching 3

14. a
15. d
16. b
17. h
18. g
19. e
20. f
21. c

### Review Questions

1. The Sellick maneuver is designed to reduce gastric distention during artificial ventilation. The Sellick maneuver will also help prevent passive regurgitation during artificial ventilation.
2. **b.** The cricoid ring is inferior to the cricothyroid membrane and is the location where pressure is applied during the Sellick maneuver.
3. **True.** Releasing the Sellick maneuver may cause the patient to vomit. The maneuver must be maintained until an endotracheal tube is inserted and the position of the tube is confirmed.
4. Indications for adult endotracheal intubation include when you cannot ventilate a patient who is apneic, when the patient is unresponsive, when a patient has no gag reflex or coughing, or when a patient cannot protect the airway.
5. **a.** Open end; **b.** 15-mm adapter; **c.** pilot balloon; **d.** inflation valve; e. syringe; f. open end; g. Murphy's eye; h. inflatable cuff.
6. **b.** Although you should evaluate every patient individually, most men will require an 8.0- to 8.5-mm internal diameter tube; most women will require a 7- to 8-mm internal diameter tube. In an emergency, a 7.5-mm tube will work for almost any adult patient.
7. A stylet is inserted into the tube to make it stiff and help it maintain shape during the intubation procedure. The pilot balloon indicates whether the cuff at the distal end of the tube has been inflated; if the pilot balloon is inflated, the cuff is inflated. Murphy's eye is an opening at the end of the endotracheal tube that decreases the chance of obstruction if the tip of the tube is blocked.
8. The straight, or *Miller* blade, lifts the epiglottis directly, allowing the EMT–Basic to visualize the vocal cords. The tip of the curved, or *MacIntosh,* blade is inserted into the vallecula and lifts just in front of the epiglottis to help visualize the cords.
9. **False.** Tape can be used to secure the tube in place, or a commercial device may be used. Discuss the methods for securing an endotracheal tube in place with your medical director, and be sure to know what methods are approved in your region. A bite block should also be inserted to prevent the patient from biting on the tube.

10. **c.** The infant patient may require padding to be placed under the upper back to elevate the shoulders, which will help bring the structures of the airway into alignment for intubation. The adult patient's head should be placed in a sniffing position before intubation. The endotracheal tube should be inserted until the cuff just passes the vocal cords (Murphy's eye is distal to the cuff on the endotracheal tube). The Sellick maneuver should be performed on all patients before intubation to decrease the risks of gastric distention and vomiting.
11. **c.** When gurgling sounds in the stomach during ventilation can be heard, the endotracheal tube is most likely in the esophagus and should be removed immediately. Esophageal intubation means that the patient is receiving no oxygen when ventilated.
12. **b.** When breath sounds are heard only on the right side following intubation, the tube is most likely in the right mainstem bronchus. Deflate the cuff with the syringe and pull the tube back until breath sounds are equal bilaterally. Reinflate the cuff and secure the tube in place.
13. **c.** No more than 30 seconds should elapse between the time the last ventilation is delivered and when the next ventilation is delivered through the endotracheal tube. If the intubation procedure cannot be completed in 30 seconds, ventilate the patient with high-flow oxygen before attempting to intubate.
14. Complications of intubation include esophageal intubation, chipped teeth and trauma to soft tissue, decreased heart rate, hypoxia, mainstem intubation, vomiting, and self-extubation.
15. **d.** Patients without a gag reflex are candidates for esophageal tracheal combitubes. Placing the head and neck in the sniffing position to visualize the vocal cords is unnecessary.
16. **False.** The esophageal tracheal combitube is designed to be used for ventilation when inserted into either the trachea or the esophagus.
17. The large cuff of the combitube is designed to hold 100 ml of air; the small cuff is designed to hold 10 to 15 ml of air.
18. **c.** If you hear gurgling when ventilating through the white port, you should ventilate through the blue port and reassess breath sounds.
19. The two indications for tracheal suctioning for the EMT–Basic are secretions seen coming out of the endotracheal tube and poor compliance when ventilating.
20. **d.** Nasogastric tubes are indicated for patients who cannot be ventilated because of gastric distention. A nasogastric tube will relieve the pressure, making ventilation more successful.
21. Infants and children should be intubated when prolonged artificial ventilation is needed (making gastric distention likely), when artificial ventilation cannot be achieved by any other method, when the patient is apneic, or when the patient is unresponsive, without a cough or a gag reflex.
22. **a.** The formula, (16 plus age in years) divided by 4, is an excellent guide for endotracheal tube selection in children. The child must be older than 2 years of age, and the age used in the formula must be in years, not months.
23. A child's airway size can be approximated by using the size of the little finger and the inside diameter of the nostril. Formulas and charts are available to help determine the correct size for airway equipment. Be sure to have a tube 0.5 mm smaller and larger than the estimated correct tube size.
24. **False.** A slow heart rate in a child is a sign of hypoxia.
25. **b.** The risk of a mainstem intubation is greater in infants and children because of the short distance from the vocal cords to the carina.
26. **a.** Endotracheal intubation is the most effective way to manage a patient's airway and is the best way to ventilate an apneic patient who has no gag reflex. Endotracheal intubation minimizes the risk of aspiration and allows for better oxygen delivery to the lungs, provides complete control of the airway, and allows for suctioning of the trachea and bronchi. **b.** When performing endotracheal intubation, you will need a laryngoscope handle, curved and straight blades, Magill forceps, endotracheal tube, stylet, lubrication, oropharyngeal airway, and tape. **c.** The tube most likely has been inserted too far and has come to rest in the right mainstem bronchi. You should deflate the cuff and slowly withdraw the tube while continuing to ventilate until you hear breath sounds. Ensure that right and left chest sounds are equal and reinflate the cuff.

## Division Eight Examination

1. **a.** The Sellick maneuver is used to prevent passive regurgitation when a patient cannot protect his or her own airway. The maneuver also reduces gastric distention.
2. **b.** The cricoid ring is inferior to the cricothyroid membrane. To locate the cricoid ring, find the thyroid cartilage and the depression just below it (the cricothyroid membrane). The cricoid ring is just below the cricothyroid membrane.
3. **d.** EMT–Basics use orotracheal intubation techniques, which means that the endotracheal tube is passed through the patient's mouth and into the trachea.
4. **c.** EMT–Basics should intubate apneic patients who cannot be ventilated and patients who are unresponsive to any painful stimuli and have no gag reflex. EMT–Basics should also intubate any patient who cannot protect his or her own airway for any reason.
5. **b.** A 7.5-mm internal diameter endotracheal tube will work for most patients in an emergency setting. Adult men usually require a 8.0- to 8.5-mm internal diameter tube, and adult women usually require a 7.0- to 8.0-mm internal diameter endotracheal tube.
6. **c.** The tip of the curved blade is placed into the vallecula, the anatomic space between the base of the tongue and the epiglottis. When the blade is lifted, the epiglottis is lifted also. The tip of the straight blade is used to lift the epiglottis out of the way to allow you to visualize the vocal cords.
7. **c.** A water-soluble lubricant should be used to lubricate the distal end of the endotracheal tube so that it will slide easily into the trachea. The stylet can also be lubricated if necessary so that it will slide into and out of the endotracheal tube easily.
8. **b.** The tip of the stylet should be approximately 0.25 inches from the distal end of the cuff or the proximal end of Murphy's eye. This distance will prevent the tip of the stylet from extending beyond the endotracheal tube and causing damage to the patient's airway structures.
9. **a.** The laryngoscope handle is held in the left hand. The laryngoscope blade is inserted into the right side of the patient's mouth, and the tongue is swept to the left and out of the line of sight.
10. **b.** From 5 to 10 cc of air should be inserted into the cuff. The air is injected through an inflation valve that also inflates the pilot balloon. The pilot balloon serves as a reminder if the cuff is inflated.
11. **d.** After intubation, auscultate over the epigastrium first. If you hear gurgling noises, the endotracheal tube is in the esophagus and should be removed immediately.
12. **c.** If gurgling is heard over the epigastrium, the tube is in the esophagus and should be removed immediately. When the endotracheal tube is in the esophagus, the patient is not being ventilated. Ventilate the patient for 2 to 5 minutes after removing the tube, and then intubate again if indicated.
13. **a.** If the endotracheal tube is in the mainstem bronchus, the EMT–Basic will hear breath sounds over only one side of the chest. The cuff of the tube should be deflated, and the tube should be pulled back while the EMT–Basic listens to breath sounds. When breath sounds are heard equally over both sides, the cuff should be reinflated and the tube secured in place.
14. **c.** The cuff of a properly placed endotracheal tube should lie just beyond the vocal cords. The EMT–Basic should watch the tube pass through the vocal cords while intubating.
15. **b.** Complications of intubation include esophageal intubation, trauma to soft tissue and teeth, decreased heart rate, hypoxia, mainstem intubation, vomiting, and self-extubation.
16. **d.** When suctioning the nasopharynx or inside the endotracheal tube, a soft catheter should be used. For tracheal suctioning, insert the suction catheter approximately 25 cm and withdraw in a twisting motion while applying suction.
17. **c.** A nasogastric tube is inserted into the stomach through the nose and the esophagus. The stomach can then be decompressed for easier ventilation. The nasogastric tube can also be used for gastric lavage, administering medications or nutrition, and diagnosing trauma patients in the hospital setting. An endotracheal tube is used for ventilation; a Foley catheter is used for urinary bladder catheterization.

18. **c.** The straight blade, or Miller blade, is preferred when intubating pediatric patients because it provides for greater displacement of the tongue when visualizing the vocal cords. Children have proportionally larger tongues compared with adults, which can make intubation difficult if not controlled properly by the blade.
19. **a.** To determine the appropriate size endotracheal tube for a pediatric patient older than 2 years of age, add 16 to the age in years and divide by four. The size also can be estimated by comparing the tube with the size of the patient's little finger or the inside diameter of the nostril.
20. **b.** Pediatric endotracheal tubes generally have one or more black rings that serve as vocal cord markers. The markers help ensure that the tip of the tube is placed halfway between the vocal cords and the carina. Pediatric endotracheal tubes are also uncuffed because the narrow cricoid ring provides a seal for the tube.